W0081169

Orthopaedics
for **Undergraduates**

Second Edition

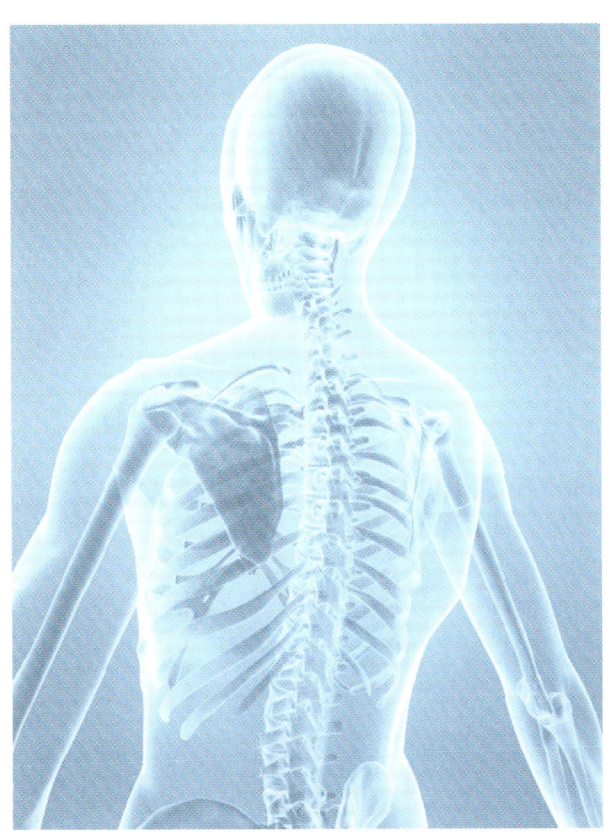

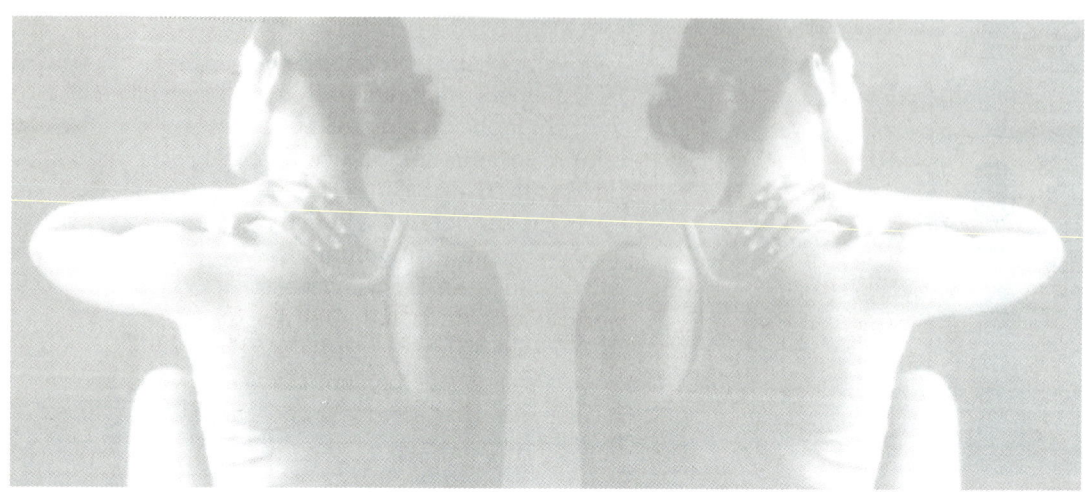

Orthopaedics
for Undergraduates

Second Edition

HS Varma

MS (Ortho) DNB (Ortho) PhD

Professor
Department of Orthopaedics
Bundelkhand Medical College
Sagar, MP

Sachin Upadhyay

MS (Ortho)

Assistant Professor
Department of Orthopaedics
NSCB Medical College
Jabalpur, MP

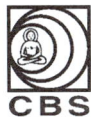

C B S

CBS Publishers & Distributors Pvt Ltd

New Delhi • Bengaluru • Pune • Kochi • Chennai

Disclaimer

Science and technology are constantly changing fields. New research and experience broaden the scope of information and knowledge. The authors have tried their best in giving information available to them while preparing the material for this book. Although, all efforts have been made to ensure optimum accuracy of the material, yet it is quite possible some errors might have been left uncorrected. The publisher, printer and the authors will not be held responsible for any inadvertent errors or inaccuracies.

ORTHOPAEDICS
for Undergraduates

ISBN: 978-81-239-1911-9

Copyright © Authors and Publishers

Second Edition: 2011

First Edition: 2004

All rights reserved. No part of this book may be reproduced or transmitted in any form or by any means, electronic or mechanical, including photocopying, recording, or any information storage and retrieval system without permission, in writing, from the authors and the publishers.

Published by Satish Kumar Jain and produced by Vinod K. Jain for

CBS Publishers & Distributors Pvt Ltd

CBS Plaza, 4819/XI, Prahlad Street, 24 Ansari Road, Daryaganj, New Delhi 110 002, India
Website: www.cbspd.com
Ph: 23289259, 23266861/67   Fax: +91-11-23243014   e-mail:delhi@cbspd.com
                                                                  cbspubs@vsnl.com
                                                                  cbspubs@airtelmail.in

Branches

- *Bengaluru:* Seema House 2975, 17th Cross, K.R. Road,
  Banasankari 2nd Stage, Bengaluru 560 070, Karnataka
  Ph: +91-80-26771678/79   Fax: +91-80-26771680   e-mail: bangalore@cbspd.com

- *Pune:* Bhuruk Prestige, Sr. No. 52/12/2+1+3/2 Narhe, Haveli
  (Near Katraj-Dehu Road Bypass), Pune 411 051, Maharashtra
  Ph: 020-32404169   e-mail: pune@cbspd.com

- *Kochi:* 36/14 Kalluvilakam, Lissie Hospital Road,
  Kochi 682 018, Kerala
  Ph: +91-484-4059061-65   Fax: +91-484-4059065   e-mail: cochin@cbspd.com

- *Chennai:* 20, West Park Road, Shenoy Nagar,
  Chennai 600 030, Tamil Nadu
  Ph: +91-44-26260666, 26208620Fax: +91-44-45530020   e-mail: chennai@cbspd.com

Printed at: Magic International Private Limited, Greater Noida, UP

to

the loving memory of my beloved father
Shri Shantilal Kalidas Varma
whose simplicity, sincerity, kindness and forgiveness
have inspired me all my life

H S Varma

my family,
who have always been there for me,
and have never doubted my dreams,
no matter how crazy they might be

Sachin Upadhyay

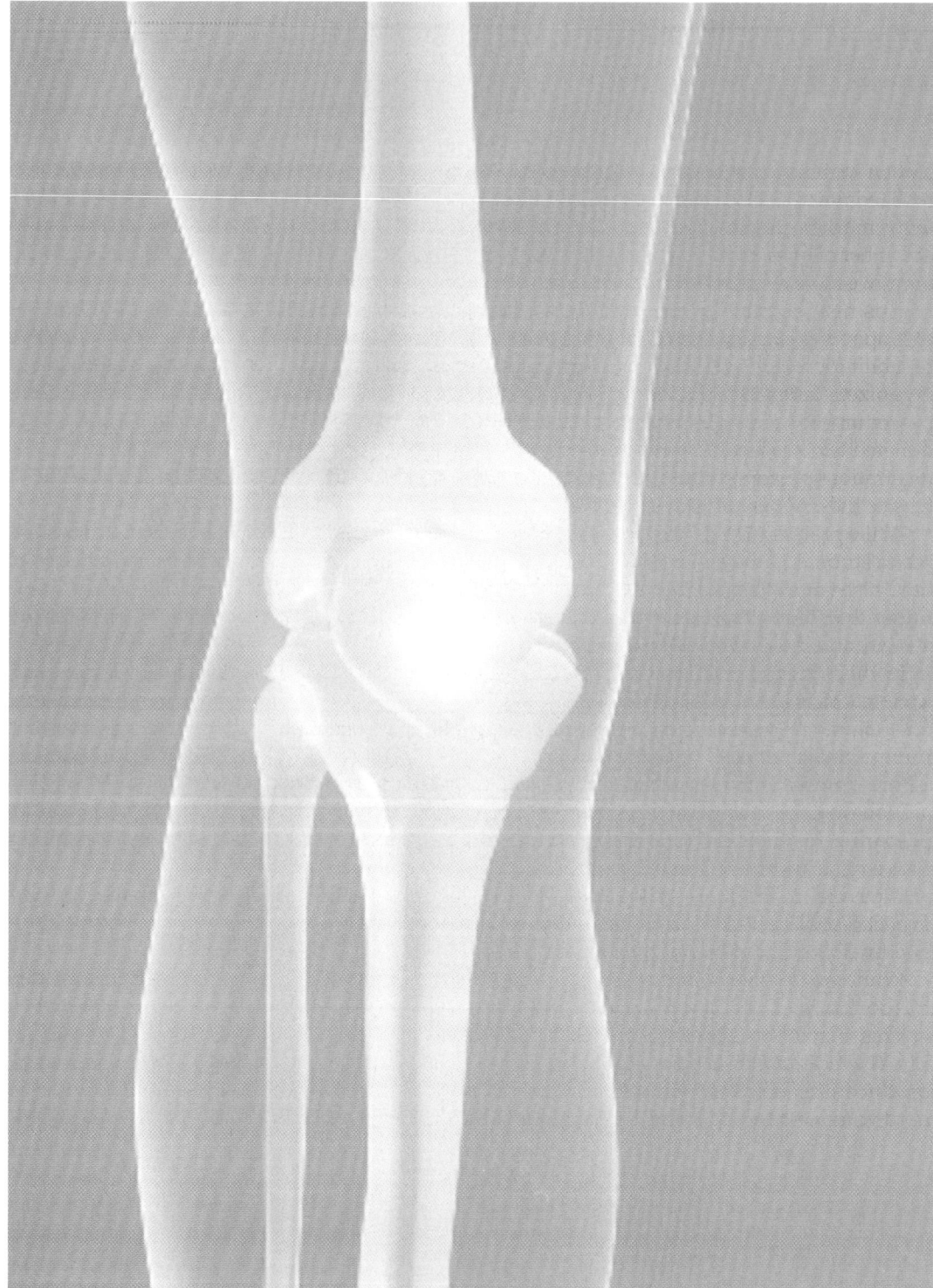

Preface to the Second Edition

When we initially considered writing and editing a completely new book on orthopaedics, we realized that it would be a great job as there are several other excellent books already available in the market. However when we reviewed the existing text thoroughly we felt that there were a number of missing facts that would be helpful to our students preparing for the exams. At this point we have decided to shape our vision into an ideal textbook on orthopaedics.

This new edition is organized into well-defined chapters comprising fundamentals of orthopaedics, upper extremity and lower extremity, spine and pelvis, and postsurgical rehabilitation of the extremities. Each chapter covers a large amount of relevant material but is organized very well with clear objectives. Basic science knowledge is integrated with clinical procedures to provide an evidence-based approach to practice. Figures, illustrations, tables and bulleted text are used extensively throughout to enforce concepts and improve retention. The illustrations principally consist of simple line drawings enhanced by minimal shading and stipple to give the effect of depth.

While preparing this new edition, we have strictly adhered to listing the common conditions that a student will encounter to maintain practical value and clarity. For the same reason, we have also endeavored to describe the useful and frequently performed clinical procedures only rather than the battalion of possible tests that exist for all conditions and that too described in an easy and interesting way.

In this edition, relevant new information has been added and all chapters revised and updated, maintaining the general format of the book. We have added an entirely new chapter on anatomy of bones and muscles, types of joints, fundamental principles of resuscitation in trauma, imaging in orthopaedics, WHO classification of bone tumours, new advances in trauma, sutures, physical therapy, sterilization and autoclaving. We have also incorporated a separate section on commonly asked questions in the form of MCQs in view of helping the students preparing for their postgraduate entrance exams. The two colour presentation should also prove to be appealing to the students.

We hope that this book will meet all the requirements of the readers and come up to their expectations. This book would take the readers from a state of dilemmas and doubts to clarity and finally to their respective destinies.

While we do not claim any perfection, we request all the teachers and the students reading this book to tell us about any shortcomings and give us suggestions in improving the book further.

This is a major achievement that was only made possible by the excellent cooperation by Mr YN Arjuna, Senior Director—Publishing, Editorial and Publicity, and the editorial/production staff of CBS Publishers & Distributors. We would like to thank all of them for their hard work and dedication in meeting the tight deadlines required to make this a reality.

HS Varma
Sachin Upadhyay

My greetings to Dr
Hasmukh S. Varma for producing
this informative & imaginative
book.

KC Dholakia.

28-XII-01

Prof KT Dholakia

Preface to the First Edition

It has been my long cherished dream come true with the release of this book *Orthopaedics for Undergraduates*. In the previous years photocopies of my handwritten and subsequently typed pages were handed over to my students in an endeavour to pass on what little I knew about orthopaedics. With every year the enthusiasm and interest of my students stimulated me to come out with this compact book. This is in fact intended for undergraduates and young budding orthopaedic surgeons, to give them a bird's-eye view of the clinical aspect of common orthopaedic problems.

I am extremely grateful to my revered ever-inspiring teacher, Prof RH Balchandani, Dr SL Mukerjee, Prof. KT Dholakia, Prof U. Holz, Padmabhusan Prof KH Sancheli, Prof PK Dave, Prof HKT Raza, from whom I learnt my clinical and surgical skills and the art of treating patients. I am thankful to staff members of my department, all my undergraduates and postgraduate students who have helped me to write this book. I am short of words to express my gratitude to Dr A Bhatt, my son Dr Bhavuk and the moral support of my family members, Mr SK Jain, Dr Girish Varma and colleagues without whom this book would not have been in its present shape.

HS Varma

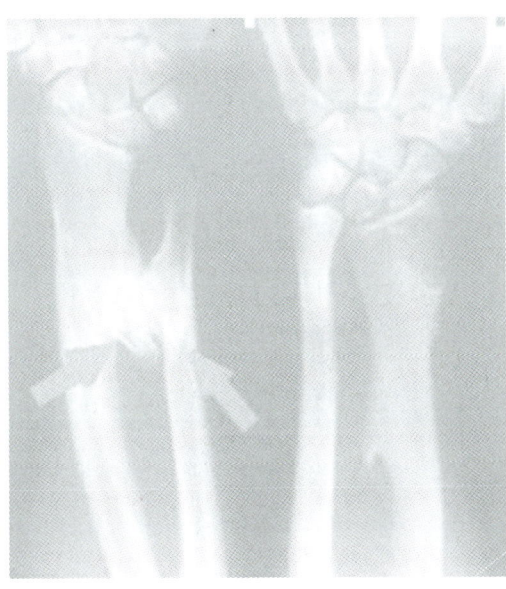

Acknowledgements

I am extremely grateful to my revered ever-inspiring teacher, Prof RH Balchandani, Prof HKT Raza, staff members of my department with special mention of Dr Alok C Agrawal for his contribution of chapter on 'bone tumours', Dr Ashish Sethi for the chapter on 'fundamental principles of resuscitation in trauma', Dr Sandeep Srivastava and Dr Gopal Pole for the X-rays, and all my undergraduate and postgraduate students who have helped me in writing this book.

I thank Mr Ajay Pitre and Mr Ravi Sarangpani of Sushrut Surgicals for their kind permission to place the figures of instruments in this book.

I am thankful to Miss A Kaur, Dr (Mrs) VL Mehta, Dr Dubey and Dr Pole for their contribution to the radiological aspects.

I am short of words to express my gratitude to Dr Sachin Upadhyay, my son Dr Bhavuk and the moral support of my family members and colleagues without whom this book would not have been in its present shape.

I am grateful to Mr YN Arjuna, Senior Director—Publishing, Editorial and Publicity, CBS Publishers & Distributors, for his valuable suggestions and all the help in the production of this book.

HS Varma

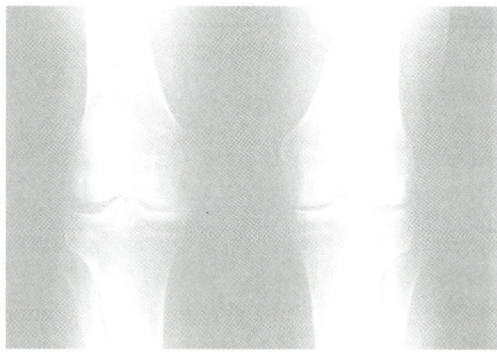

Introduction

Orthopaedics is the art and science of managing problems associated with the musculoskeletal system. This was known to the ancient Indians, records of which are available in *Rig Veda*. We had the knowledge of wide ranging herbal medicines for a variety of ailments. The highest order of clinical sense, the physician could analyse the persons, dietary intake, state of heart and all major systems by simple pulse examination. Very specific surgeries were performed by the ancient Indian surgeon Sushruta way back in 600 BC.

The word *orthopaedics* was first coined by a French physician Nicolas Andry in 1741; he wanted to straighten the bent bones of a ricketic child and that's how the two words *orthos* and *paedeos* came together. It was by the pioneering work of Sir HO Thomas, that basic principles of orthopaedics were laid down. The surgical skills were propounded by Sir Robert Jones, who subsequently established an orthopaedic training centre at Liverpool. It was a milestone in the first aid management of trauma patients by the introduction of plaster of Paris by the famous military surgeon Antonius Mathesen, a century ago. Better understanding of metallurgy laid foundation for the highly advanced material being used as implants today. In today's scenario, the patient can return to his daily routine within no time due to excellent fixation material and techniques available. It is indeed the modern age.

By the untiring efforts of surgeon's like Prof KT Dholakia, we are abreast of the clinical and surgical skills which are among the best in the world today. In spite of our instrumental handicaps, the Indian orthopaedic surgeon commands respect in any part of this globe because of our training and wide ranging exposure to a variety of orthopaedic problems prevalent in this country. Some of the best surgeons in USA, UK and many other parts of this world are Indians.

Today, orthopaedics has become a very big speciality with a wide range of subspecialities to cater to specific regional problems of the osteoarticular system. With the advances in science and technology, treatment of patients has improved with the jet speed. Today a patient can engage in a conference with the doctor across the globe and computer-aided robots have started performing surgery.

HS Varma

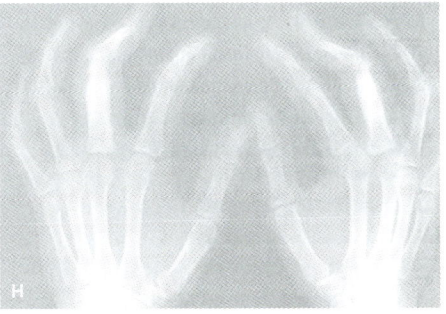

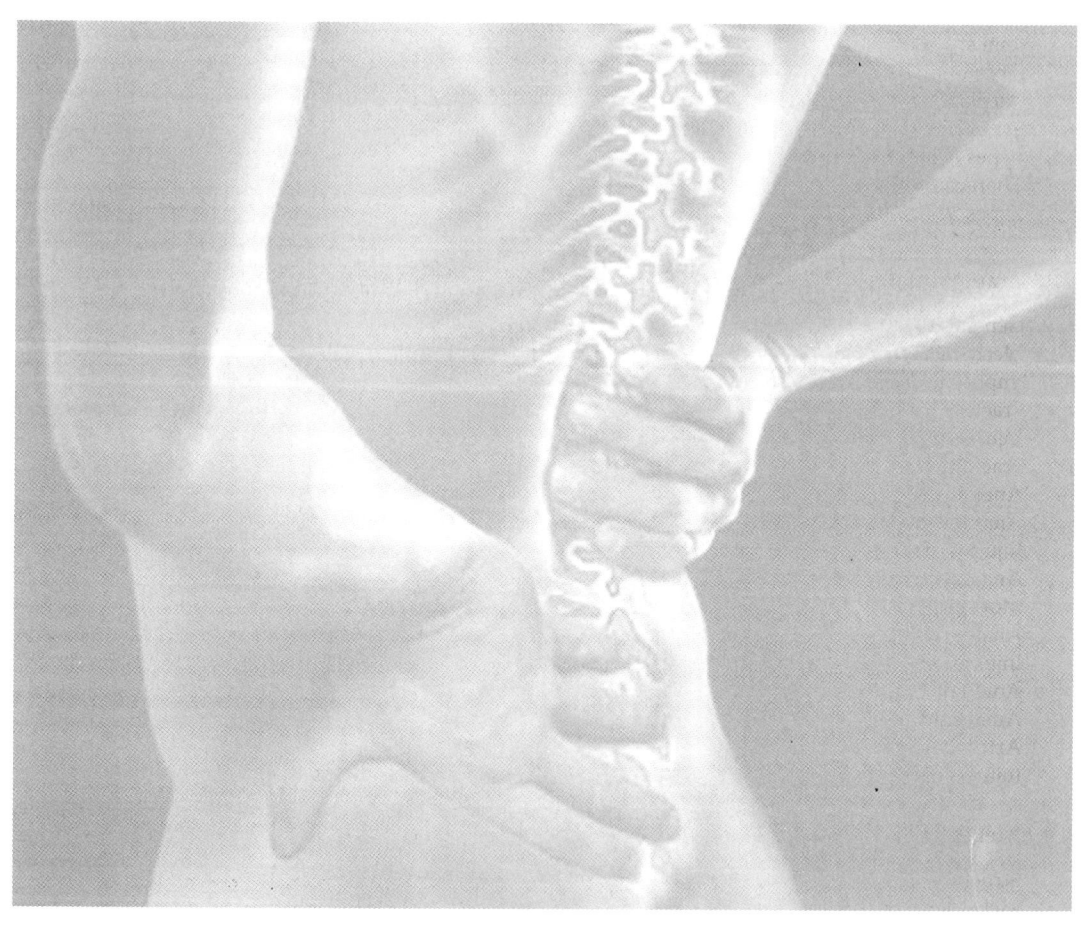

Contents

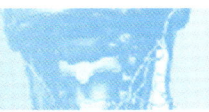

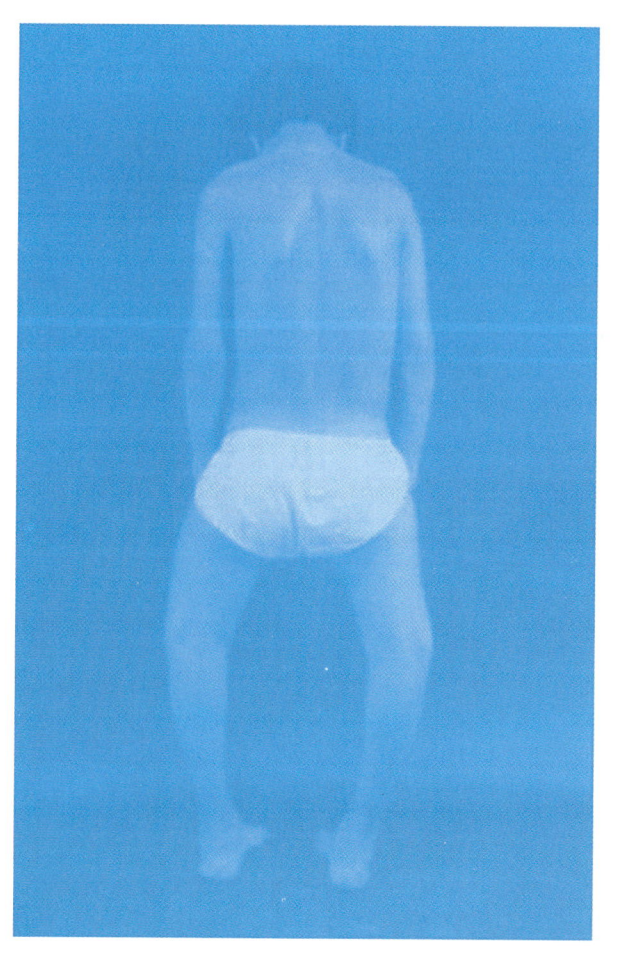

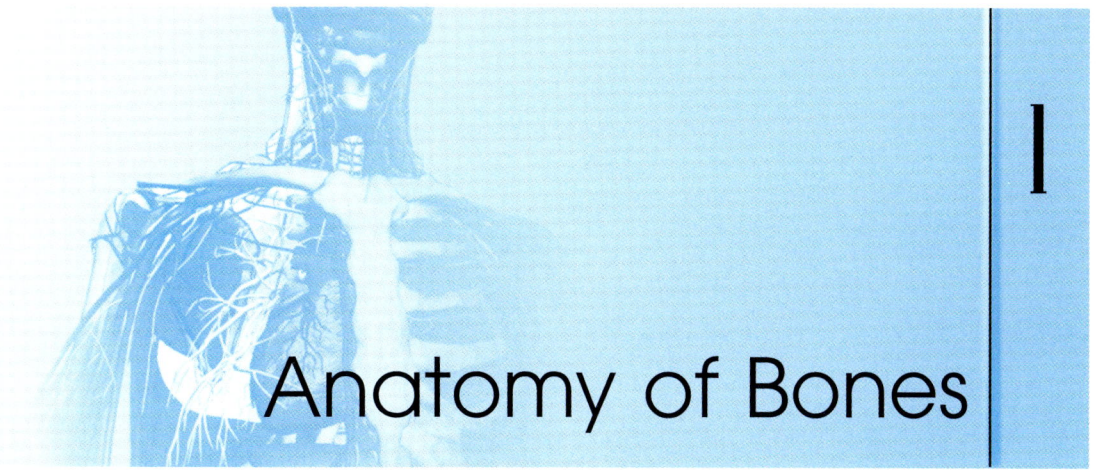

Anatomy of Bones

The bone develops from either (1) membranous sheets, e.g. the facial and cranial bones, or (2) cartilage models which subsequently ossify, a process called enchondral ossification, e.g. femur.

There are 206 bones in the adult human skeleton 80 of which are in the axial skeleton.

Type: The bones are divided as per their shape into (a) long, e.g. femur, (b) short—metacarpals, (c) flat—scapula, (d) irregular-vertebra, (e) sesamoid—patella.

The first bone appears in the 7th embryonic week, its the vertebra. The clavicle is the first bone in the skeleton to ossify.

Bone is a connective tissue, impregnated with calcium salts. The *inorganic* calcium salts (mainly calcium phosphate, partly calcium carbonate, and crystal of hydroxyapatite $Ca_{10}(PO_4)_6(OH)_2$ traces of other salts) make it hard and rigid, which can afford resistance to compressive forces of weight-bearing and impact forces of jumping. The *organic* connective tissue (collagen fibres) makes it tough and resilient (flexible), which can afford resistance to tensile forces. In strength, bone is comparable to iron and steel.

Despite its hardness and high calcium content the bone is very much living tissue. It is highly vascular, with a constant turn-over of its calcium content. It shows a characteristic pattern of growth. It is subject to disease and heals after a fracture. It has greater regenerative power than any other tissue of the body, except blood. It can mould itself according to changes in stress and strain it bears. It shows disuse atrophy and overuse hypertrophy.

Functions

1. Bones give shape and support to the body, and resist all forms of stress.
2. They provide surface for the attachment of muscles, tendons, ligaments, etc.
3. They serve as levers for muscular actions.
4. The skull, vertebral column and thoracic cage protect brain, spinal cord and thoracic viscera, respectively.
5. Bone marrow manufactures blood cells.
6. Bones store 97% of the body calcium and phosphorus.
7. Bone marrow contains reticuloendothelial cells which are phagocytic in nature and take part in immune responses of the body.
8. The larger paranasal air sinuses affect the timber of the voice.

Structural Classification

- Macroscopically, the architecture of bone may be compact or cancellous.

1

1. Compact bone is dense in texture like ivory, but is extremely porous. It is best developed in the cortex of the long bones. This is an adaptation to bending and twisting forces (a combination of compression, tension and shear).
2. Cancellous spongy, or trabecular bone is open in texture, and is made up of a meshwork of trabeculae (rods and plates) between which are marrow containing spaces. The trabecular meshworks are of three primary types, namely (a) meshwork of rods, (b) meshwork of rods and plates, and (c) meshwork compressive forces.

Bones are marvelously constructed to combine strength, elasticity and lightness in weight. Though the architecture of bone may be modified by mechanical forces, the form of the bone is primarily determined by heredity.

According to *Wolff's law* (Trajectory Theory of Wolff, 1892), the bone formation is directly proportional to stress and strain. The tensile force favours bone formation, whereas compressive force favours bone resorption. This theory has been severely criticized and is no longer accepted without reservation. In fact, both the tensile and compressive forces can stimulate bone formation in proper conditions.

The architecture of cancellous bone is often interpreted in terms of the trajectorial theory. Thus the arrangement of bony trabeculae (lamellae) is governed by the lines of maximal internal stress in the bone. Pressure lamellae are arranged parallel to the line of weight transmission, whereas tension lamellae are arranged at right angles to pressure lamellae. The compact arrangement of pressure lamellae forms bony buttresses for additional support, like calcar femoral.

- Microscopically, the bone is of four types, namely lamellar (including both compact and cancellous), fibrous, dentine and cement.
1. **Lamellar:** Most of the mature human bones, whether compact or cancellous, are composed of thin plates of bony tissue called lamellae.
2. **Fibrous:** It is found in young fetal bones, but are common in reptiles and amphibia.
3. Dentine
4. Cement occurs in teeth.

Mineralized bone could be either *Woven Bone* (immature) or *Lamellar Bone* (mature). The basic microscopic unit of bone is an *Osteon*. *Haversian canals* run through the entire length of the bone carrying blood vessels. They are interlinked to each other through the *Volkmann's canals*. On a transverse section of the bone each of these haversian canals is surrounded by a grouped of *lacunae*, which lodge an *Osteocytes*. The entire group of osteocytes link to each other and to the centrally located haversian canal through cytoplasmic extensions that run through tiny channels called **canaliculi** (Fig. 1.1).

The osteocytes derive their nutrition through their cytoplasmic extensions from the vessels in the haversian canal. In mature bone the osteons are arranged in layers (lamellar bone) while in developing bone they are arranged randomly (woven bone). Lamellar bone makes up the compact or cortical bone in the skeleton. When the same lamellar bone is loosely arranged it makes up trabecular bone. It is called trabecular bone because of the trabecular pattern. Woven bone is found on the growing ends of an immature skeleton or at the site of fracture healing.

GROSS STRUCTURE OF AN ADULT LONG BONE

Naked eye examination of the longitudinal and transverse sections of a long bone (Fig. 1.2) shows the following features:
1. **Shaft:** From without inwards it is composed of periosteum, cortex and medullary cavity.
   a. *Periosteum* is a thick fibrous membrane covering the surface of the bone. It is made up of an outer fibrous layer, and an inner

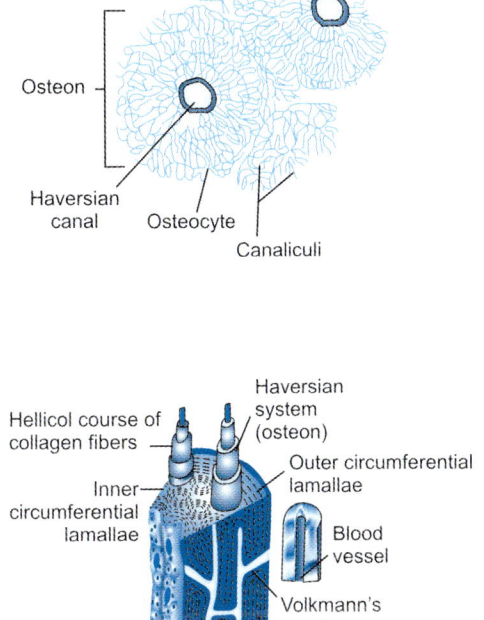

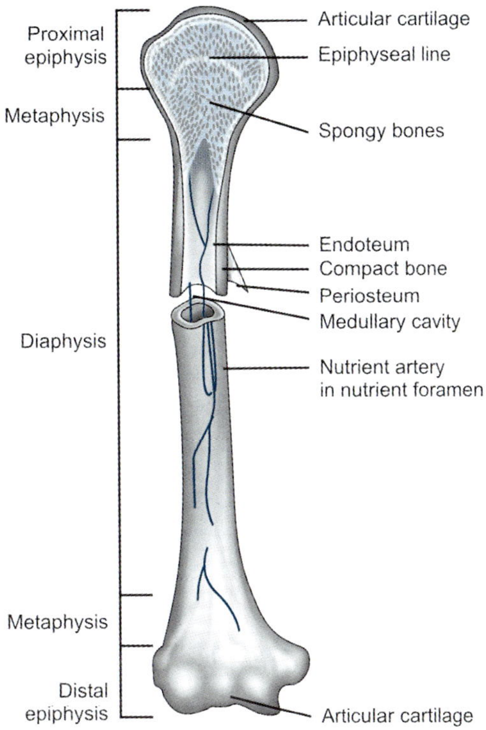

Fig. 1.2: Gross and cut section anatomy of a long bone

Fig. 1.1: Transverse section of decalcified bone

cellular layer, which is osteogenic in nature. Periosteum is united to the underlying bone by Sharpey's fibres, and the union is particularly strong over the attachments of tendons and ligament. At the articular margin the periosteum is continuous with the capsule of the joint. The abundant arteries nourish the outer part of the underlying cortex also. Periosteum has a rich nerve supply, which makes it the most sensitive part of the bone.

b. *Cortex* is made up of a compact bone, which gives it the desired strength to withstand all possible mechanical strains.

c. *Medullary cavity* is filled with red or yellow bone marrow. At birth the marrow is red everywhere with widespread active hemopoiesis. As the age advances the red marrow at many places atrophies and is replaced by yellow, fatty marrow, with no power of hemopoiesis. Red marrow persists in the cancellous ends of long bones. In the llium, sternum, ribs, vertebrae and skull bones the red marrow is found throughout life.

2. The two ends of a long bone are made up of cancellous bone covered with hyaline cartilage (articular cartilage).

PARTS OF A YOUNG BONE

A typical long bone ossifies in three parts, the two ends from secondary centres, and the intervening shaft from a primary centre. Before ossification is complete the following parts of the bone can be defined.

1. **Epiphysis:** The tips and ends of a bone ossify from secondary centers are called epiphyses. These are of the following types:
   a. *Pressure epiphysis:* It is articular and participates in transmission of the weight. *Examples:* Head of femur, lower end of radius, condyles of tibia, etc.
   b. *Traction epiphysis:* It is also known as apophysis it is extra-articular and does not participate in the transmission of the weight. It always provides attachment to one or more tendons, which exert traction on the epiphysis. The pressure epiphyses ossify earlier than traction epiphyses. *Examples:* Trochanters of femur, tibial tuberosity tubercles of humerus, mastoid process, etc.
   c. *Atavistic epiphysis:* It is phylogenetically an independent bone, which in man becomes fused to another bone. *Examples:* Coracoid process of scapula and os trigonum.
   d. *Aberrant epiphysis:* It is not always present. *Examples:* Epiphysis at the head of the first metacarpal and at the base of other metacarpal bones.
2. **Diaphysis:** It is the elongated shaft of a long bone, which ossifies from a primary centre.
3. **Metaphysis:** The ends of a diaphysis are called metaphysis. Each metaphysis is the zone of active growth. Before epiphysial fusion, the metaphysis is richly supplied with blood through and arteries forming *hair-pin* bends. This is the commonest site of osteomyelitis in children because; the bacteria or emboli are easily trapped in the hair-pin bends, causing infraction. After the epiphysial fusion, vascular communications metaphysis contains no more end arteries, and is no longer subject to osteomyelitis.
4. **Epiphysial plate of cartilage:** It separates epiphysis from metaphysis. Proliferation of cells in this cartilaginous plate is responsible for lengthwise growth of a long bone. After the epiphysial fusion the bone can no longer grow in length. The growth cartilage is nourished by both the epiphysial and metaphysial arteries.

BLOOD SUPPLY OF BONES

1. **Long bones:** The blood supply of a long is derived from the following sources.
   a. Nutrient artery enters the shaft through the nutrient foramen, runs obliquely through the cortex, and divides into ascending and descending branches in the medullary cavity. Each branch divides into a number of small parallel channels which terminate in the adult metaphysis by anastomosing with the epiphysial, metaphysial, and periosteal arteries. The nutrient artery supplies medullary cavity, inner two-thirds of cortex and metaphysis (Fig. 1.3).

   The nutrient foramen is directed away from the growing end of the bone; their directions are indicated by a jingle, *'To the elbow I go, from the knee' I flee.*

   The oblique direction of nutrient foramina opposite to the growing end of the bone is best explained by the growing-end hypothesis. There are several alternative hypotheses such as 'periosteal slip theory', 'vascular theory' and 'asymmetrical muscular development theory'.
   a. Periosteal arteries are especially numerous beneath the muscular and ligamentous attachments. They ramify beneath the periosteum and enter the

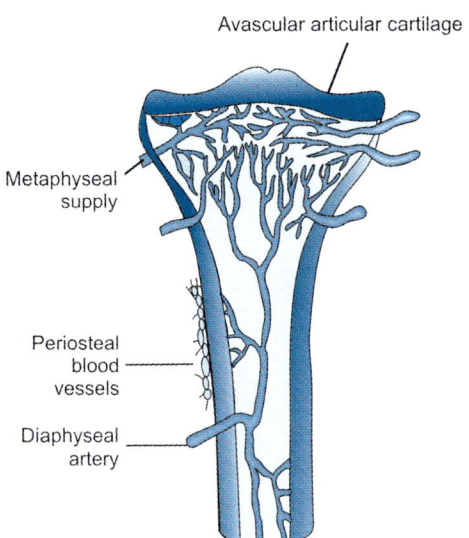

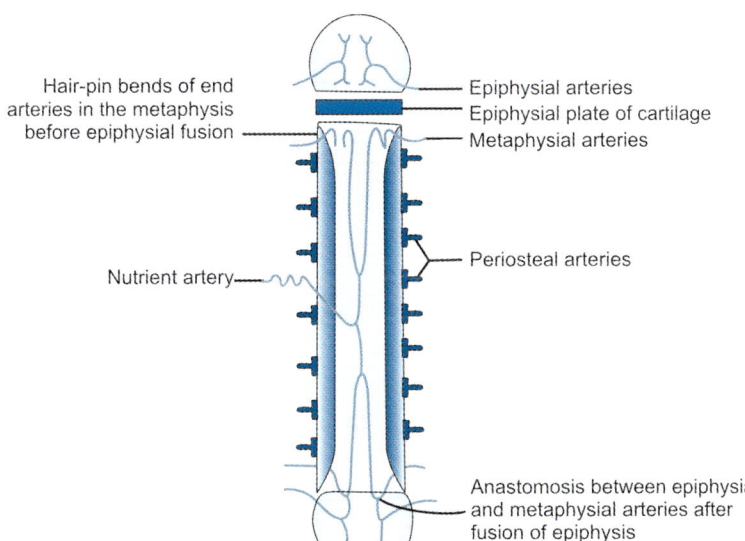

Fig. 1.3: Transverse section of decalcified bone

Volkmann's canals to supply the outer one-third of the cortex.

b. Epiphysial arteries are derived from periarticular vascular arcades (circulus vasculosus) found on the nonarticular bony surface.

c. Metaphysial arteries are derived from the neighbouring systemic vessels. They pass directly into the metaphysis and reinforce the metaphysial branches from the primary nutrient artery.

In miniature long bones, the infection begins in the middle of the shaft rather than at the metaphysis because; the nutrients artery breaks up into a plexus immediately upon reaching the medullary cavity. In the adults, however, the chances of infection are minimized because the nutrient artery is mostly replaced by the periosteal vessels.

2. **Other bones:** Short bones are supplied by numerous periosteal vessels which enter their non-articular surfaces. In a vertebra, the body is supplied by anterior and posterior vessels, and the vertebral arch by large vessels entering the bases of transverse processes. Its marrow is drained by two large basivertebral veins. A rib is supplied by: (a) the nutrient artery which enters it just beyond the tubercle, and (b) the periosteal arteries.

Veins are numerous and large in the cancellous, red marrow bones (e.g. basivertebral veins). In the compact bone, they accompany arteries in the Volkmann's canals.

Lymphatics have not been demonstrated within the bone, although some of lymphatic do accompany the periosteal blood vessels, which drain to the regional lymph nodes.

NERVE SUPPLY OF BONES

Nerves accompany the blood vessels. Most are sympathetic and vasomotor in function. Few are sensory which are distributed to the articular ends and periosteum of the long bones, to the vertebra, and to large flat bones.

DEVELOPMENT AND OSSIFICATION OF BONES

Bones are first laid down as mesodermal (connective tissue) condensations. Conversion of mesodermal models into bone is called intra membranous or mesenchymal ossification and the bones are called membrane (dermal) bones.

However, mesodermal stage may pass through cartilaginous stage by chondrification during 2nd month of intrauterine life. A conversion of cartilaginous model into bone is called *intracartilaginous* or *endochondral ossification* and such bones are called cartilaginous bones.

Ossification takes place by centres of ossification. The centres of ossification may be primary or secondary. The primary centres appear before birth, usually during 8th week of intrauterine life; the secondary centres appear after birth, with a few exceptions. Many secondary centres appear during puberty.

A primary centre forms diaphysis, and the secondary centres form epiphyses. Fusion of epiphysis with the diaphysis starts at puberty and is complete by the age of 25, after which no more bone growth can take place. The law of ossification states that secondary centres of ossification which appear first are last to unite. The end of a long bone where epiphysial fusion is delayed is the growing end of the bone.

GROWTH OF A LONG BONE

1. Bone grows in length by multiplication of cells in the epiphysial plate of cartilage.
2. Bone grows in thickness by multiplication of cells in the periosteum.
3. Bone grows by deposition of new bone on the surface and at the ends. This process of bone deposition of osteoblasts is called *appositional growth or surface accretion*. However, in order to maintain the shape the unwanted bone must be removed. This process of bone removal by osteoclasts is called remodelling. This is how marrow cavity increases in size.

Types of Joints, Movements and Range

JOINT STRUCTURE

1. **Fibrous joints** (synarthroses, immovaable)
   1. Sutures (in the skull)
   2. Syndesmoses
   3. Gomphoses.
2. **Cartilaginous joints** (amphiarthroses partially moveable)
   1. Synchondroses (hyaline cartilage)
   2. Symphyses (fibrocartilage)
3. **Synovial joints** (diarthroses freely moveable)
   1. Uniaxial
      - Ginglymus (hinge)
      - Trochoid (pivot)
   2. Biaxial
      - Condyloid
      - Saddle
   3. Triaxial
      - Ball and socket
      - Planar*

FIBROUS JOINTS

Fibrous (synarthrodial): This type of joint is held together by only a ligament. Examples are (a) sutures in the sagittal and partial bones of skull, (b) where the teeth are held to their bony sockets (Gomphoses) and at (c) both the radio-ulnar and tibiofibular joints (syndesmosis) (Fig. 2.1).

CARTILAGINOUS JOINTS

Cartilaginous (synchondroses and symphyses): These joints occur where the connection between the articulating bones is made up of cartilage for example between vertebrae in the spine (Fig. 2.2) sacroiliac joint.

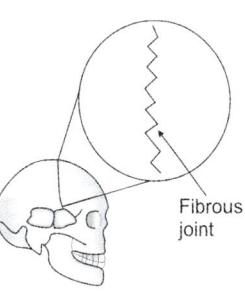

Fig. 2.1: Fibrous joint (synarthrodial): Skull suture

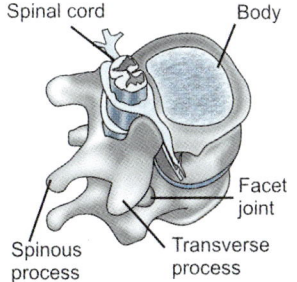

Spinal cord   Body

Facet joint

Spinous process   Transverse process

Fig. 2.2: Cartilaginous (synchondroses): Intervertebral joint

7

Synchondroses are temporary joints which are only present in children, up until the end of puberty. For example the epiphyseal plates in long bones. *Symphysis* joints are permanent cartilaginous joints, for example the pubic symphyses.

SYNOVIAL JOINTS

Synovial (diarthrosis): Synovial joints are by far the most common joint within the human body. They are highly moveable and all have a synovial capsule (collagenous structure) surrounding the entire joint, a synovial membrane (the inner layer of the capsule) which secretes synovial fluid (a lubricating liquid) and cartilage known as hyaline cartilage which pads the ends of the articulating bones. There are 6 types of synovial joints which are classified by the shape of the joint and the movement available.

Synovial joints are most evolved, and, therefore, most mobile type of joints (Figs 2.3 and 2.4).

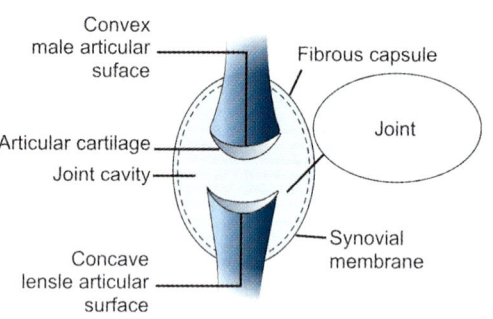

Fig. 2.3: A synovial joint

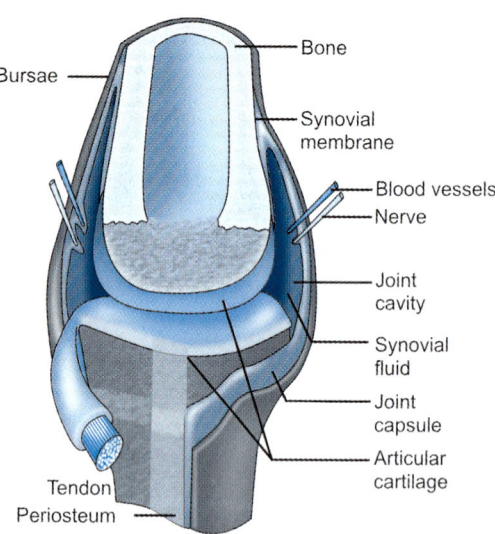

Fig. 2.4: A typical synovial joint

Table 2.1: Classification of synovial joints and their movements	
Type of joint	*Movements*
A. Plane or gliding type	Gliding movement
B. Uniaxial joints	
a. Hinge joint	Flexion and extension
b. Pivot joint	Rotation only
C. Biaxial joints	
a. Condylar joint	Flexion and extension, and limited rotation
b. Ellipsoid joint	Flexion, extension, abduction, adduction, and circumduction
D. Multiaxial joints	
a. Saddle joint	Flexion, and extension, abduction, adduction, and conjunct rotation
b. Ball-and -socket joint	Flexion, extension, abduction, and adduction, circumduction, and rotation

TYPES OF MOVEMENT

1. *Gliding:* two opposing surfaces slide past one another
2. *Flexion:* movement in the anterior-posterior plane that reduces the angle between the bones
3. *Extension:* movement in the anterior-posterior plane that increases the angle between the bones
4. *Abduction:* movement away from the longitudinal axis of the body in the frontal plane
5. *Adduction:* movement toward the longitudinal axis of the body in the frontal plane
6. *Rotation:* rotation to the right or left
7. *Internal (medial) rotation:* arm movement so the anterior side of the arm moves toward the ventral surface of the body
8. *External (lateral) rotation:* an outward turning movement of the arm (opposite of internal rotation)
9. *Pronation:* movement of the wrist and hand from palm-facing anterior to palm-facing posterior
10. *Supination:* movement of the wrist and hand from palm-facing posterior to palm-facing anterior

CHARACTERS

1. The articular surfaces are covered with hyaline (articular) cartilage (occasionally fibrocartilage in certain membrane bones). Articular cartilage is avascular, non-nervous and elastic. Lubricated with synovial fluid, the cartilage provides slippery surfaces for free movements, like 'ice on ice'.
2. Between the articular surfaces there is a joint cavity filled with synovial fluid. The cavity may be partially or completely subdivided by an articular disc or meniscus.
3. The joint is surrounded by an articular capsule, which is made up of a fibrous capsule lined by synovial membrane. Because of its rich nerve supply, the *fibrous capsule* is sensitive to stretches imposed by movements. This sets up appropriate reflexes to protect the joint from any sprain. This called the 'watch –dog' action of the capsule. The *synovial membrane* lines whole of the interior of the joint, except for the articular surfaces covered by hyaline cartilage. The membrane secretes a slimy viscous fluid called the synovia or synovial fluid, which lubricates the joint and nourishes the articular cartilage. The viscosity of fluid is due to hyaluronic acid secreted by cells of the synovial membrane.
4. Varying degrees of movements are always permitted by the synovial joints.

TYPES

1. **Plane synovial joints**
   Articular surfaces are more or less flat (plane). They permit gliding movements (translations) in various directions (Figs 2.5 and 2.6).

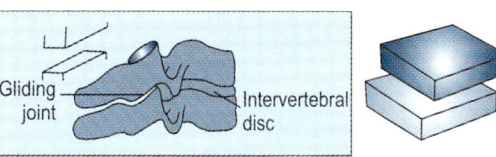

Fig.2.5: Superior and inferior articular facet of vertebrae

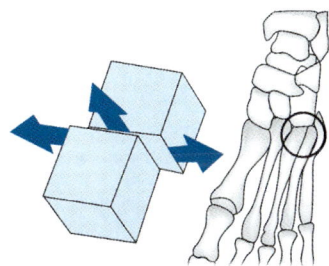

Fig. 2.6: Plane synovial joint between intertarsal bones of foot (as shown)

Examples:

a. Intertarsal joints
b. Facet between superior and inferior articular process of vertebrae
c. Intercarpal joints
d. Jaw: Temporomandibular joint

2. **Hinge joints (ginglymi)**

Articular surfaces are pulley-shaped. There are strong collateral ligaments. Movements are permitted in plane around a transverse axis (Fig. 2.7).

Examples:

a. Elbow joint
b. Ankle joint
c. Interphalangeal joints.

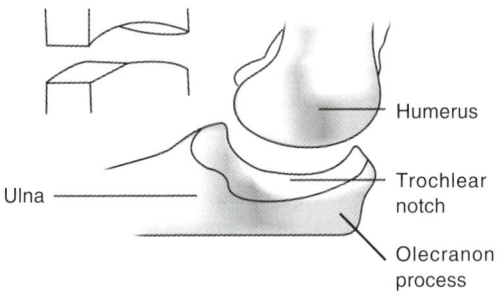

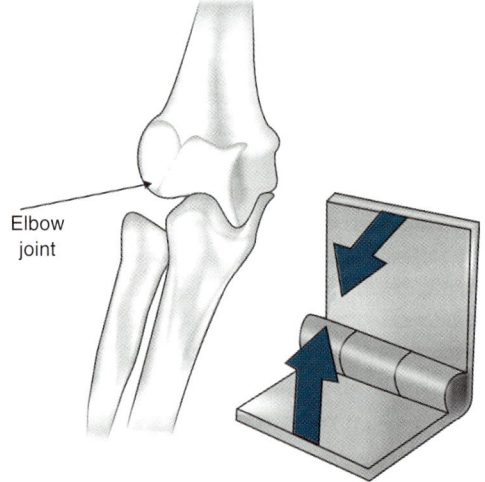

Fig. 2.7: Hing joint: Elbow joint (distal humerus and proximal end of ulna)

3. **Pivot (trochoid) joints**

Articular surfaces comprise a central bony pivot (peg) surrounded by an osteo-ligamentous ring. Movements are permitted in one plane around a vertical axis (Figs 2.8a and b).

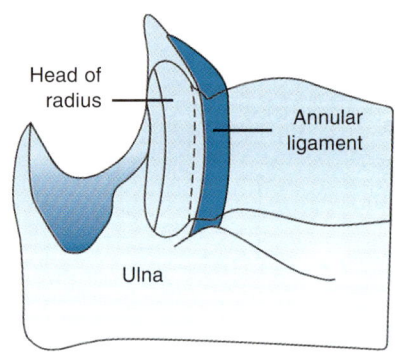

Fig. 2.8a: Superior radio-ulnar joint (pivot joint between the head of radius and radial notch of ulna)

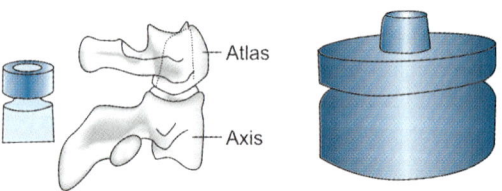

Fig. 2.8b: Pivot joint: Atlanto-axial joint

Examples:

a. Median atlanto-axial joint;
b. Superior and inferior radio-ulnar joints

4. **Condylar (bicondylar) joints**

Articular surfaces include two distinct condyles (convex male surfaces) fitting into reciprocally concave female surfaces (which are also, sometimes, known as condyles, such as in tibia). These joints permit movements mainly in one plane around a transverse axis (Figs 2.9a and b).

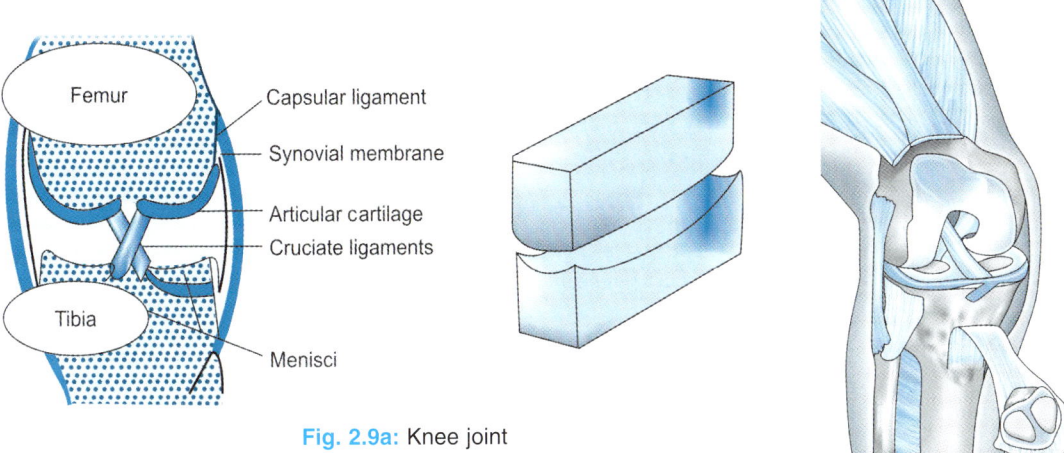

Fig. 2.9a: Knee joint

Fig. 2.9b: Knee joint

Examples:
a. Knee joint
b. Temporomandibular joints
5. **Ellipsoid joints** (Fig. 2.10)
   Articular surfaces include an oval, convex, male surface fitting into an elliptical, concave female surface. Free movements are permitted around both the axes, flexion and extension around the transverse axis and abduction and adduction around the anteroposterior axis. Combination of movements produces circumduction. Typical rotation around a third (vertical) axis does not occur.

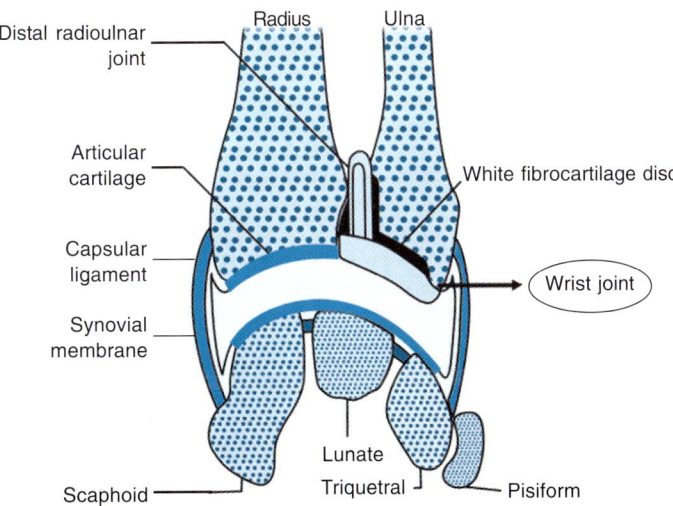

Fig. 2.10: Ellipsoidal joint between the distal end of radius and proximal rows of carpels

Examples:
a. Wrist joint
b. Metacarpophalangeal joints
c. Atlanto-occipital joints.

6. Saddle (sellar) joints

Articular surfaces are reciprocally concavoconvex. Movements are similar to those permitted by an ellipsoid joint, with addition of some rotation (conjunct rotation) around a third axis which, however, cannot occur independently (Fig. 2.11).

Examples:
a. First carpometacarpal joint
b. Sternoclavicular joint
c. Calcaneocuboid joint.

7. Ball- and-socket (spheroidal) joints

Articular surfaces include a globular head (male surface) fitting into a cup-shaped socket (female surface). Movements occur around an indefinite number of axes which have one common center. Flexion, extension, abduction, medial rotation, lateral rotation, and circumduction, all occur quite freely (Fig. 2.12).

Examples:
a. Shoulder joint
b. Hip joint
c. Talocalcaneonavicular joint

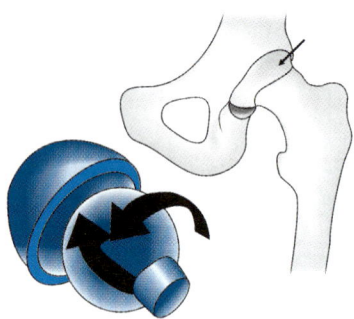

Fig. 2.12: Hip joint (arrow) (head of femur and acetabulum)

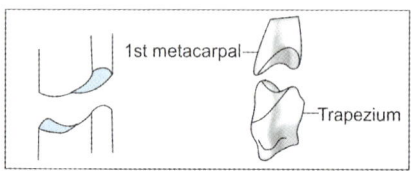

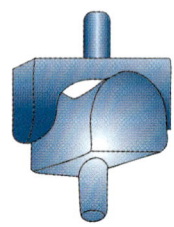

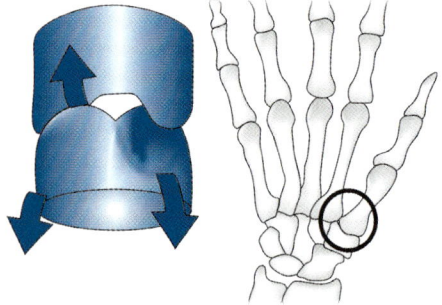

Fig. 2.11: Saddle joint: Carpometacarpal joint (marker)

Major joints of the body	
Joint	*Type*
Vertebrae	Amphiarthroidial
Hip	Ball-and-socket
Shoulder	Ball-and-socket
Knee	Condyloid
Wrist	Ellipsoid
Metacarpophalangeal (fingers)	Ellipsoid
Carpometacarpal (thumb)	Saddle
Elbow	Hinge
Radioulnar	Pivot
Atlantoaxial	Pivot
Ankle	Hinge
Interphalangeal	Hinge

Contd.

Contd.

Range of movement at the joints

Movement	Range	Knee flexion	
Wrist flexion	90°	Standing	113°
Wrist extension	99°	Kneeling	159°
Wrist adduction	27°	Prone	125°
Wrist abduction	47°	Knee rotation	
Forearm supination	113°	Medial	35°
Forearm pronation	77°	Lateral	43°
Elbow flexion	142°	Hip flexion	113°
Shoulder flexion	188°	Hip adduction	31°
Shoulder extension	61°	Hip abduction	53°
Shoulder adduction	48°	Hip rotation (sitting)	
Shoulder abduction	134°	Medial	31°
Ankle flexion	35°	Lateral	30°
Ankle extension	38°	Hip rotation (prone)	
Ankle adduction	24°	Medial	39°
Ankle abduction	23°	Lateral	34°

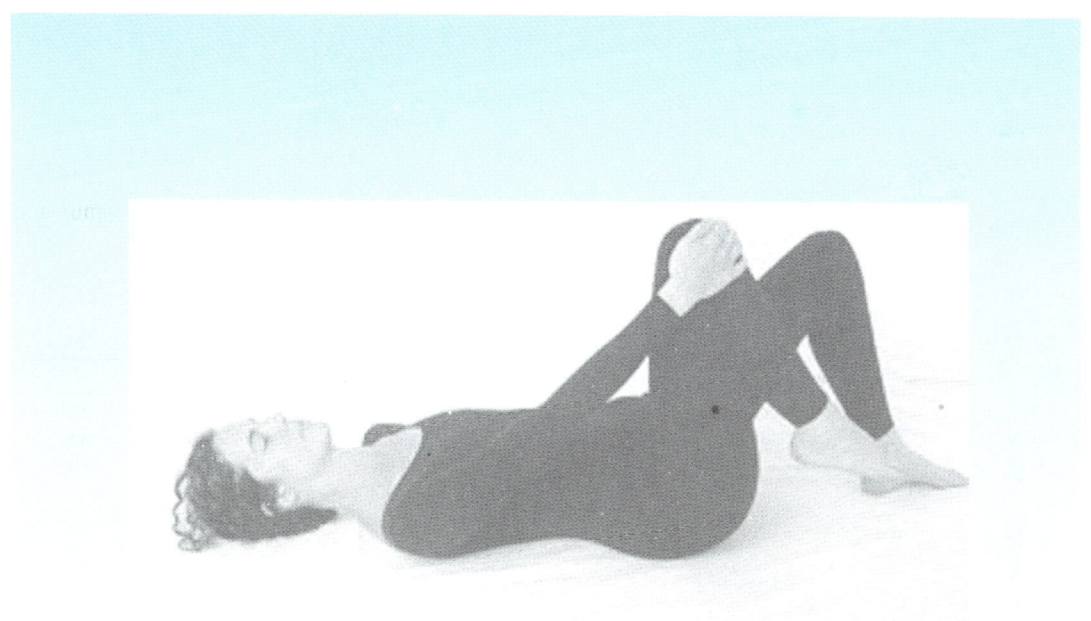

3

Traumatology

GENERAL

Definitions

- *Fracture:* It is the breach in the continuity of bone or damage to the trabecular pattern, as a result of accidental implication of force with or without associated injuries.
- *Subluxation:* This is partial loss of contact of two articulating surfaces of a joint.
- *Dislocation:* This is total loss of contact of the articulating surfaces of a joint, due to complete tear of the joint capsule and damaged supporting ligaments.
- *Osteoclasis:* If the surgeon breaks the bone, by bending a deformed one, it is called osteoclasis.
- *Osteotomy:* When the surgeon cuts the bone with an osteotome, for correction of a deformity, it is called osteotomy.
- *Osteoporosis:* Bone mass loss.
- *Osteomalacia:* Bone mineral loss.
- *Osteopenia:* Reduction in bone density.
- *Arthrodesis:* Surgical fusion of a joint to abolish movements (intra-articular/extra-articular).
- *Arthroplasty:* Surgical refashioning of a joint to relieve pain or restore mobility. This can be done by excision, interposition or replacement of the joint (partial or total).
- *Ankylosis:* Loss of movements of a joint due to underlying pathology. It may be
  a. Bony, leading to loss of all movements and is painless.
  b. Fibrous, showing some movements on stress and is painful.

Classification of Fractures

- Simple
- Compound
- Complicated
- Miscellaneous
- Epiphyseal injuries.

Simple

When there is a fracture, but the overlying soft tissue and the skin is intact and there is no associated vital tissue damage (Fig. 3.1).

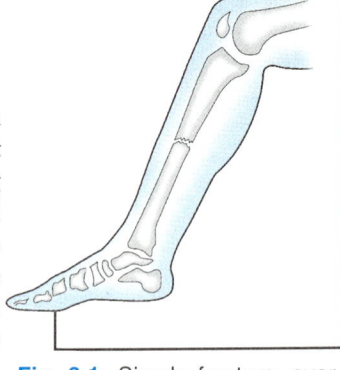

Fig. 3.1: Simple fracture, overlying soft tissue and skin is intact

14

Compound

When the fracture haematoma communicates with the exterior atmosphere, through an overlying wound in the skin and soft tissue. Evaluation and treatment depends on extent of soft tissue damage and level of wound contamination (Figs 3.2a and b).

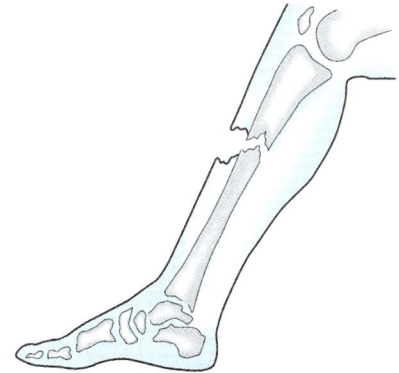

Fig. 3.2a: Compound fracture

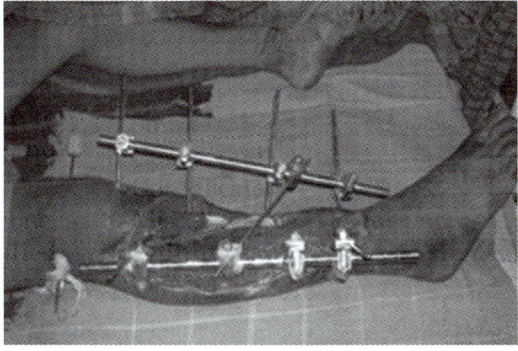

Fig. 3.2b: Open fracture fix with external fixator

The well accepted classification of open fracture is as follows:

Gustilo's Classification of Compound Fractures

Type 1 : Clean wound of size < 1 cm
Type 2 : Lacerated wound > 1 cm but without extensive soft tissue damage, skin flaps or avulsions.

Type 3A : Extensive soft tissue lacerations/ flaps, but maintain adequate soft tissue coverage of bone or they result from high-energy trauma regardless of the size of wound especially segmental/severely comminuted fractures.
Type 3B : Extensive soft tissue damage with periosteal stripping and bony exposure, usually massively contaminated.
Type 3C : Open fractures with an arterial injury that requires repair regard-less of size of wound.

Complicated

When the fracture is associated with injury to vital tissue, viscera, vessels and nerves related to the bone, e.g. fracture of mid shaft humerus with radial nerve palsy, fracture pelvis with rupture of urethra.

Miscellaneous

Stress Fracture

Cyclic application of minor trauma over a prolonged period causing cracks in the long bones, e.g. fracture tibia, second metatarsal fracture seen in army recruits (*March fracture,* Fig. 3.3a).

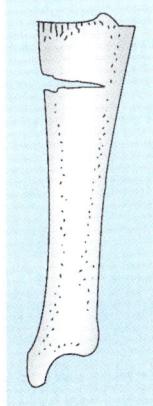

Fig. 3.3a: Stress fracture

Comminuted Fracture

When bone breaks into multiple pieces as in crush injuries, commonly seen in run over accidents (Fig. 3.3b).

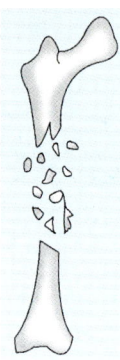

Fig. 3.3b: Comminuted fracture

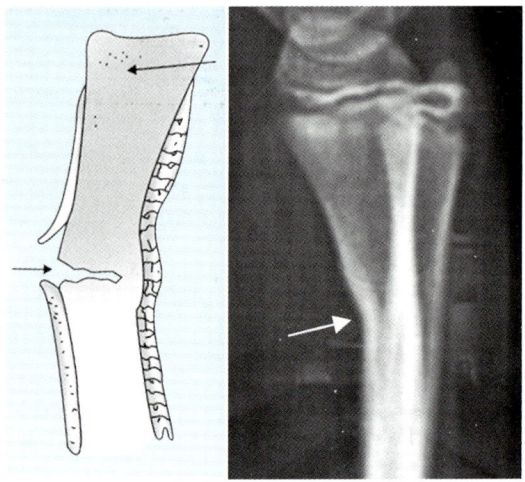

Figs 3.3d and e: Greenstick fracture

Segmental Fracture

When the long bone breaks at two places, proximal and distal with a free-floating middle fragment.

Torus Fracture

Here both cortices are buckled, due to vertical compression, with intact periosteum, hence the fragments are undisplaced (Fig. 3.3f).

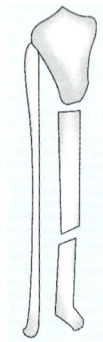

Fig. 3.3c: Segmental fracture

Greenstick Fracture

In a child, the bones are pliable and elastic hence they bend under pressure, with or without a breach in the cortex. Greenstick fracture has intact periosteum on the concave side, where the bone buckles while the other cortex bends and breaks at the convex side (Figs 3.3d and e).

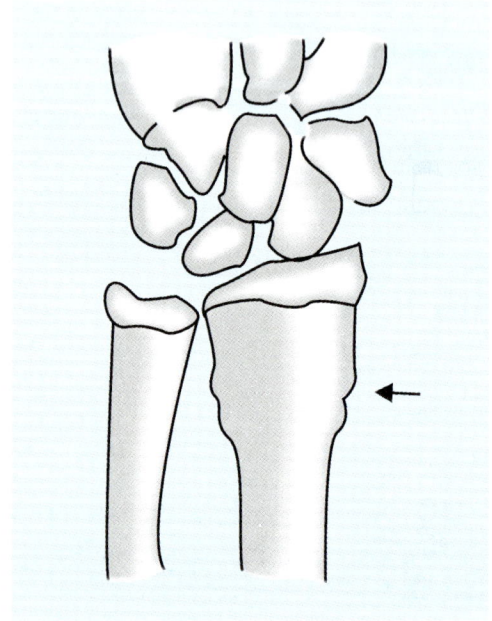

Fig. 3.3f: Torus fracture

Epiphyseal Injuries

These are fractures in children at the epiphyseo-metaphyseal area, classified as shown below :

Salter-Harris Classification.

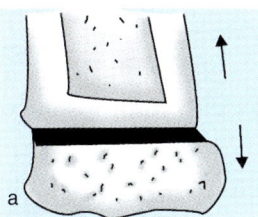

Type 1: Complete separation of epiphysis from metaphysis without any X-ray evidence of a metaphyseal fragment attached to displaced epiphysis (Fig. 3.4a).

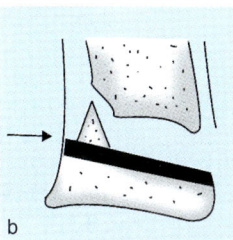

Type 2: Fracture plane travels transversely across the growth plate for a variable distance and then through the metaphysis producing a triangular-shaped fragment the *"Thurston-Holland"* sign (Fig. 3.4b).

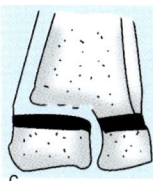

Type 3: Fracture plane passes along the growth plate and across the epiphysis (intra-articular), seen around the knee and elbow (Fig. 3.4c).

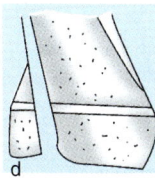

Type 4: Fracture line is vertical passing across the epiphysis, growth plate and metaphysis (intra-articular) (Fig. 3.4d).

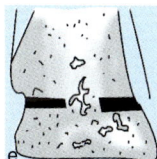

Type 5: Compression injury, destruction of growth plate, and growth disturbances (Fig. 3.4e).

Figs 3.4a to e: Types of epiphyseal injuries

MECHANISM OF INJURY

- **Severe trauma :** Enough to cause a fracture (single or repeated).
- **Trivial injury :** As in pathological fracture.

Severe Trauma

Single Episode of Injury

Direct injuries

Always associated with (in adults) overlying soft tissue damage. The force passing through the soft tissue to the bone.

i. *Tapping force*: Transverse fracture shaft of long bones, depressed fracture of skull (Gutter fracture), fissure fracture of flat bones (scapula, pelvis fracture) (Fig. 3.5a).

ii. *Crushing injuries:* Comminuted fracture with extensive soft tissue damage. The damaging force passes through the skin and muscles down to the bone, crushing all the tissue along its path (Fig. 3.5b).

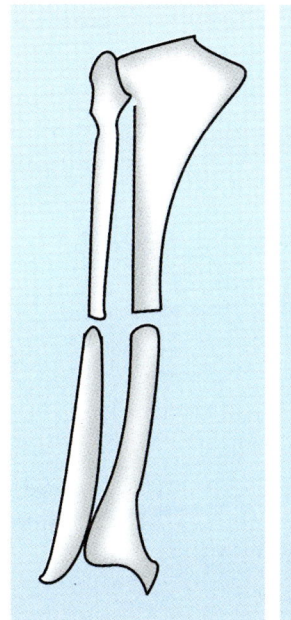
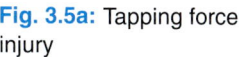
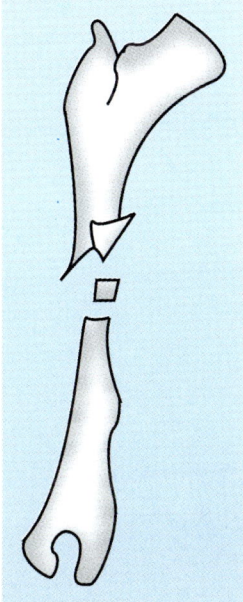

Fig. 3.5a: Tapping force injury

Fig. 3.5b: Crushing injuries

iii. *Missile injuries:* Splintering fracture, seen in war, as bullet and blast injuries. This high energy force passes through the bone, blasting it into several pieces (Fig. 3.5c).

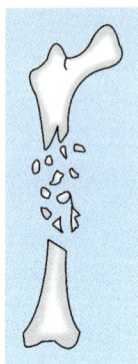

Fig. 3.5c: Splintering fracture

Indirect injuries

The soft tissue escapes the line of force and hence is often undamaged.

i. *Twisting force:* Spiral fracture (Fig. 3.6a).
ii. *Angulation force:* Transverse fracture without soft tissue damage (Fig. 3.6b).

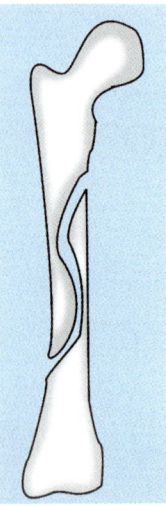

Fig. 3.6a: Spiral fracture

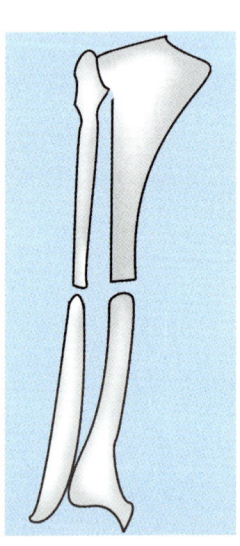

Fig. 3.6b: Transverse fracture

iii. *Angulation + axial compression:* Fracture with butterfly piece (Fig. 3.6c).
iv. *Angulation + axial compression + rotation:* Short oblique fracture (Fig. 3.6d).

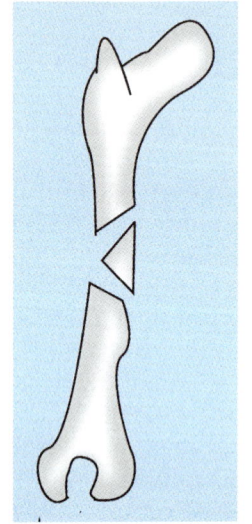

Fig. 3.6c: Angulation/axial compression fracture

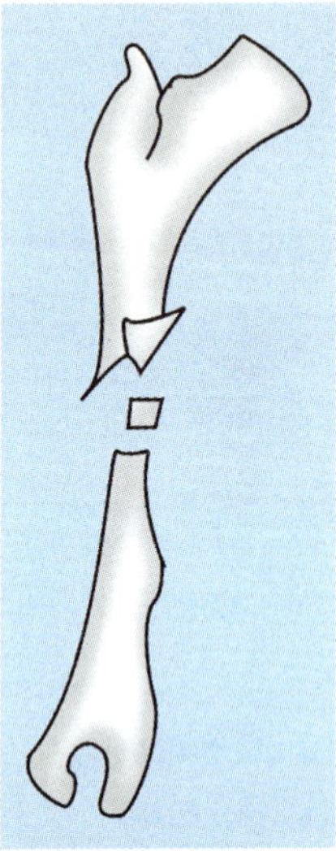

Fig. 3.6d: Short oblique fracture

Vertical compression

Wedge/collapse as in vertebrae and calcaneum (Fig. 3.6e).

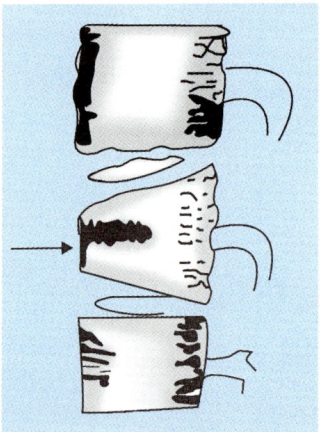

Fig. 3.6e: Wedge/collapse in vertebrae (arrow)

Traction

Due to violent muscular contraction it causes avulsion of bone, e.g. fracture patella (seen in epileptics and tetanus) (Fig. 3.6f)

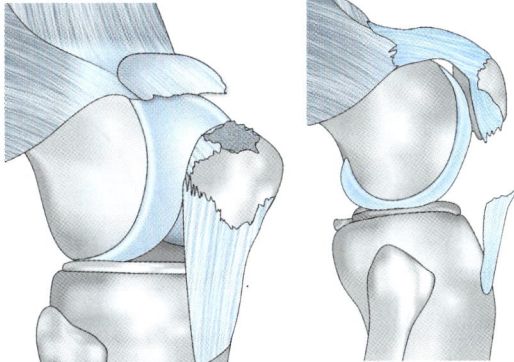

Fig. 3.6f: Fracture patella (avulsion of bone)

Repeated Episodes of Injury

Stress fracture

This is due to repeated, cyclic minor trauma over a long period of time, e.g. **March fracture** in military recruits (Fig. 3.7).

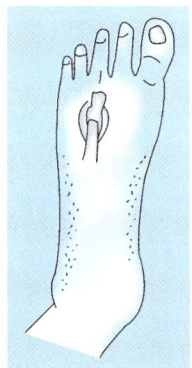

Fig. 3.7: March fracture

Trivial Injury

Fracture occurs as a result of underlying pathology.

- **Hereditary:** Osteogenesis imperfecta, brittle bone disease.
- **Infection:** Osteomyelitis.
- **Degenerative:** Osteoporosis.
- **Metabolic:** Osteomalacia, hyperparathyroidism.
- **Tumour:** Simple bone cyst in young (Fig. 3.8a) and secondaries in old patients (Fig. 3.8b).

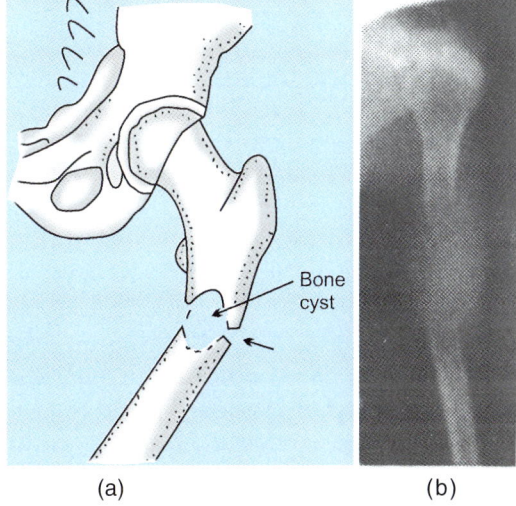

(a)   (b)

Figs 3.8a and b: Simple bone cyst in young, (b) secondaries in old patients

Diagnosis

- Careful history
- Thorough clinical examination
- Investigation.

History

Care should be taken to evaluate the fracture in view of the age, sex, occupation and previous history of fracture, mechanism of forces in injury, history of convulsions. Keep in mind the involvement of bladder, bowel habits and history of the drug allergies and addictions.

Clinical Examination

General

Posture may be typical in cervical cord injury and dislocations, etc.

Lesion at cervical segment	Attitude
• 5th cervical segment	Immobile against the trunk and completely paralysis
• 6th cervical segment	Patient lies helplessly on the back with the arm "Hands up" position abducted and externally rotated and the forearm flexed and supinated
• 7th cervical segment	Arm is partially abducted and internally rotated with the forearm flexed and pronated paralysis of intrinsic muscle as hand will used to main en griffe

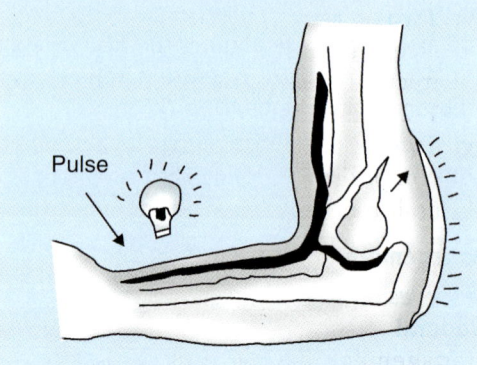

Pulse

Fig. 3.9: Supracondylar fracture of humerus with doubtful radial pulse.

Always keep in mind that the injured patient should be examined as a whole not just the injured part. The part should be well exposed for examination and compared with the normal. Always make it a point to examine head, eyes, ears, mouth, chest, its respiratory movements, abdomen, pelvis, the pelvic viscera and the functions of the spinal cord. *Record the pulse, BP and respiration.*

Local

i. Posture of the patient.
ii. Deformity of part, shortening and swelling.
iii. Bruising and blisters at fracture site.
iv. Bony crepitations, abnormal movements.
v. Loss of transmitted movements.
vi. Examination of distal sensation and pulsation for neuromuscular damage (Fig. 3.9).
vii. Always examine important related viscera , e.g. bladder, urethra in the pelvic injury and spinal cord in the vertebral injuries.
viii. Range of movements and stability of relevant joints for intra-articular injuries.

Whenever the patient comes to you, he may have 3 important complications
Following trauma each may be fatal:
Few hours – Shock
Few days – Fat embolism
Few weeks – Thromboembolism

Investigations

For diagnosis and subsequent management :
i. Radiological; X-rays, CT scan, MRI, myelography, nerve conduction study, electromyography, ultrasonography.
ii. Doppler studies for vascular injuries, arthroscopy for intra-articular injuries.
iii. Routine haematological and serological evaluation to assess the status of health.
iv. Urine routine and microscopy.
v. Synovial fluid for synovitis, haemarthrosis and arthritis.

Whenever writing a requisition for X-ray of an injured patient, following points must be kept in mind "Rule of 2".
i. Full length of bone should be clearly visible in the skiagram.
ii. **Two joints**, i.e. one above and one below the fracture should be included.
iii. **Two view**, AP and lateral (if necessary oblique also especially in hand and foot injuries).

iv. **Two occasions**, whenever in doubt as in stress fracture, scaphoid/greenstick fracture (repeat X-ray after an interval of 1–2 weeks).

v. **Two limbs**, in the epiphyseal injuries (for comparison with normal) especially in children.

Management

Principles of Treatment

General

Management of shock and haemorrhage, replace fluid and electrolytes, maintain input and output chart. Antibiotics, anti-inflammatory drugs, tetanus toxoid, etc.

Local

Care of the soft tissue and stabilization of bone.

Management of Simple Fracture

Reduced and maintained in position for 6–12 weeks.

i. **Reduction:** The fracture fragments are reduced by
   a. Closed reduction under anaesthesia.
   b. Open reduction for unstable fracture, intra-artricular fracture, complicated fracture, segmental fracture.

ii. **Maintenance** of reduction is achieved by:
   a. External support
      • Plaster, splints, tractions (Fig. 3.10a).
   b. Internal fixation (Fig. 3.10b)
      • Cortical by plates and screws.
      • Medullary fixation by nails.
   c. External fixators (Fig. 3.10c)

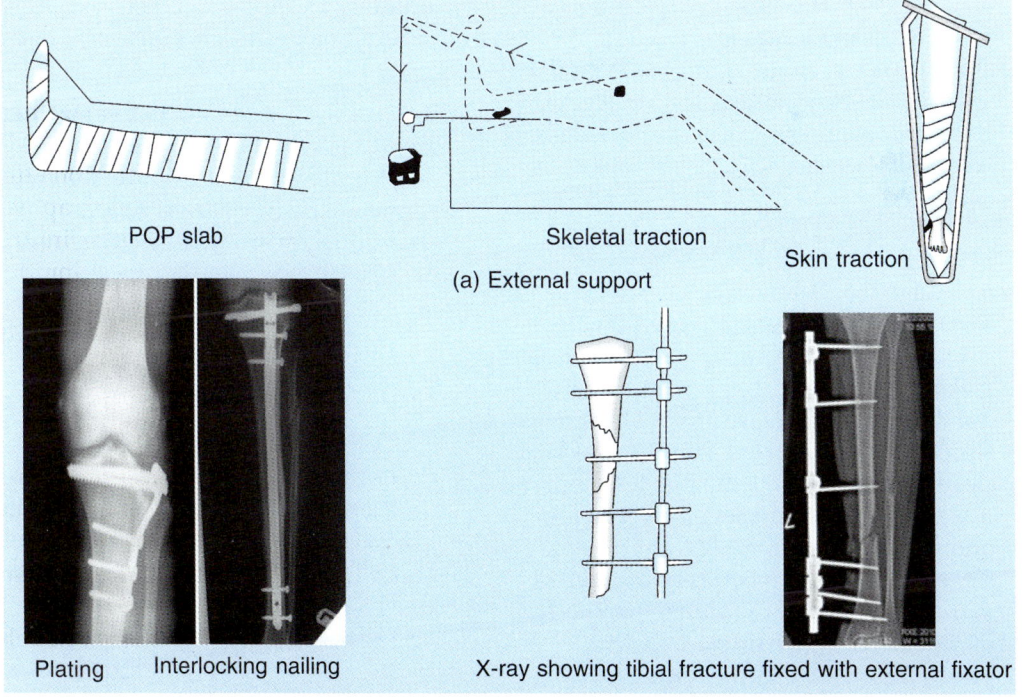

POP slab   Skeletal traction   Skin traction

(a) External support

Plating   Interlocking nailing   X-ray showing tibial fracture fixed with external fixator

(b) Internal fixation   (c) External fixator

Figs 3.10a to c: Different modalities to stabilize a fracture

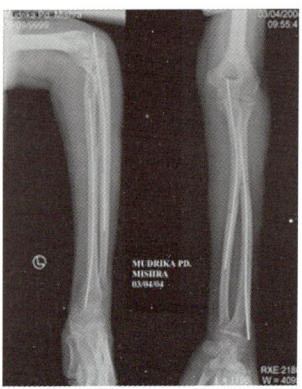 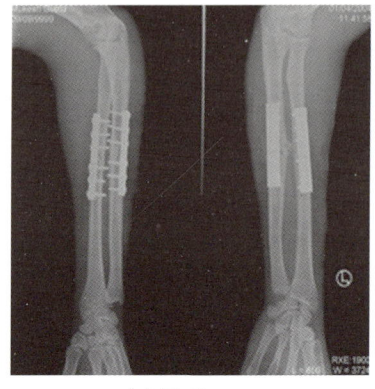 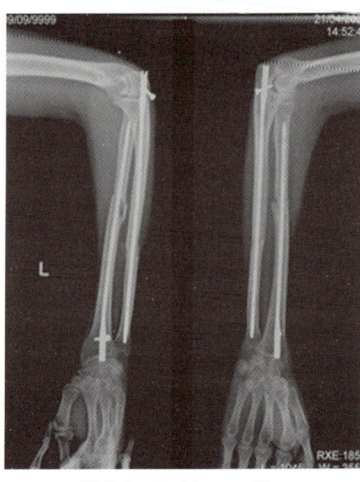

(d) Simple nailing (e) Plating (f) Interlocking nailing

Figs 3.10d to f: Different modalities to stabilize a fracture

External fixation is for temporary stabilisation of the fracture when there is :
- Potentially contaminated wound.
- Extensive soft tissue damage (Type III) to continue maintaining accurate reduction and stabilisation of bone, till healing of fracture and soft tissue cover is achieved.

Management of Compound Fractures

Principle of management is:

i. **First aid management (airway, bleeding, circulation):** Clear airway, control of haemorrhage by firm compression bandage, management of shock by quick fluid and blood replacement. Most of the deaths which occur in the first few hours are due to the mismanagement of shock and haemorrhage.
Take care during transport with cervical collar and support of injured part with maintenance of life support system.

ii. **Assessment of the patient:** Examine CNS, cardiothoracic function, abdomen, bladder, bowel status and always note down the vitals.

iii. **Supportive treatment:** Antibiotics, antitetanus protection, antigasgangrene serum, analgesics *(note all the treatments given)*.

iv. **Local (bone and soft tissue) management**
a. Wound debridement to remove all dead and devitalised tissue.
b. Stabilization of bone by external fixators initially (Fig. 3.11).

v. **Final management of wound**
a. Primary closure by suture of skin is done only if the wound is clean, and has good circulation without NV deficit. Wound age should be < 6 hours.
b. *Wound left open:* If wound > 6 hours, and potentially contaminated, delayed primary closure is preferable after few days.
c. Delayed autogenous graft using split thickness, rotational/cross leg flaps.
d. Secondary closure after five days by:
- suture
- grafting

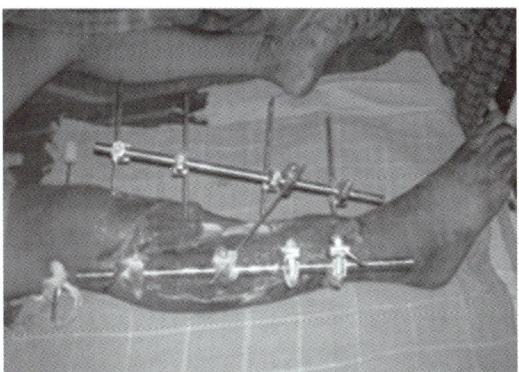

Fig. 3.11: External fixator for a compound fracture

- Split thickness over raw granulating tissue.
- Full thickness over exposed bone, tendons.
vi. Delayed repair of tendons/nerves.
vii. Final stabilization of bone by POP cast/internal fixation.

Complications of Fractures

General
i. *Early:* Shock and haemorrhage, fat embolism and fracture fever.
ii. *Late:* Thromboembolism and osteoporosis due to prolonged immobilization.

Local
i. *Immediate:*
   a. Injury to important vessels, nerves and viscera.
   b. Infections such as pyogenic, tetanus and gas gangrene.
ii. *Late:*
   a. *Bone:* Delayed union, malunion, non-union, avascular necrosis (e.g. head of femur in fracture neck), growth disturbance following epiphyseal injury in children.
   b. *Soft tissues:*
      • *Muscles:* Myositis ossificans following passive manipulation of an injured joint, muscle adhesions leading to stiffness of joints.
      • *Tendons:* Adhesions, rupture.
      • *Vessels:* Volkmann's ischaemia, contracture/atrophy due to compartmental syndrome.
   c. *Joints:*
      • Stiffness due to Sudeck's atrophy.
      • Instability due to ligament injuries.
   d. Malignancies following trauma, e.g. osteoclastoma and osteogenic sarcoma following injury to metaphyseal area.

IMPORTANT COMPLICATIONS

- Non-union, malunion, delayed union, avascular necrosis.
- MOT (Myositis ossificans traumatica).
- VIC (Volkmann's ischaemic contracture), compartment syndrome.
- Fat embolism.
- Sudeck's atrophy.
- Joint stiffness.
- Fracture disease (problems associated with rest and immobilisation following fracture).

Non-union

Definition

It is the failure of the fracture to heal after adequate time (6–9 months) by the osseous tissue, there is persistence of the fracture gap and painless abnormal mobility at the fracture site entailing surgical intervention.

Types

i. Hyper vascular non-union, elephant foot (Fig. 3.12a), horse hoof (Fig. 3.12b). This is due to inadequate immobilization of a well vascularised fractured end.
ii. Atrophic non-union (Fig. 3.12c). This is due to poor vascularity and nutrition.
iii. Avascular non-union, torsion wedge (Fig.3.12d), comminuted non-union,

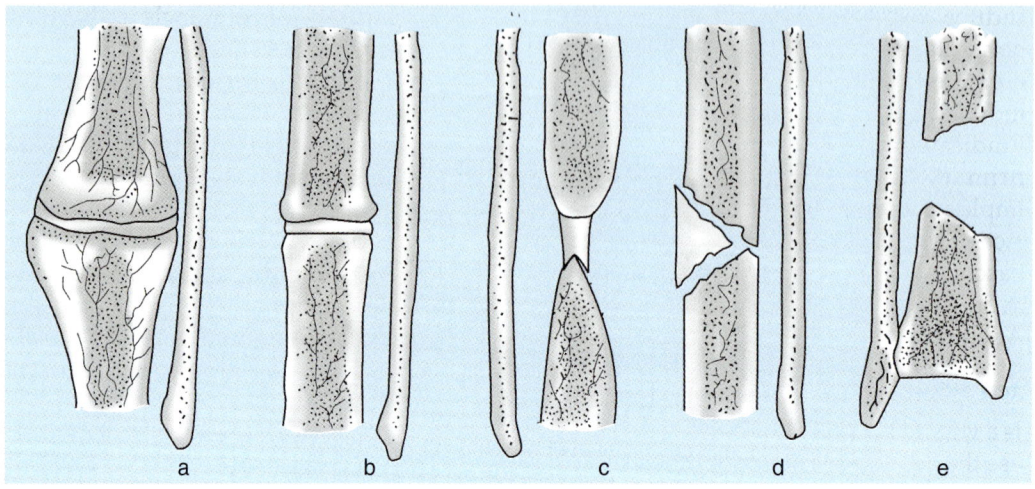

a   b   c   d   e

Figs 3.12a to e: Types of non-union fracture

defective non-union due to bone loss (Fig. 3.12e).

iv. *Pseudoarthrosis:* A false joint formation at fracture site (congenital defect, acquired due to hypermobility at fracture site).

Causes (SIX 'I')

i. **I**nadequate immobilization.

ii. **I**nfections.

iii. **I**schaemia, due to severe crushing, skin and soft tissue loss.

iv. **I**nfarction of the bone (avascular necrosis), as in fracture of neck of femur/scaphoid.

v. **I**ntervening soft tissue: Muscle, periosteum, synovial fluid (fracture of neck of femur).

vi. **I**ntact fellow bone as in Galeazzi's fracture where the intact ulna interferes with the healing of radius fracture.

Clinical Features

Painless abnormal mobility at the fractured site after 6–9 months of injury.

Radiological Features

Persistence of fracture gap after adequate time, sclerosed margins of the fracture ends with surrounding osteoporosis.

i. **Atrophic:**
   a. Conical bone ends.
   b. Medullary plug.
   c. No signs of periosteal or endosteal callus formation.

ii. **Hypertrophic:** Rounded elephant foot type of callus formation on both sides of fracture line, but fracture gap still persists.

iii. **Gap non-union:** Loss of bone at fracture sites at the time of injury so that there is loss of contact between fracture ends.

Principle of Treatment

i. Excision of sclerosed and atrophic bone to create raw bleeding surface.

ii. Removal of medullary plug, to open up medullary vascular channels.

iii. Rigid cortical or medullary fixation in the proper alignment by DCP, intramedullary locked nail or Illizarov's fixator, compression at fracture site.

iv. Induce osteogenesis by bone grafting, bone marrow injection at fracture site, electrical stimulation by magnetic induction.

v. Eradication of the infection (if this is the primary cause), removal of improper implant.

vi. Active mobilization to promote periosteal vascular inflow through muscles and to avoid stiff joints.

vii. Adequate skin and soft tissue cover.

Infected Non-union

This is a very common and difficult situation, because the problem is double fold. First, it is necessary to eradicate the infection by drugs and local debridement of all the infective tissue from skin down to the bone and remove all devitalized tissue. The next step is to change or remove the implant (which is the most common cause) and to switch over to a suitable fixator for stabilization of the fracture. Finally, after control of infection, a well-planned procedure for bone grafting and fixation of fracture is done.

Myositis Ossificans

Definition

Ossification of an injured muscle (haematoma) following a fracture or dislocation, leading to a stiff and painful joint.

Types

i. *Traumatica:* After injuries.

ii. *Progressiva:* As a hereditary disease.

iii. *Heterotrophica:* As in head injury.

Most common cause: Repeated manipulations and massage of injuries around the joint.

Most common area is around the elbow.

X-ray

i. **Active stage:** Hazy, translucent or cotton wool appearance with diffuse margins in front (in the branchialis muscle), behind (in triceps muscle), sides (common flexor/extensor muscles) of elbow.

ii. **Quiescent stage:** Bony shadow with clear margins and visible trabecular pattern.

Treatment

i. **Active stage:** Immobilization in a slab, avoid massage or any passive stretching, antiinflammatory drug like indomethacin.

ii. **Healed:** Active mobilization of joint and surgical excision of the myositis mass after it has matured (with caution, as recurrence is frequent).

Volkmann's Ischaemic Contracture (Compartment syndrome)

Definition

This is a crippling complication of fracture due to impeded blood flow, increased compartmental pressure and progressive damage of all the tissues; skin, muscles, nerves and bone which are preventable to a great extent. Commonly involving the forearm/tibial compartment; first described by Prof. Richard Volkmann, a German surgeon in 1881.

Stages

- Initial phase of ischaemia (reversible)
- Phase of contracture (irreversible and crippling).

1. **Phase of Ischaemia**
   a. **Causes:**
      i. *Upper limb:* Damage to the brachial artery following fracture supracondylar humerus, sometimes posterior dislocation of elbow and fracture of radius/ulna, causing damage to forearm vessels.
      ii. *Lower limb:* Damage to posterior/anterior tibial vessel after fracture

of tibia/fibula, usually the upper third.

b. *Occlusion of blood flow through the artery may be because of*
   i. External pressure on the vessel due to:
      • tight plaster bandage or wooden splints.
      • grossly displaced fracture fragments.
   ii. Damage to the vessel wall by cut or contusion of artery/vein.
   iii. Occlusion of lumen due to:
      • spasm
      • thrombus
      • intimal tear.

c. *Pathophysiology of ischaemia:* Vessels, nerves and muscles are compressed in tight osteofascial compartment due to oedema, with no arterial inflow and poor venous return due to rapid increase in compartmental pressure, slow tissue death and necrosis.

d. *Clinical features:* Patient presents with following clinical features.
   Five P's:
   i. **P**ain in distal parts of forearm and hand, which is excruciating, unbearable and is the earliest symptom.
   ii. **P**allor of nail bed.
   iii. **P**aresthesia, numbness and tingling.
   iv. **P**ulselessness (absent radial/dorsalis pedis pulsations).
   v. **P**aralysis of the involved muscles, in late cases.

   Most important and earliest single sign is *Griffith's sign* (passive stretching of the flexed finger causes severe pain).

e. *Principle of management:* To relieve the compression on the vascular channel and to restore the vascularity of the distal part at the earliest.

f. *Treatment:*
   i. **Decompress:**
      • Remove all external splintages and bandages immediately, do fasciotomy.
      • Cool the limb by ice packs to reduce metabolic demands.
      • If the fracture fragments are grossly displaced, do closed reduction under anaesthesia at the earliest.
      • Watch for return of capillary circulation and the pulsation.
   ii. **Repair:** If within few hours circulation does not improve, Doppler study may show the type of arterial block, exploration of the damaged vessel, decompression and necessary repair should be done.

2. **Phase of contracture**
   It is the end result of prolonged ischaemia, causing irreversible damage to muscle and nerve.
   a. **Pathophysiology of contracture:** Prolonged ischaemia leads to necrosis of muscles, nerves, atrophy of skin, bone and soft tissue. In due time necrosed muscles are replaced by fibrous tissue (bands) resulting into contracture.
   b. **Clinical features:** Patient presents with a deformed hand, which is stiff, weak and numb. The extent of involvement may be mild, moderate or severe with extensive involvement of muscles, bones and nerves.

   Deformity (Volkmann's sign is positive, as shown below).

   Fingers are flexed at interphalangeal joints due to contracture of flexor muscles of the forearm. This deformity increases with dorsiflexion (Fig. 3.13a), and diminishes with flexion of wrist; this is due to fibrotic flexor muscles (Fig. 3.13b).

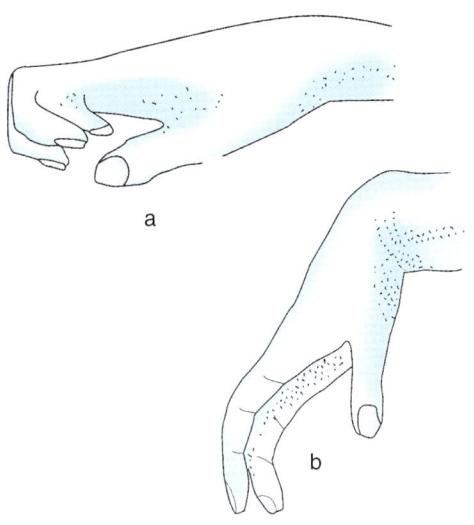

a

b

Figs 3.13a and b: Volkmann's sign

- *Joints:* Stiff and bones are atrophied.
- *Muscles:* Loss of the power of grip, small muscles of hand/forearm are wasted.
- *Nerves:* Loss of sensation affecting the median and ulnar nerves.
- *Skin:* Skin becomes atrophic and so do nails and hair.
- c. **Treatment:** Depending on the extent of the involvement:
  - i. *Mild:* Muscle sliding of the common flexors (MaxPage).
  - ii. *Moderate to severe:* Excision of the dead fibrotic muscle, tendon transfers, nerve grafting, proximal row carpectomy, wrist arthrodesis.

Fat Embolism
- Seen within 2–3 days after fracture of major bones.
- Following liposuction for cosmetic surgery.
- Polytrauma and crush injuries.

Clinical Features
Depends on the organ involved, i.e. brain, lungs, heart, kidney, etc.

The patient suddenly becomes restless, disoriented, feverish, comatose, dyspnoeic, has retention of urine and transient rash over neck and chest, might have conjunctival haemorrhage, hypertension with tachycardia. Fundoscopy may show characteristic findings.

Investigations
  i. The sputum and urine contains fat globules.
  ii. X-ray chest, shows **snow storm** pattern and bilateral infiltration of lungs.
  iii. PO_2 is always less than 60.

Management
Hyperbaric oxygen to combat hypoxia. Steroids to manage cardiac and respiratory distress, maintain adequate renal perfusion.

FRACTURE HEALING

Primary
Seen when accurate reduction and firm fixation is done. Fracture heals without external callus formation, the stage of cartilage formation is absent and direct endosteal bone formation occurs. There is no periosteal cuff of callus.

Secondary
Healing occurs both by periosteal as well as endosteal callus.

Fracture Healing Time (Table 3.1)
Perkin's Rule of "6"

Table 3.1: Healing time (in weeks)			
	Spiral fracture	*Transverse fracture*	*Consolidation time*
Upper limb	6	12	24
Lower limb	12	24	48

Stages of Fracture Healing

(Classic stages as described by Hunter).

Stage 1 : Haematoma
Stage 2 : Granulation
Stage 3 : Soft callus
Stage 4 : Hard callus
Stage 5 : Remodelling
Stage 6 : Final healing

Stage of haematoma

When a bone breaks, the gap is filled with blood from the ruptured periosteal and endosteal vessels. This blood distends to the soft tissues and clots to form a haematoma. This process takes about one to two days (Fig. 3.14a).

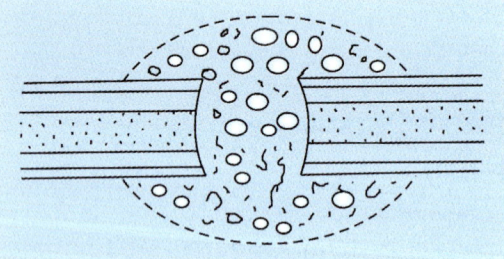

Fig. 3.14a: Formation of haematoma

Stage of granulation tissue

The margins of the bone undergo aseptic necrosis. The soft tissues in the region undergo the usual changes of acute aseptic inflammation with vasodilatation and exudation of plasma and leucocytes. The clotted blood is invaded by fine capillaries and young connective tissue and is converted into granulation tissues in about two weeks. The multipotent cells can differentiate into fibroblast, chondroblast and osteoblast (Fig. 3.14b).

Stage of soft callus formation

The granulation tissue matures into fibro-cartilaginous mass, which subsequently is

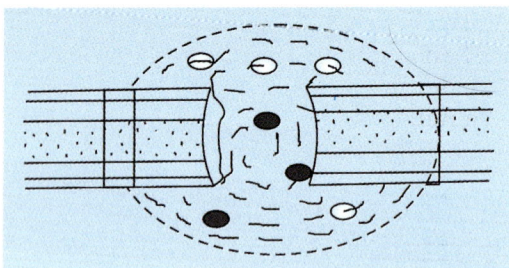

Fig. 3.14b: Formation of granulation tissues

converted into spongy immature bone. First, a bridge of callus develops in the subperiosteal zone, this is called external callus. Subsequently, medullary callus formation starts, which is called the internal callus (Fig. 3.14c).

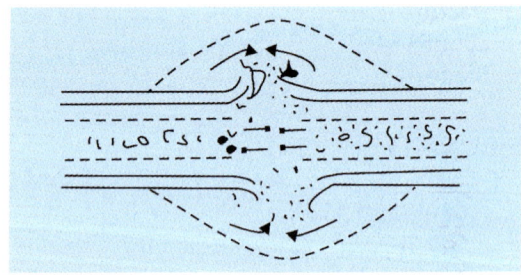

Fig. 3.14c: Soft callus formation

Stage of hard callus formation

The spongy bone gets converted into matured lamellar bone (Fig. 3.14d).

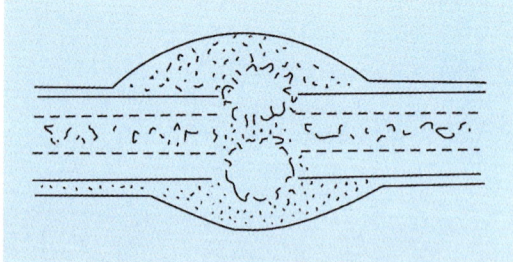

Fig. 3.14d: Hard callus formation

Stage of remodelling (Fig. 3.14e)
The new formed bone starts arranging itself under stress and strain into sheets of new lamellae. The initially deformed bone

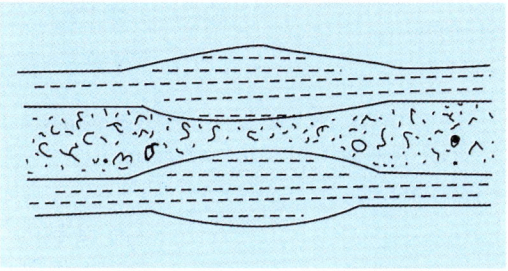

Fig. 3.14e: Stage of remodelling

undergoes the process of reorganisation and contouring. The extra callus which is formed gradually gets absorbed. The fracture is clinically well united and takes about 3 to 6 months.

Stage of final healing (Fig. 3.14f)

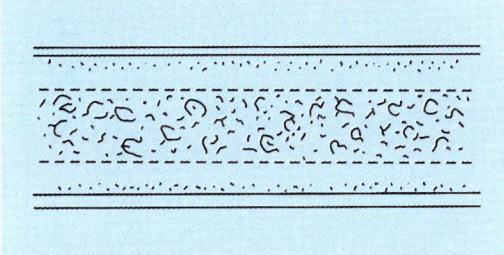

Fig. 3.14f: The final healing stage

The original bone structure is restored and extra callus formation is completely reabsorbed. This takes about a year.

Factors Affecting the Healing

General
i. *Age:* In children quick healing is due to the high osteogenic potential, whereas it is, poor, in old age and debilitated persons.
ii. *Nutritional status:* Protein, calorie and calcium are required for good callus formation.
iii. *Associated diseases:* Diabetes, tuberculosis, malignancies (they all decrease the rate of healing).

Local
i. Type of fracture, apposition of bone at fracture site, adequacy of immobilization, vascularity of the part, status of soft tissue around and infections. Soft tissue damage and infection leads to delayed healing.
ii. Compression/distraction can induce osteogenesis as stated by Wolff's law that "new bone is laid down along stress and compression lines".
iii. Status of the muscles acting across the joint, active mobilization and weight bearing, encourages rapid healing and remodelling of fracture, by encouraging inflow of blood through the muscles and laying down of bone along stress lines.

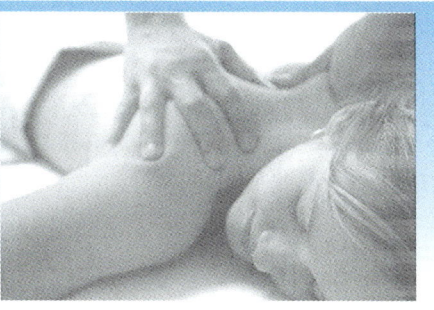

THERE ARE 206 BONES IN THE HUMAN SKELETON OF WHICH 80 ARE SINGLE, SITUATED IN THE MEDIAN PLANE AND 63 ARE PAIRED OCCUPYING THE LIMBS. THERE ARE 639 MUSCLES.

SOME IMPORTANT FRACTURES

INJURIES OF THE UPPER LIMB

FRACTURE—CLAVICLE

It is the most common bone fracture in body as well as in baby.

Commonest Site

Junction of two curves, i.e. lateral one-third and medial two-thirds.
- Lateral fragment is pulled:
  - Down by the weight of limb.
  - Medially by the pull of pectoral muscle.
- Medial fragment is pulled up by sterno-mastoid muscle.

Mechanism of Injury

- Pulling out the foetus during the breech presentation (shoulder dystocia).
- Fall on the outstretched hand.
- Direct blow to the shoulder by stick or boxing.
  In spite of the fact that this bone is subcutaneous throughout its length, compound fracture is very uncommon because skin overlying is freely mobile.

Clinical Features

- Painful lump involving the clavicle after trauma.
- Palpable bony crepitus.
- Inability to move the upper limb, especially in neonates (pseudoparalysis).
  Always examine the pulsation and the sensations to rule out the possibility of underlying subclavian vessel and brachial plexus injury.

If the patient has surgical emphysema then the apical zone of lung has been damaged.

Treatment
- **Neonates and infants:** (Reassurance of the parents) Triangular sling with arm to chest bandage, for a few days.
- **Adults:**
  - *Simple fracture:* Figure of '8' bandage with good axillary cotton padding for 3 to 4 weeks, with cuff and collar sling or Meck's clavicle brace (Figs 3.15a to d).

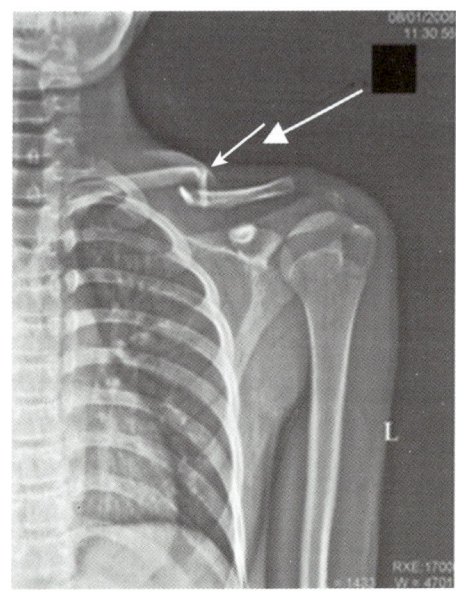

Fig. 3.15a: X-ray showing fracture clavical (arrow)

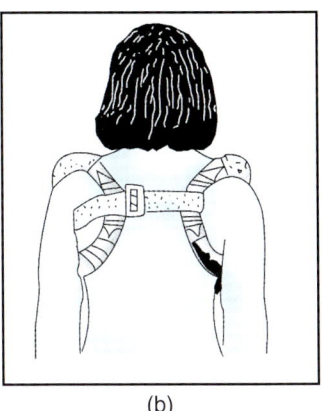
(b)

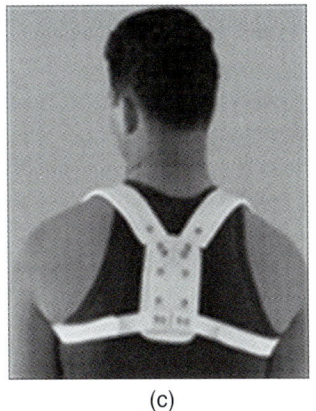
(c)

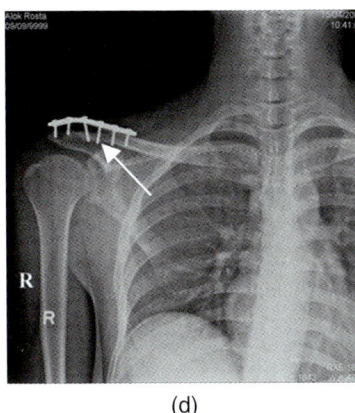
(d)

Figs 3.15b to d: (b) Figure of '8' bandage (c) Meck's clavicle brace (d) X-ray showing fracture clavicle fix with cortical plate and screw

– *Compound fracture:* Intramedullary fixation with K-wires, cortical plates and screws, if necessary with bone grafting (Fig. 3.15).

Complications
- **Bone:** Malunion (unavoidable, lump) but remodelling occurs later. Non-union is seen in comminuted fracture.
- **Nerve:**
  – Damage to the medial cord of the brachial plexus.
  – Entrapment of the middle branch of the supraclavicular nerve in the callus causing paresthesia over the pectoral region.
- **Vessels:** Damage to the subclavian vessel *(patient may bleed to death on the spot).*
- **Lungs:** Emphysema due to pulmonary injury involving the apical lobe.

Acromio-Clavicular Dislocation

This is as a result of fall on the shoulder. If only the acromioclavicular ligament is torn then subluxation occurs, if in addition, the coracoclavicular ligament ruptures then dislocation is seen. The displacement is best visualized clinically by asking the patient to hold weights in both the hands and radiologically, by taking AP view of both the shoulder joints, the clavicle is seen lifted up laterally.

Treatment
- Subluxation is treated in a triangular sling for 4 weeks.
- Dislocation requires surgical fixation of clavicle to the coracoid by screw or threaded pin through the acromio-clavicular joint with repair of the coraco-clavicular ligaments.

ANATOMY OF SHOULDER JOINT

The glenohumeral joint, commonly known as the shoulder joint, is a synovial ball and socket joint and involves articulation between the glenoid fossa of the scapula (shoulder blade) and the head of the humerus (upper arm bone).

On the lateral angle of the scapula is a shallow pyriform, articular surface, the glenoid cavity (or glenoid fossa of scapula), which is directed lateral ward and forward and articulates with the head of the humerus; it is broader below than above and its vertical diameter is the longest. The surface is covered with cartilage in the fresh state; and its margins, slightly raised, give attachment to a fibrocartilaginous structure, the glenoid labrum, which deepens the cavity (Fig. 3.16).

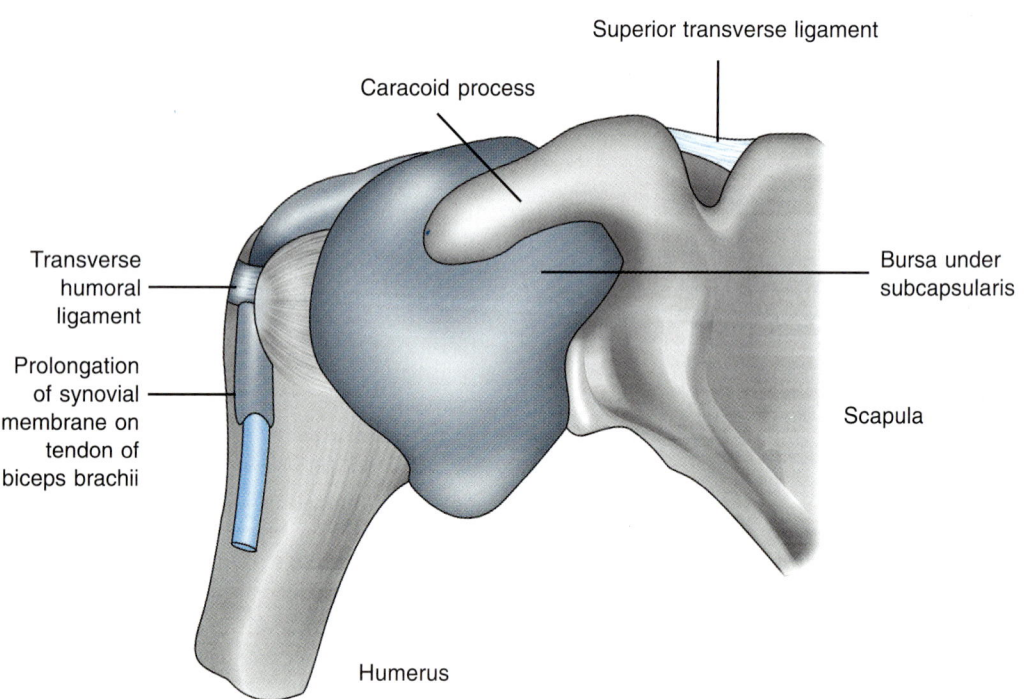

Fig. 3.16: Anatomy of shoulder joint

Movements of Shoulder Joint

Active movements permitted at the shoulder joint are: flexion (180°) and extension (40°), abduction and adduction, circumduction, medial and lateral rotations (80°). These movements are analysed with reference to the body of scapula, rather than the conventional planes of the trunk. Abduction is first 90 degrees at the shoulder joint and the beyond 90 to 160 degrees is at the scapulo- thoracic zone. The clavicle plays an important role in the abduction.

Shoulder Dislocations

Type

1. **Habitual:** Can be done at will by patients (especially girls) due to ligamentous laxity as a parlour trick.
2. **Recurrent:** With trivial trauma or abduction and external rotation of shoulder, often, as a result of improper management of the initial dislocation.
3. **Acute traumatic type:** Acute single episode of the major trauma. Depending on the position of the head of humerus:
   - Anterior – Subclavicular
     – Subcoracoid (commonest)
   - Posterior – Supraspinous
     – Infraspinous
   - Inferior – Luxatio-in-erecta (Infraglenoid).

Clinical Features

Most common is anterior dislocation. Patient comes with arm abducted, forearm and elbow supported by other hand. Round contour of the deltoid is lost (flat shoulder) with positive Hamilton's ruler test. Head palpable below clavicle in abnormal position. Diminished length of the arm. Examine the sensation over insertion of the deltoid, to rule out the injury to axillary nerve. Due to spasm of muscles around the shoulder, all the movements are painfully restricted.

Tests

- **Hamilton's ruler test:** Loss of round shoulder contour. Normally, a ruler kept on the lateral side of the arm, does not touch the acromion above and the lateral epicondyle below, due to the deltoid muscle (Fig. 3.17a) but if there is dislocation of the head of humerus, the deltoid becomes flat, now a ruler kept on the lateral side of the arm, will touch the acromion above and the lateral epicondyle below.

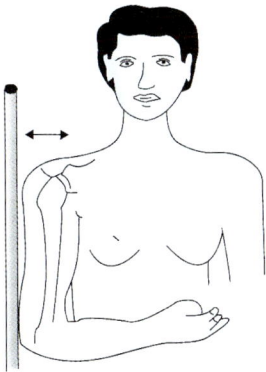

Fig. 3.17a: Hamilton's ruler test

- **Positive Duga's sign:** Inability to keep the elbow adducted in front of abdomen and palm touching the opposite shoulder (internal rotation) (Fig. 3.17b)

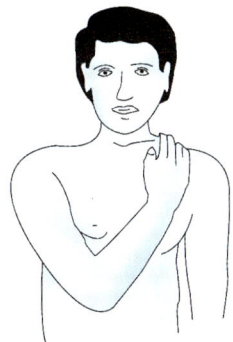

Fig. 3.17b: Duga's position

X-ray

AP and lateral view of the shoulder to see the type of the dislocation and to rule out associated fractures.

Management

- **Reduction:** Done under GA
  a. *Kocher's technique:*
    - Counter traction given by the assistant who pulls through well padded axillary sling.
    - The surgeon pulls and manipulates in 4 steps—**TEAM**
      T : Traction in the line of the deformity with the elbow flexed.
      E : External rotation.
      A : Adduction so that the tip of the elbow comes in front of the abdomen.
      M: Medial rotation, so that palm touches the opposite shoulder (Duga's position).
  b. *Hippocrates' method:* The traction is applied with forearm extended and the surgeon pulling against the pressure of the foot in the axilla (it is now obsolete and dangerous).
  c. *Stimson's method:* If patient is unfit for the anaesthesia then the patient is kept prone and appropriate traction is applied in forearm with the forearm hanging down. This is more so for the post dislocation of the shoulder.

  - **Maintenance:** Arm is strapped to the chest with the elbow in front of the umbilicus and the palm touching the opposite shoulder (Duga's position) for 3 weeks.

  - **Rehabilitation:** Start gentle active movements of the shoulder and build up the power of the rotator cuff after 3–4 weeks.

Complications

- **Bone** : Associated fracture, greater tuberosity, surgical neck of humerus.
- **Joint** : Recurrent dislocation, old unreduced dislocation, stiff shoulder.
- **Tendon** : Rupture of the supraspinatus.
- **Muscle** : Rotator cuff injury.
- **Nerve** : Brachial plexus, axillary nerve injury.

Recurrent Dislocations

It occurs as a result of the damage to anterior part of the capsule and rotator cuff or detachment of the glenoid labrum (Bankart lesion). Sometimes defect in the postero-superior quadrant of the head of humerus (Hill-Sachs lesion).

Even trivial injury or abduction and external rotation of the shoulder causes recurrent dislocations.

Clinical Features

Positive apprehension test: Abduction and external rotation movement causes pain and insecure feeling.

Treatment

- *Conservative:* Develop the power of the muscles of rotator cuff by physiotherapy.
- *Surgical:*
  - **Bankart operation:** Suturing of the detached labrum glenoidale to margins of glenoid cavity by sutures/staples.
  - **Putti Platt's operation:** Double breasting of the capsule and subscapularis tendon in front of the shoulder joint.
  - **Bristow's operation:** Especially for athletes (anterior bone block). Coracoid with its attachment is reposed in front of anterior rim of glenoid margin.

Fracture–Neck of Humerus

- **In children:** Due to fall on outstretched hand, pathological (due to bone cyst).
- **In old age:** Due to the osteoporosis or secondaries.

Clinical Features

Pain, swelling and tenderness, bony crepitation and loss of transmitted movements. All movements are painful and restricted, extensive bruising and ecchymosis over arm, especially in old patients.

Treatment

- **Children and old-age:** Undisplaced and impacted fracture is immobilized in a triangular sling.
- **Adults:**
  - In displaced fractures: Reduction under GA and immobilization in 'U slab' with arm to chest bandage for 3 weeks.
  - For irreducible fracture open reduction and internal fixation by K-wire or T-plate.

Fracture–Shaft Humerus

Displacement

Proximal fragment is abducted by deltoid, overriding of fragments due to contraction of the biceps and the triceps.

Clinical Features

Pain, swelling and deformity of arm, bony crepitus, loss of transmitted movements and shortening. All movements restricted by pain. **Always examine distal pulsations and sensations especially radial nerve in mid shaft fracture (may cause wrist drop).**

Treatment

- **Conservative:**
  - In neonates arm to chest bandage.
  - In adults hanging 'U' cast (weight of limb and plaster acts as reducing forces).

- **Surgical:** Open reduction and internal fixation for irreducible and unstable fracture.
  - *Children:* Rush nail fixation.
  - *Adults:*
    * Cortical fixation by plates and screws (Figs 3.18 a to d).
    * Intramedullary by 'V' nails and interlocked nails (Fig. 3.18b).
    * External fixators is done whenever there is extensive soft tissue damage and risk of contamination (Fig. 3.18c).

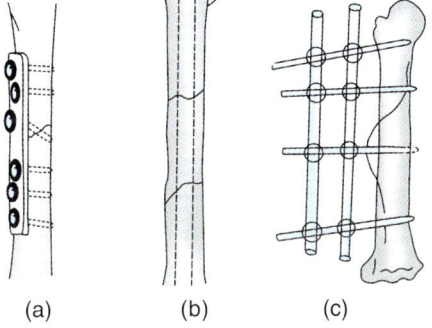

(a) (b) (c)

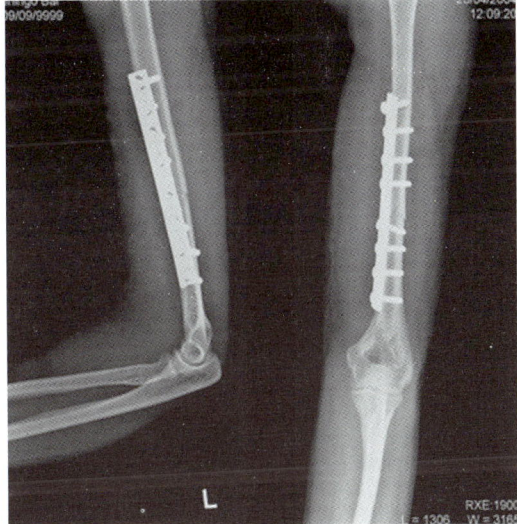

(d) X-ray showing cortical fixation with DC plating and screws

Figs 3.18a to d: Different modalities of internal fixation for fracture humerous

Complications

- **Bone:** Delayed union, non-union due to muscle entrapment, malunion.
- **Joint:** Shoulder and elbow stiffness.
- **Nerve:** Radial nerve injury (wrist drop).
- **Vessel:** Injury to brachial artery (VIC).

Fracture–Supracondylar Humerus

Most common and most serious fracture in childhood as it is often associated with complication. It is the fracture occurring through the supracondylar zone (metaphysis) of humerus. If any child comes with injury and swelling around the elbow, always think of this fracture unless or until proved otherwise.

Types

According to the position of the distal fragment in relation to the proximal fragment.

i. **Extension/posterior type (95%):** Fall on outstretched hand with elbow extended and forearm pronated. The distal fragment carrying the elbow with it gets displaced posteriorly, laterally, shifted proximally and gets pronated (Fig. 3.19a).

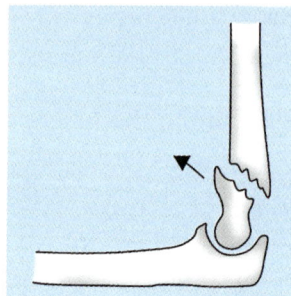

Fig. 3.19b: Flexion/anterior type

ii. **Flexion/anterior type (5%):** Mechanism of injury fall on point of flexed elbow. Distal fragment with elbow displaced proximally, anteriorly, laterally and supinated.

Clinical Features

Pain, swelling, deformity following injury. All movements painfully restricted. Relationship of three bony prominences of elbow maintained. Shortening of the arm length, palpable bony crepitus, often elbow is grossly swollen with blisters all over (Fig. 3.20).

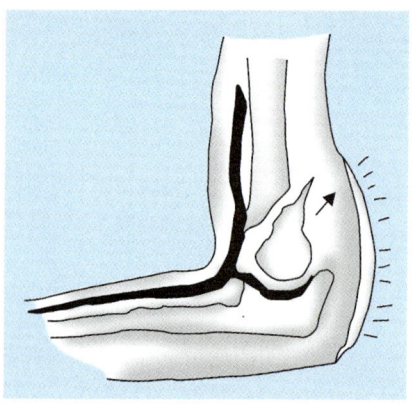

Fig. 3.19a: Extension/posterior type supracondylar humerus fracture

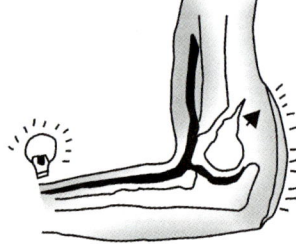

Fig. 3.20: Not to forget to examine the distal pulsion

Always examine the distal pulsations as well as sensations and make a note of it, after comparing it with the other side.

X-ray

To see the type of fracture, displacement and to rule out associated injury.

- *AP view:* Remember normal carrying angle is about 10°.
- *Lateral view:* Anterior inclination of condyle about 45° in relation to the shaft humerus.
- Normal epiphysis should not be confused with the fracture line.

If in doubt always compare the X-rays with that of the uninjured elbow.

Gross displacement of distal fragment is invariably seen. At times X-ray may show no fracture line on 1st day, but a positive fat pad sign is indicative of hairline fracture without displacement.

Principles of Treatment

- To restore accurate anatomical reduction.
- Good range of elbow movement.
- Emergency care of the injured vessels.

There is extensive oedema following fracture hence it is always advisable to keep a fair margin and treat the patients in a well padded posterior slab, sling and avoid cast application, advise the patient to keep a watch on nail bed colour and report immediately if there is paresthesia or pallor.

Management

When the elbow is flexed beyond 90°, the triceps provides a posterior splinting effect and stabilizes the fracture.

- Hairline fracture and fracture with minimal displacement. Posterior above elbow slab with cuff and collar sling for 21 days.
- Displaced fracture without neurovascular deficit- closed reduction under anaesthesia, with a posterior above elbow POP slab in more than 90° flexion at elbow with compatible radial pulse and nail bed circulation for 3 weeks.
- Displaced fracture with massive oedema and blisters.
  - Olecranon pin traction.
  - Dunlop traction (Fig. 3.21a).
- Irreducible simple fracture.

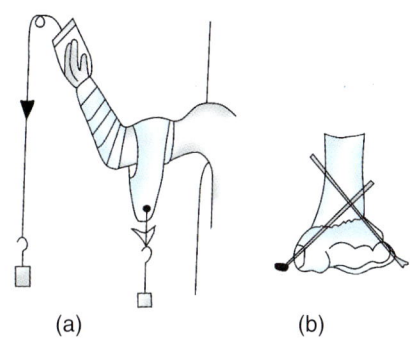

(a)   (b)

Figs 3.21a and b: (a) Dunlop traction (b) Open reduction by posterior exposure with K-wire fixation

- Open reduction by posterior exposure with K-wire fixation (Fig. 3.21b).
- Complicated fracture management of vascular injury—elevation, ice-pack and if necessary exploration of vessel and repair.

Elbow is mobilized after 3–4 weeks, by gentle active elbow exercise.

No passive stretching or massage whatsoever to avoid myositis and stiff elbow.

Complications

- **Bone:** Malunion in
  a. Anteroposterior plane causing limitation of flexion/extension.
  b. Mediolateral plane:
     This can be of two types:
     - Cubitus varus showing gunstock deformity.
     - Cubitus valgus showing increased carrying angle.
  c. Rotational plane.
     (Remodelling occurs in ant/post, side to side but not for rotational malunion)
- **Muscles:** Myositis ossificans traumatica, usually follows manipulations/massage.
- **Joints:** Elbow stiffness.
- **Nerves:** Median nerve injury, tardy ulnar nerve palsy (Cubitus valgus).

- **Vessel:** Volkmann's ischaemia due to kinking of brachial artery between fracture fragments or due to oedema after tight splintage by quacks.

Fracture–Lateral Condyle of Humerus

This is avulsion injury involving the lateral condyle of the humerus in children (Fig. 3.22a). Since it is a type-IV epiphyseal fracture, it is important to accurately reduce and fix the fragment, if displaced, by open/closed reduction and K-wire fixation (Fig. 3.22b).

Complication

- Nonunion
- Cubitus valgus (due to malunion of a fractured lateral condyle result in late ulnar nerve palsy (tardy ulnar nerve palsy).

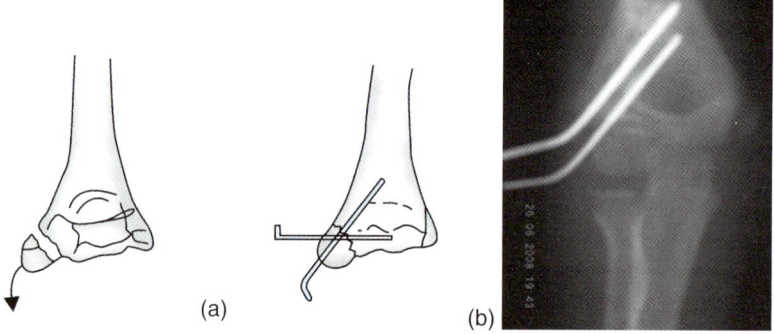

(a) (b)

Figs 3.22a and b: (a) Fracture-lateral condyle humerus (b) X-ray showing 'K' wire fixation of lateral condyle fracture.

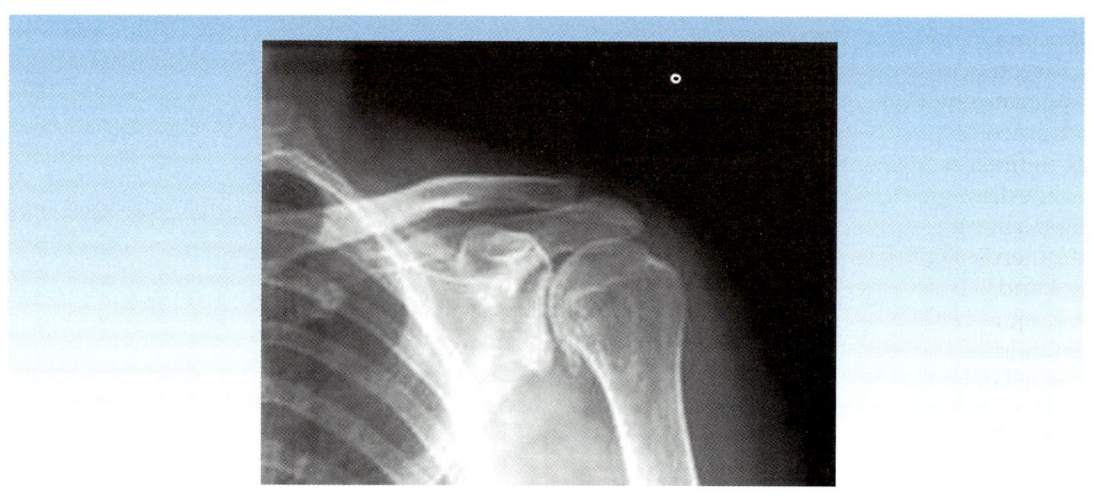

ANATOMY OF ELBOW JOINT

The elbow-joint is a ginglymus or hinge-joint. The trochlea of the humerus is received into the semilunar notch of the ulna, and the capitulums of the humerus articulates with the fovea on the head of the radius. The articular surfaces are connected together by a capsule, which is thickened medially and laterally, and, to a less extent, in front and behind. These thickened portions are usually described as distinct ligaments under the following names: anterior and posterior ligament, ulnar and radial collateral ligament.

The synovial membrane is very extensive. It extends from the margin of the articular surface of the humerus, and lines the coronoid, radial and olecranon fossa on that bone; it is reflected over the deep surface of the capsule and forms a pouch between the radial notch, the deep surface of the annular ligament, and the circumference of the head of the radius. Projecting between the radius and ulna into the cavity is a crescentic fold of synovial membrane, suggesting the division of the joint into two; one the humeroradial, the other the humeroulnar (Fig. 3.23).

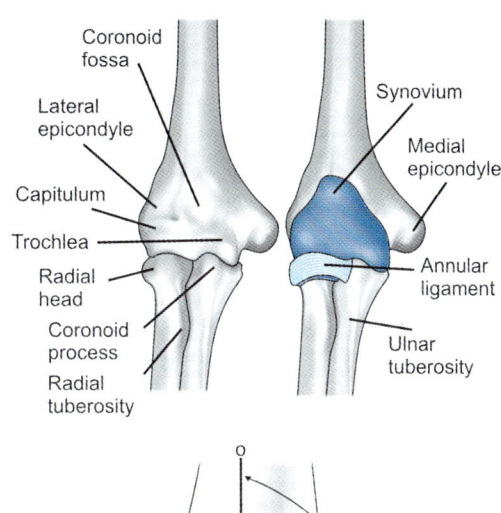

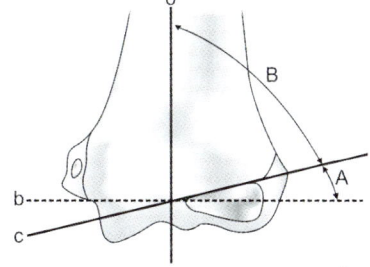

Fig. 3.23: Anatomy of elbow joint and Bowman's angle (A)

Bauman's Angle

Bauman's angle is measured on a true AP projection of the elbow and may be helpful in determining the adequacy of reduction of a supracondylar fracture. The angle (Fig. 3.23) is defined as that created by the intersection of a line drawn along the physis of the capitellum and a line perpendicular to the long axis of the humerus. This angle should be approximately 70 and within 4 of that of the contralateral uninjured elbow. This angle is of limited value in children less than 3 years of age in whom the bony landmarks are difficult to define.

Movements of Elbow Joint

The chief movements at the elbow joint are flexion and extension.

Dislocation of Elbow

This is due to fall on outstretched hand or on the elbow:

Types

Depending on the position of the olecranon and head of radius—(i) Anterior (ii) Posterior.

It may be isolated or part of complex injury with associated fracture of olecranon, (Fig. 3.24a) coronoid process, head/neck of radius or side swipe injury (Figs 3.24a and b).

Clinical Features

a. The most common is posterior dislocation and is diagnosed by obvious posterior prominence of olecranon elbow flexed at

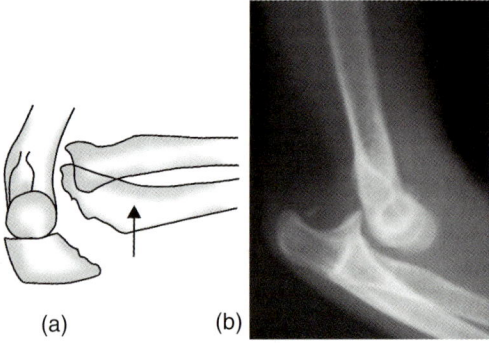

(a)   (b)

Figs 3.24a and b: (a) Anterior dislocation of elbow with fracture of olecranon (b) Posterior dislocation of elbow

130°, with severe pain, spasm and immobility. The three bony points relationship is reversed, there is often associated median nerve palsy. Always look for damage to ulnar and median nerve.

b. Anterior dislocation is often associated with fracture olecranon.

Management

- Closed reduction under GA by traction in the line of deformity and gradual flexion of elbow, beyond 90°.
- POP post-slab for three weeks and followed by active physiotherapy.
- Unreduced dislocation may require open reduction by post approach.
- Fixation of associated fracture of ulna and dislocation.

Complications

- **Bones:** Associated fracture are olecranon, coronoid, supracondylar humerus and head of radius.
- **Joint:** Unreduced dislocation, stiff elbow.
- **Muscle:** Myositis ossifican due to repeated manipulation and massage by bone setters.
- **Vessel:** Damage to brachial artery leading to VIC.
- **Nerve:** Damage to median and ulnar nerve.

Olecranon Fracture

Types

(a) Avulsion, (b) Transverse, (c) Comminuted (Figs 3.25a to c).

- Isolated.
- Part of complex injury: Fracture olecranon with anterior dislocation of elbow (Fig. 3.25b), side swipe injury (associated fracture of ulna and humerus).

Mechanism of Injury

- Injury to elbow due to fall or blow to a flexed elbow.
- Epileptic seizures.

Clinical Features

Pain, boggy swelling over posterior side of elbow, palpable gap in the posterior border of olecranon, three bony points of elbow are disturbed and inability to extend the elbow.

X-ray

To see the type of fracture and decide appropriate treatment, to rule out associated injuries. Always keep in mind—'Patella cubitae' (where developmentally two separate centres of ossification are present) and may be

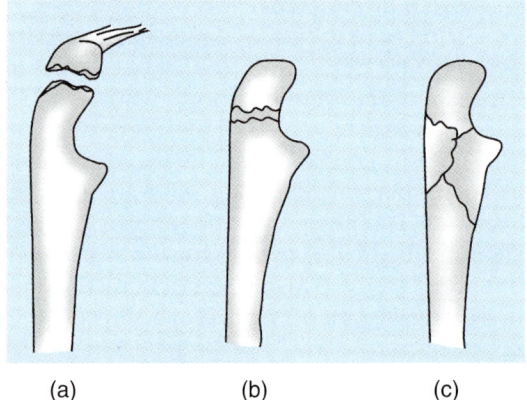

(a)   (b)   (c)

Figs 3.25a to c: Types of olecranon fractures: (a) Avulsion; (b) transverse; (c) comminuted

mistaken for fracture in a child. In such situation, it is always advisable to take X-rays of the other uninjured elbow.

Principles of Treatment (Accurate Reduction and Early Mobilisation)

To provide a stable elbow with good range of motion and power of extension.

Treatment

- **Avulsion fracture:** Excision of fragments with triceps repair. Immobilize by posterior slab in 45° extension for 3 weeks followed by gentle active elbow movements.
- **Transverse fracture:** Tension band wiring, cancellous olecranon screw fixation (Fig. 3.26a).
- **Comminuted fracture:** Plate fixation and early mobilization (Fig. 3.26b).

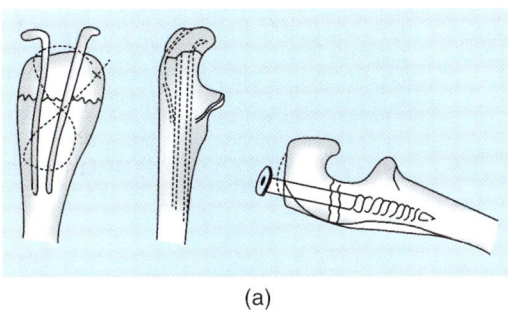

(a)

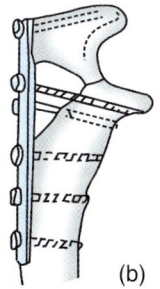

(b)

Figs 3.26a and b: Different modalities of olecranon fracture fixation

Radius–Head and Neck (Fig. 3.27)

Head

Types

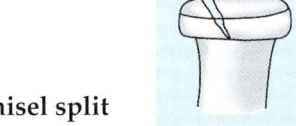

- **Chisel split**

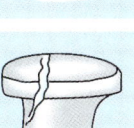

- **Marginal**

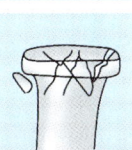

- **Comminuted**

Fig. 3.27: Types of radial head fracture

Neck (Fig. 3.28)

- Epiphyseal injuries of childhood – Type II.
- Fracture in adults with or without displacement.

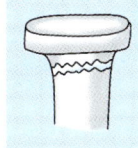

Fig. 3.28: Radial neck fracture

Mechanisms of Injuries

Fall on the outstretched hand.

Clinical Features

Fullness of radial fossa, lateral to the triceps insertion, swollen painful elbow, limitation of forearm movements, palpable bony crepitus and pain felt as thumb is pressed over the head of radius when forearm is rotated.

X-ray

- To see the type of fracture and extent of displacement.

- Skiagram AP and lateral view in full pronation/supination to see the head all over.

Treatment

- **Children:** Reduction of the displaced epiphysis (head of radius) open or closed and fixation with K-wire if necessary. Excision of radial head should never be advised in children because it is a growing end, as growth occurs the radius is liable to ride up toward the humerus with consequent disturbance of its relationship to the ulna, the inferior radioulnar joint subluxates and rotation become limited.
- **Adults:**
  - *Post slab for 3 weeks if:* Chisel split, undisplaced marginal fracture of head and fracture neck with tilt <15°.
  - *Excision of head if:* Comminuted fracture, displaced fracture head and neck in adults.

Complications

- Joint stiffness
  - *Radioulnar:* Limitation of supination and pronation.
  - *Radio humeral:* Limitation of flexion and extension.
- Myositis ossificans around the head of radius and stiff elbow.
- Proximal migration of radius with subluxation of wrist, following excision of head of radius, hence it is always better to wait for a few days to allow the interosseous ligament to recover and then do excision.

Radius and Ulna

Types

- **Children:** Greenstick fracture (Fig. 3.3d).
- **Adults:**
  - Transverse, spiral, displaced, comminuted, segmental.
  - Single bone.

- Both bones.
- Fracture of one bone with dislocation of proximal/distal radioulnar joint.

Mechanism of Injury

Fall on outstretched hand, direct blow, crushing injury.

Clinical Features

- Deformity of forearm, shortening, swelling, painful restriction of all movements, palpable crepitus.
- Always examine the distal pulsation and sensation.

X-ray

Full length of radius and ulna, including the elbow and wrist joint AP and lateral view (Fig. 3.29).

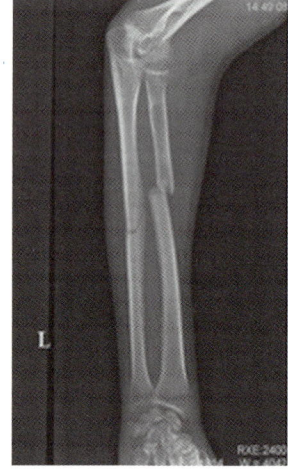

Fig. 3.29: Fracture shaft as ulna and radius

Principles of Treatment

- To restore accurate anatomical alignment of both bones and joints.
- Maintenance of interosseous space.
- Full range of hand and forearm movements with adequate power.

Always note While Treating a Fracture Radius, in AE POP Cast

- **Fracture of upper third:** The proximal fragment is supinated due to the strong supinators, hence *immobilize the forearm in full supination* so that the two fragments are well aligned.
- **In lower third**, as there are strong pronators, *immobilize in pronation.*
- **In middle third**, as there is balance between the supinators and the pronators *midprone position* should be kept for immobilisation in AE POP cast.

In any case when the forearm is in the cast, active movements of the shoulder and the fingers should be encouraged to avoid stiffness.

Treatment

- **Children with greenstick fracture:** Correction of the deformity under anaesthesia and AE POP cast for 6 weeks.
- **Adults:** Even in spite of good position the chances of displacement are there, hence open reduction and internal fixation is always best.
  - **Simple:** Intramedullary square nail for distal one-third ulna and proximal two-thirds radius (narrow medullary canal). Plating is best for, upper third of ulna and lower third of radius (wide marrow cavity). It provides rigid fixation and can withstand rotational distortion (Fig. 3.30).
  - **Compound:** External fixators (JESS).

Complications

- **Bone:**
  - Delayed union.
  - *Non-union:* Due to soft tissue entrapment or bone loss.
  - *Malunion:*
    - Angulatory.
    - Rotational.

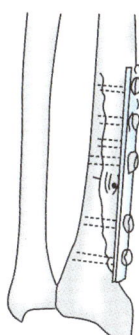

Fig. 3.30: Plating for lower third fracture radius

- *Cross union:* Union through the interosseous space between radius and ulna.
- **Joint:** Stiffness of hand and fingers.
- **Vessels:** VIC, compartmental syndrome.
- **Muscle:** Myositis.
- **Tendons:** Entrapment of the tendons in between the fracture fragments.

Note: Never accept isolated fracture of one bone in the forearm unless both the proximal and distal R/U joints are visualised.

Monteggia's Fracture Dislocation

First described by Monteggia as fracture of the upper third ulna and dislocation of head of radius in 1814 (Figs 3.31a and b).

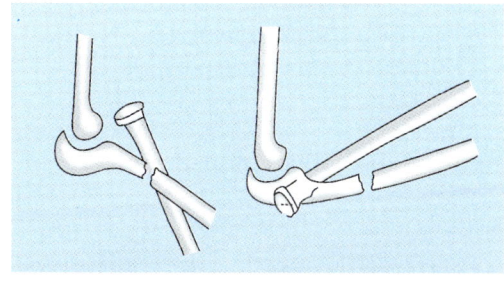

(a) Anterior   (b) Posterior

Figs 3.31a and b: Monteggia's fracture with anterior and posterior dislocation displacements radial head

Mechanism of Injury

Direct blow in front or behind the upper third, fall on outstretched hand with forearm pronated.

Clinical Features

Deformity of proximal ulna, head of radius palpable in abnormal position (anterior, posterior, lateral). Movements of elbow and forearm restricted, painful with shortening of forearm.

X-ray

Full length forearm with elbow (AP and lateral view).

Treatment

(Anterior type) which is the most common.
• Close reduction under anaesthesia— immobilization in A/E slab with forearm fully supinated with 90° flexion at the elbow.
• If closed reduction fails then open reduction of head of radius and DCP fixation of ulna should be done.
• In old unreduced dislocation, excision of head of radius and realignment of ulna and fixation by dynamic compression plate should be done.

Complications

• **Bone:** Malunion, non-union of ulna, persistence of the dislocation of head of radius.
• **Traumatic ossification** around head of radius.
• **Joint stiffness:** Loss of flexion/extension at elbow, supination/pronation of forearm.

Galeazzi Fracture Dislocation

Fracture of the lower third radius with subluxation of inferior radioulnar joint (Figs 3.32a and b).

Clinical Features

Deformity of the forearm in the lower third and subluxation of inferior radioulnar joint so that the two styloid processes come to lie in the same plane. There is bony crepitus and loss of transmitted movements of the radius.

X-ray

To see the type of fracture and decide the line of treatment.

Treatment

Since conservative treatment is not predictable, open reduction and dynamic compression plate fixation of the fracture of radius should be done (Fig. 3.32b).

Complications

• **Bone:**
  – Non-union of the radius,
  – Malunion leading to loss of supination and pronation of forearm.
• **Joint:** Persistence of subluxation of inferior radioulnar joint.

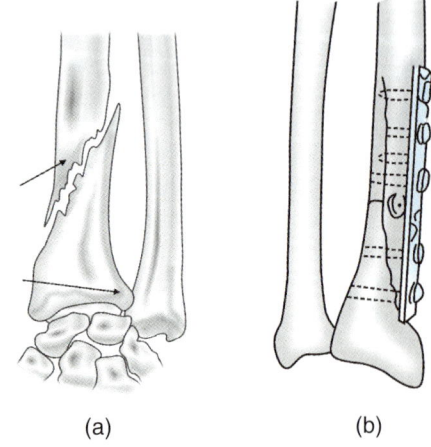

(a)   (b)

Figs 3.32a and b: (a) Glaeazzi fracture: Fracture of the lower third radius with subluxation (arrow) of inferior radioulnar joint (b) DCP plate fixation

Colles' Fracture

Described by Abraham Colles in 1814. This is the most common of all fractures after the age of 40, invariably associated with osteoporosis.

Definition

Fracture of lower end of the radius, within an inch of the distal articulating surface with subluxation of inferior radioulnar joint with or without fracture of ulnar styloid.

Clinical Features

Commonest fracture in elderly patients due to osteoporosis and occurs after fall on outstretched hands (Fig. 3.33).
- Pain, swelling and dinner fork deformity (Fig. 3.34).
- Loss of all movements of wrist and hand.
- Both the styloid comes to lie at the same level due to impaction and proximal shift of the fracture end of the radius (normally radial styloid is lower than ulnar).

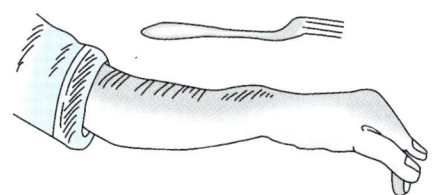

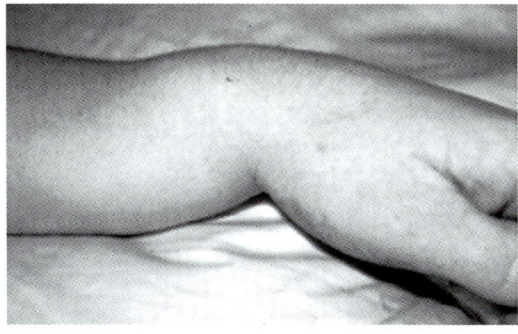

Fig. 3.34: Dinner fork deformity

X-ray

Normal anatomy of the wrist joint (Fig. 3.35)

1. Radial angulation – 23°
2. Radial length – 12 mm
3. Palmar angulation –110°
   - *Normal values*

X-ray is done

To see the displacement and the associated fracture (Fig. 3.36). Classical displacement of the distal fragment are
- Impaction.
- Dorsal tilt and shift.
- Lateral tilt and shift.
- Supination.

Additional findings may be, fracture ulnar styloid, subluxation of inferior radioulnar joint (Figs 3.36a and b).

Management

- *Fresh fracture:* Closed reduction under G/A, well moulded and padded below elbow POP cast extending up to the proximal palmar crease for 4–6 weeks (Fig. 3.37).

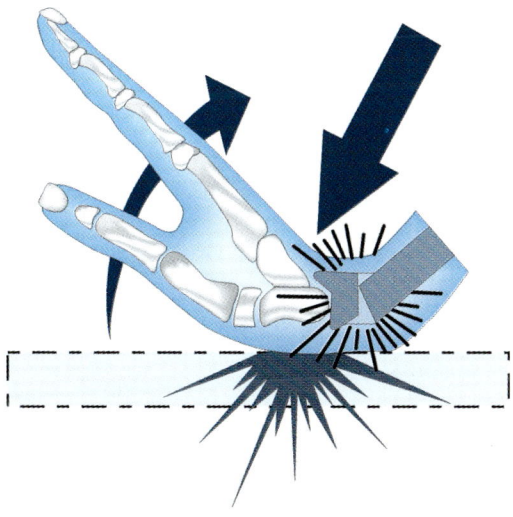

Fig. 3.33: Mechanism of injury

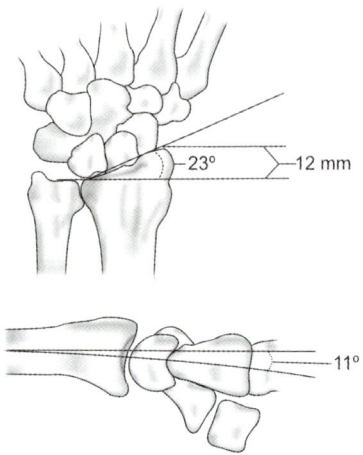

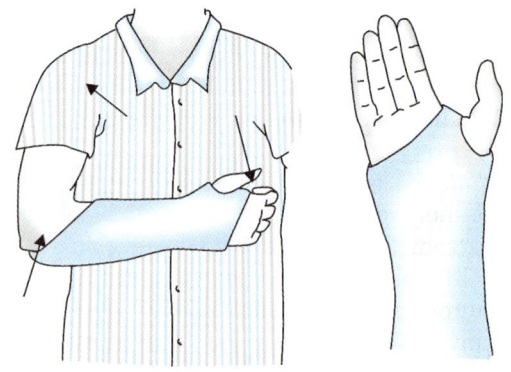

Figs 3.37a and b: (a) Well moulded and padded Colles' cast (b) Colles' fracture stabilised with JESS distractor

Fig. 3.35: Anatomy of wrist joint

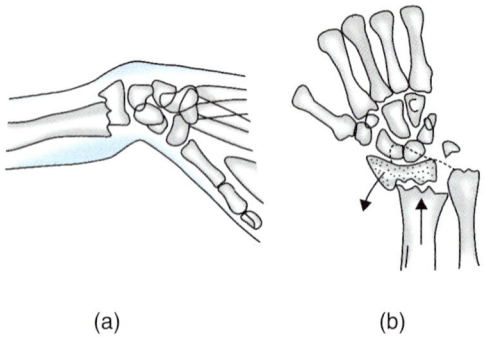

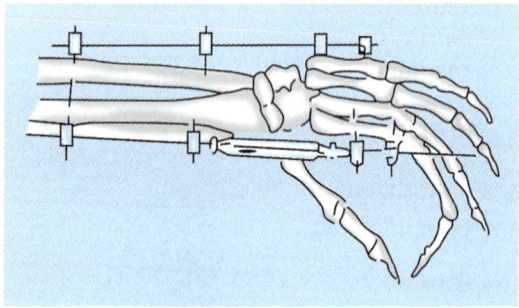

(a)   (b)

(a) JESS distractor

Figs 3.36a and b: Colles' fracture associated with fracture ulnar styloid, subluxation of inferior radioulnar joint

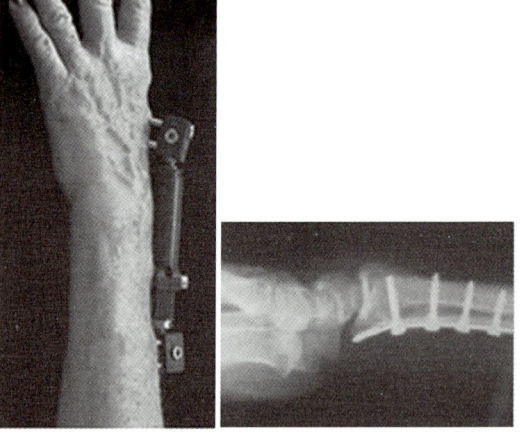

- *Unstable fractures:* JESS Distractor, AO Distractor (Figs 3.38a and b), K-wire fixation. Buttress plating (Fig. 3.38c).
- *Malunited fracture* with painful limitation of wrist movement and pronation/supination is treated by Darrach's excision of distal ulna.

(b) AO distractor   (c) Buttress plate

Fig. 3.38a to c

Complications

- **Bone:** Malunion of radius, non-union of ulnar styloid/subluxation of inferior radio-ulnar joint.
- **Joint:**
  Sudeck's atrophy (this is painful reflex sympathetic osteodystrophy and presents as extremely painful and swollen hand and stiff fingers. X-ray shows patchy osteoporosis around the wrist). This is treated by physiotherapy and exercises.
  Shoulder hand syndrome, the hand and shoulder is stiff after the injury due to immobilization.
- **Tendon:** Rupture of extensor pollices longus after a few weeks, due to friction at fracture site, near the Lister's tubercle.
  - *Nerve:* Carpal tunnel syndrome due to median nerve entrapment at the wrist.
  - *The most important complication is stiffness of wrist, fingers and malunion.* Finger stiffness is the commonest complication while non-union is least common.

Juvenile Colles'

In children, this is type 2 epiphyseal fracture (Fig. 3.39). The management is the same as fracture Colles'.

Smith's Fracture

This is reverse of Colles' fracture (Fig. 3.40a), the distal fragment is displaced in the volar direction, and needs reduction and mobilization in above elbow POP cast kept in, supination of the forearm and dorsiflexion of the wrist or open reduction and internal fixation by small T (Ellis) plate (Fig. 3.40b). JESS distractor frame is useful for comminuted fracture.

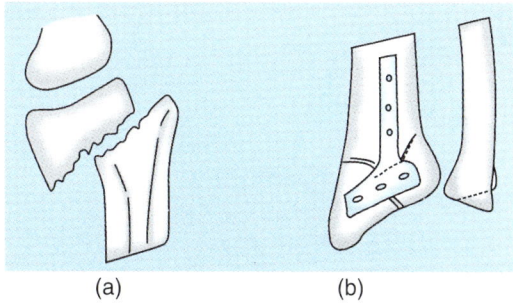

Figs 3.40a and b: (a) Smith's fracture (b) Smith's fracture is fixed with Ellis plate

Barton's Fracture (Fig. 3.41)

This is a vertical fracture of the distal articular end of the radius, the fragment carries with it, the carpus. The treatment is the same as Smith's fracture.

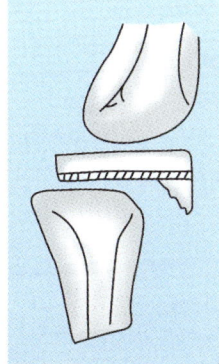

Fig. 3.39: Type 2 epiphyseal fracture

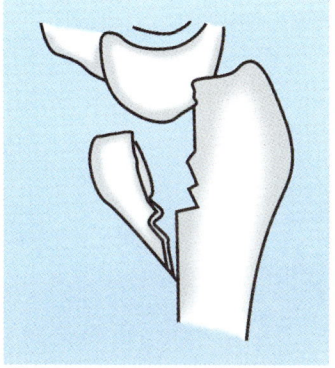

Fig. 3.41: Barton's fracture

Chauffeurs Fracture (Fig. 3.42)

This is an intra-articular fracture of the radial styloid, the fracture line passing vertically upwards (Fig. 3.42), and was very commonly seen during the era of old cars which had to be started manually by a **Z** handle. It is treated in below elbow cast with incorporation of the thumb for 4 weeks, or closed K-wire fixation.

Scaphoid Fracture

This is due to fall on the outstretched hands (Fig. 3.43).

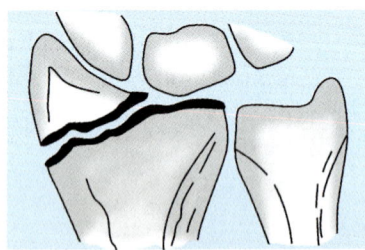

Fig. 3.42: Chauffeurs fracture

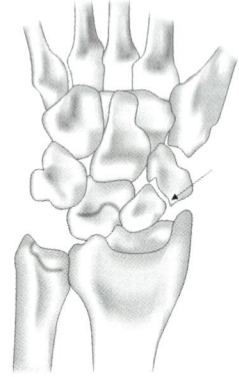

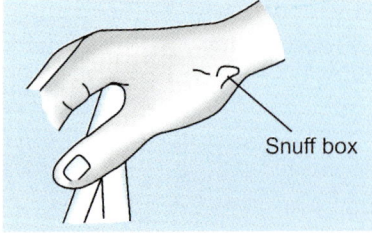

Fig. 3.43: Scaphoid fracture

Clinical Features

Pain, swelling and tenderness in the anatomical snuff box, loss of grip, wrist movements are painful.

X-rays

At least 3 views: Anteroposterior, lateral and oblique. Even if the X-ray is negative and the patient has tenderness in the anatomical snuff box he is treated as fracture scaphoid. X-ray repeated after 2 weeks which may show a fracture.

Treatment

- *Fresh fracture:* Below elbow POP cast, incorporating the proximal phalanx of thumb with wrist dorsiflexed and hand in glass holding position for 6 weeks. Review after 6 weeks and if evidence of delayed union is seen, one more cast for another 6 weeks.
- *Non-union:* Herbert screw fixation with bone grafting (Fig. 3.44).

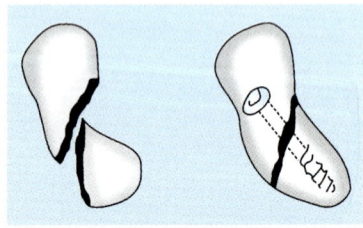

Fig. 3.44: Herbert screw fixation with bone grafting

- *Painful OA of wrist:* Arthodesis of wrist or proximal row carpectomy.

Complications

- *Bone:* Delayed union, non-union, avascular necrosis of the proximal pole (the vascular supply of scaphoid is distal to proximal, hence fracture waist of scaphoid causes AVN of the proximal pole, Fig. 3.45).

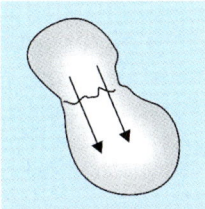

Fig. 3.45: Direction as flow as vascular supply from distal to proximal

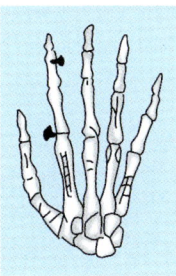

Fig. 3.47: ORIF with plating/screws/K-wires

- *Joint:* Osteoarthritis of the wrist and intercarpal joints causing loss of power of grip.

Bennett's Fracture Dislocation

This is fracture dislocation of base of 1st metacarpal with intra-articular extension.

Treatment

- *Conservative:* Reduction and B/E spica POP cast with incorporation of thumb.
- *Operative:* Closed/open reduction and internal fixation by K-wire.

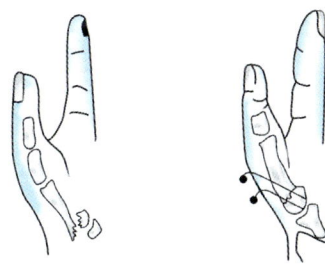

(a)   (b)

Figs 3.46a and b: (a) Bennett's fracture dislocation (b) Fixed with two K wires

Metacarpal Fracture

- **Undisplaced**
  Dorsal slab, finger cott, ball and bandage.
- **Displaced**
  ORIF with K-wires/fixators/mini-plate and screws.

Phalanx Fracture

- **Undisplaced**
  Strap 2 fingers together (injured + normal), finger splint/ball and bandage.
- **Displaced**
  ORIF K-wire, with JESS frame for compound fracture (Fig. 3.48).

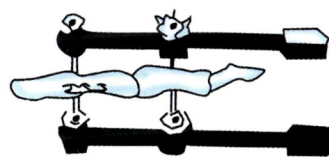

Fig. 3.48: Phalangeal fracture fixed with K-wire and JESS

It is important to move all the fingers to avoid stiffness of fingers.

Mallet Finger

This is due to avulsion of the extensor tendon at the base of the distal phalanx causing inability to extend the distal phalanx, which in due course ends up with a flexion deformity of the terminal phalanx (Figs 3.49a and b).

It is best treated in a frog splint (Fig. 3.49c) which keeps the proximal interphalangeal joints in flexion and the distal joint in hyperextension so as to repose the avulsed tendon along with its bony insertion in the distal phalanx. This is kept for 3 weeks.

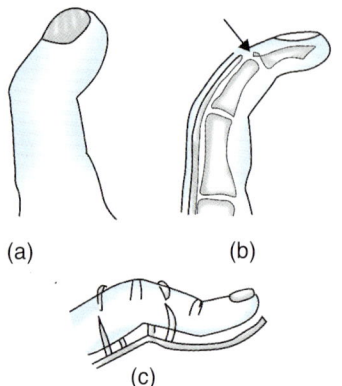

(a) (b)

(c)

Figs 3.49a to c: Frog splint keeps the proximal inter phalangeal joint in flexion and distal interpharangeal joint in extension

If the avulsed bone piece from the base of the distal phalanx is large enough, fixation may be done.

Trigger Finger

Tenosynovitis involving long flexor of thumb or finger causing locking of finger in flexion due to entrapment of the nodular tendonitis within its sheath. It is often seen in diabetics. Patient has to straighten it passively. Treatment is local steroid injection into the sheath of the tendon and at times excision of the synovial sheath around the nodular tendonitis may have to be done.

Hand Injuries

Mechanism of injury

Crush, blast, mutilating injuries.

Principles of Management

- Debride all devitalized tissue and salvage remaining parts.
- Stabilize in functional position by K-wires or JESS frame.
- Mobilize uninjured joints.
- Prevent infection.
- Promote primary healing by primary/ secondary skin cover.
- Repair of tendons and nerves.
- Restores function of pinch, grasp and grip.

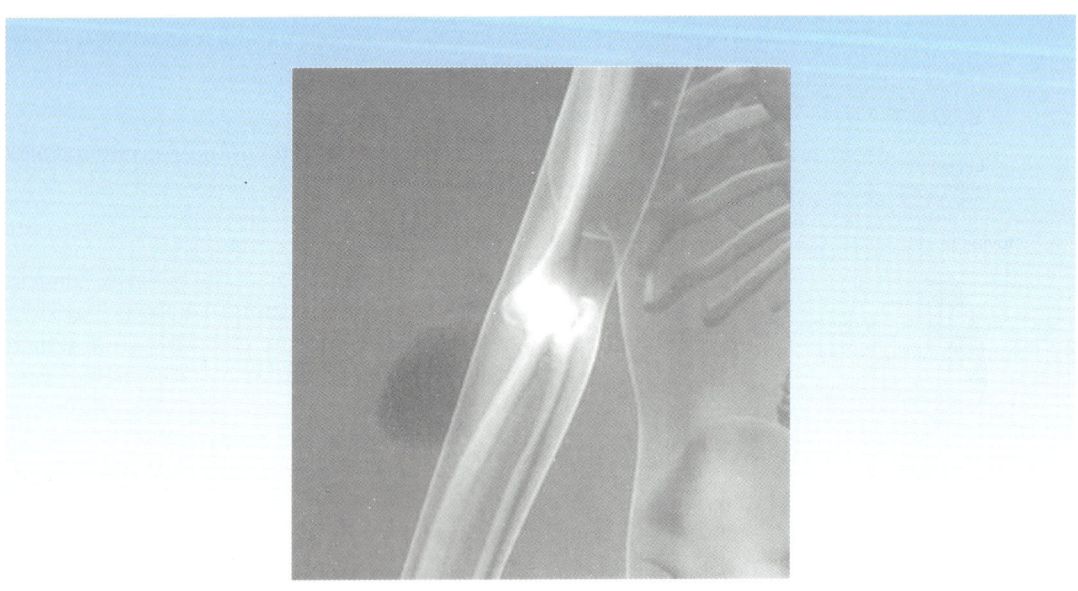

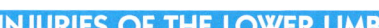

INJURIES OF THE LOWER LIMB

ANATOMY OF HIP JOINT

The hip joint is the articulation between the hemispherical head of the femur and the cup-shaped acetabulum of the hip bone. The cavity of the acetabulum is horseshoe-shaped and is deficient at the acetabular notch. The cavity of the acetabulum is deepened by the presence of a fibrocartilaginous rim called the acetabular labrum. The articular surfaces are covered with *hyaline cartilage*. It is a type of synovial ball and socket joint. The capsule encloses the joint and is attached to the acetabular labrum medially. Laterally, it is attached to the intertrochanteric line of the femur in front and halfway along the posterior aspect of the neck of bone behind. Synovial membrane lines the capsule and is attached to the margins of the articular surfaces. There are various ligaments, i.e. *iliofemoral (ligament of Bigelow), pubo-femoral, ischio-femoral ligament,*

transverse acetabular ligament and ligament of the head of the femur which are responsible for the stability of the joint.

The neck of the femur is placed at an angle of 135° to the shaft and it projects 10–12° anteriorly to the coronal plane (Fig. 3.50).

MOVEMENTS OF HIP JOINT

Active movements permitted at the hip joint are flexion and extension, abduction and adduction, circumduction, medial and lateral rotation.

Dislocation of Hip

Types

Based on position of the head of femur:

- Posterior: 75% (most common)
- Anterior
- Central

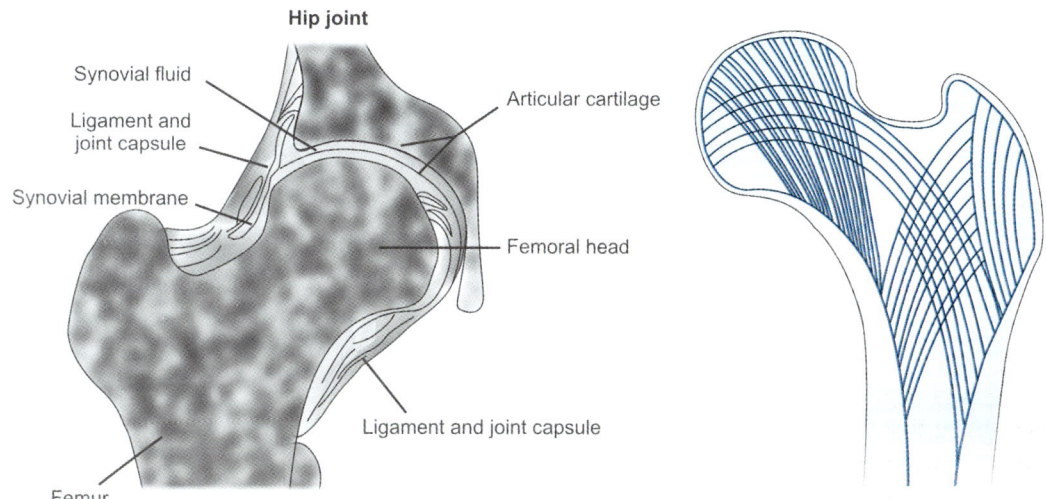

Fig. 3.50: Anatomy of hip joint and normal trabecular pattern

Posterior Dislocation

Usually as a result of dashboard injuries, especially when the limb is flexed and adducted.

Clinical Features

Attitude: Flexion, adduction and internal rotation at hip. True shortening of the thigh is present. Femur head palpable in gluteal area. All movements are painful and restricted due to muscle spasm. Trochanter is shifted proximally (change in Bryant's triangle). In dislocation of hip, the femoral artery pulsations are feeble due to lack of posterior bony support, i.e. vascular sign of Narath (positive).

Anterior Dislocation

Clinical Features

Attitude: Flexion, abduction and externally rotated leg with lengthening of thigh. Head palpable in the femoral triangle.

X-ray

To see the type of dislocation and associated injuries.
- Break in Shenton's line.
- Head seen in abnormal position.
- Associated fracture of neck, greater trochanter, acetabulum, shaft femur and at times, fracture patella with knee injuries.

Treatment

- **Reduction under anaesthesia:**
  - *Closed:* Patient is supine on the floor, assistant holding pelvis, to give counter traction, surgeon gives vertical traction to the femur with hip and knee flexed to achieve reduction, the head reduces with a snap, the leg is then extended and both the legs are then brought parallel to make sure, that reduction is achieved.
  - *Open:* If dislocation is irreducible by closed manipulation (often due to fracture of posterior lip of acetabulum).

- *Maintenance:* The reduction achieved is maintained by above knee skin traction or skeletal traction through the upper tibial pin for 3 weeks and avoid weight bearing for further 3 weeks.

Complications

- *Bone:* Associated fractures of posterior lip of acetabulum, a large piece requires open reduction and screw fixation for a stable hip reduction, head and neck femur, upper third shaft of femur, avulsion of greater trochanter. Avascular necrosis of the head of femur.
- *Joint:* Unreduced dislocation, early secondary osteoarthritis.
- *Muscle:* Myositis ossificans around the hip joint.
- *Nerve:* Sciatic nerve palsy.

Central Dislocation

Head bursts through the floor of acetabulum and moves into the pelvis (Fig. 3.51a).

Clinical Features

Shortening and external rotation, gross limitation of abduction and rotational movements.

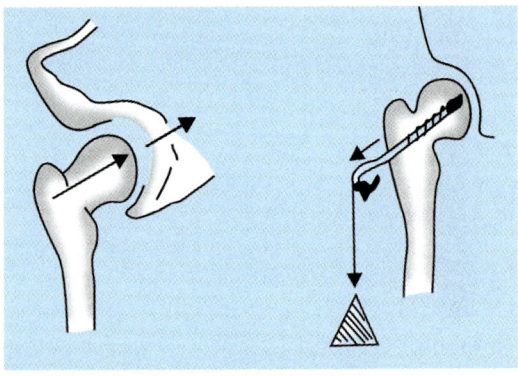

(a)　　　　　　(b)

Figs 3.51a and b: (a) Central dislocation (b) Lateral traction through a hook passed into head and neck of femur

Treatment

This is best treated by lateral traction through a hook screw passed into the head and neck of femur (Fig. 3.51b).

Fracture: Neck of Femur

Causes

- In young children and adults due to trauma.
- In old age (above 60 years) pathological fracture, due to senile osteoporosis or secondaries from prostate, cervix, breast, etc. may occur.

Classification

- **Anatomical** (Fig. 3.52)
  a. Subcapital
  b. Transcervical
  c. Basal

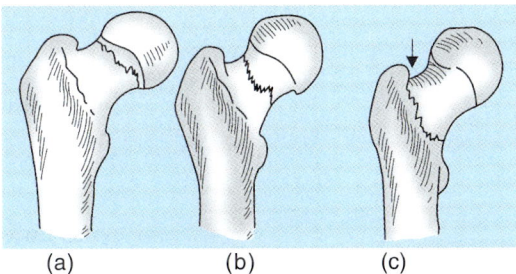

(a)   (b)   (c)

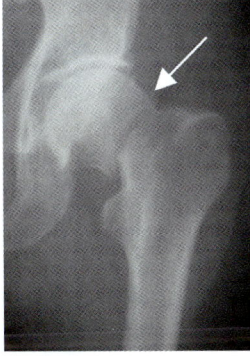 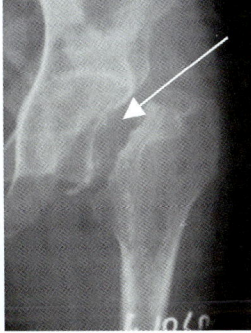

Garden's grade III fracture neck femur. partial displacement (arrow)

(d) X-ray showing Garden's grade IV Complete fracture with and rotation (arrow)

Figs 3.52a to d

- **Garden's classification:**
  Grade I : Incomplete fracture with one cortex intact.
  Grade II : Complete fracture with no displacement.
  Grade III : Complete fracture with partial displacement.
  Grade IV : Complete fracture with displacement and rotation.

Clinical Features

- Usually seen in the old patients, if he slips in bathroom or after a very trivial injury falls to the floor and is unable to stand up or bear weight on the injured limb.
- Children and adults : There is always history of major trauma/trivial in pathological fracture (bone cyst).
  - Limb shortened slightly and externally rotated by 45° (Fig. 3.53).

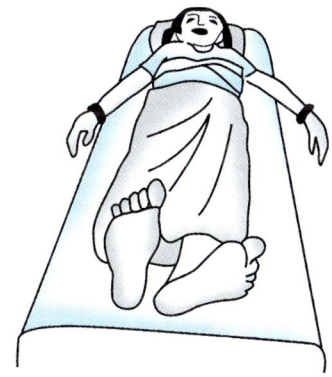

Fig. 3.53: Patient with injured limb in external rotation position

  - Inability to raise the leg against the resistance.
  - Tenderness over mid-inguinal point.
  - Bitrochanteric compression test positive.
  - Trendelenburg sign and pump handle test is positive (in old fracture), supratrochanteric shift seen in Bryant's triangle, Nelaton's line and Shoemaker's

line deviates as compared to the normal side.

X-ray

To see type of fracture, extent of displacement, break in Shenton's line. Status of bone is seen in X-ray to decide the line of treatment.

Management

• **Children**
  – Undisplaced and impacted injury requires hip spica for 6 weeks.
  – Displaced (save the head), closed reduction under general anaesthesia and fix the neck by Austin Moore's pins or Knowle's pins or cannulated cancellous screws (Figs 3.54a to c).
• **Adult**
  – *Fresh case:* Reduction and fixation by:

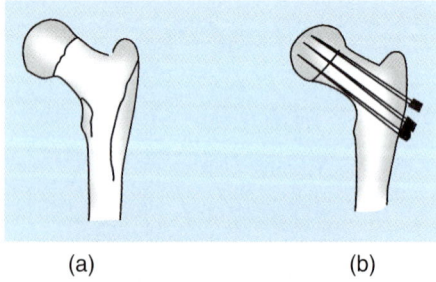

(a)   (b)

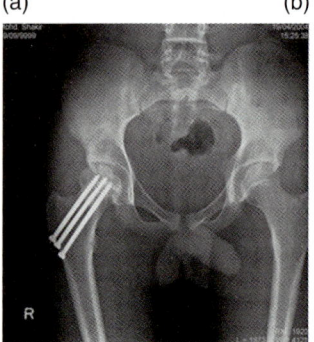

(c) X-ray showing cannulated cancellous screws

Figs 3.54a to c: (a) Undisplaced fracture, (b) fracture fixed with Moore's pin, (c) X-ray showing fracture fixation by cannulated cancellaous screws

  – Knowle's pin,
  – Dynamic hip screw.
– *Old case:* Up to 3 months.
  – McMurray's osteotomy with hip spica for 8 weeks, valgus sub-trochanteric osteotomy and fixation with a plate.
  – Vascularised muscle pedicle bone grafting with fixation of fracture neck (Meyer's quadratus femoris graft), Sartorius graft.
• **Old age (above 60 years):** Partial hip replacement:
  – If 2 cm calcar is present, Austin Moore's prosthesis is used (Fig. 3.55a).

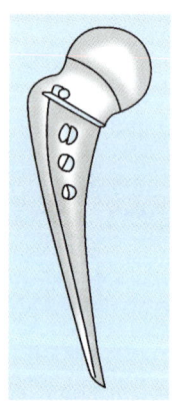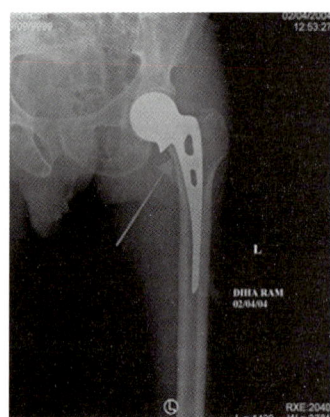

Fig. 3.55a: X-ray showing Austin Moore's prosthesis in old patients with at least 2 cm of calcar (arrow)

  – If no calcar then Thomson's prosthesis, and use bone cement if necessary.
  – Early OA changes of hip then bipolar prosthesis (Fig. 3.55b) is required. These prosthesis may be augmented by using Bone cement if the pt is osteoporotic
  – In women with sedentary house living, excision arthroplasty in which the head of femur is removed as shown below (Fig. 3.55c). This causes shortening and instability but provides a good range of painless mobility.

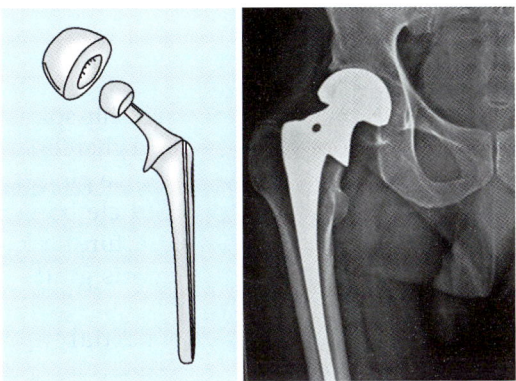

Fig. 3.55b: X-ray showing bipolar prosthesis (uncemented)

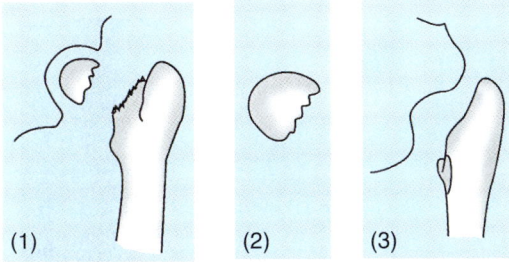

(1) (2) (3)

Fig. 3.55c: Excision arthroplasty: (1) Fracture neck femur; (2) Head of femur; (3) After excision arthroplasty

– Fracture neck with AVN or severe OA changes of hip joint then total hip replacement (Fig. 3.55d) is required.

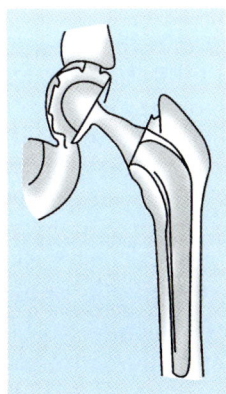

Fig. 3.55d

Stress should be made on the maintenance of the quadriceps and gluteal power by exercises for good recovery after surgery.

Complications

- Non-union of fracture leading to absorption of neck, unstable gait and shortening.
- Avascular necrosis of head of femur leading to painful motion.

Trochanteric Fracture

Classification

i. **Anatomical**
   – Cervicotrochanteric,
   – Intertrochanteric or pertrochanteric,
   – Subtrochanteric.
ii. **Surgical:** To decide the type of fixation. **Boyd's and Griffin classification in four grades as shown in Fig. 3.56.**

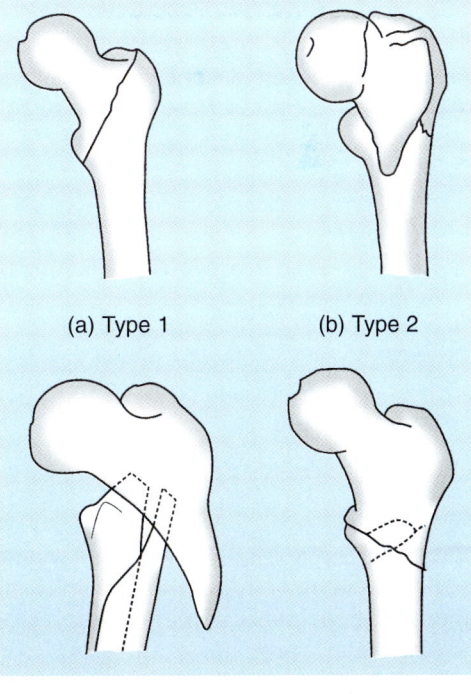

(a) Type 1 (b) Type 2

(c) Type 3 (d) Type 4

Fig. 3.56: Boyd's and Griffin classification

iii. **Mechanical:** Depending on the geometry of fracture line.
 – *Stable:* The abductors and adductors create force of compression at the fracture line (Fig. 3.57a).
 – *Unstable:* The adductors pull the distal fragment medially, while the gluteal abductors pull and rotate the proximal fragment laterally (Fig. 3.57b).

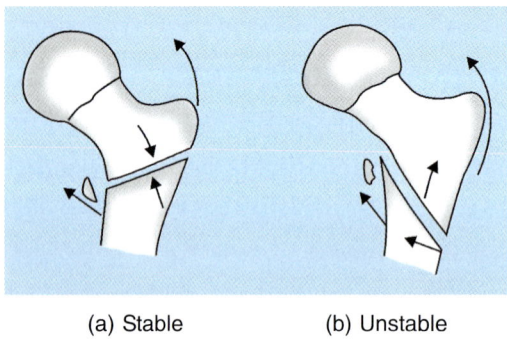

(a) Stable   (b) Unstable

Figs 3.57a and b: Line of force as abductors and adductors

Clinical Features

- Fall or severe trauma involving the trochanteric area.
- Pathological fracture as seen in
  – *Children:* Osteogenesis imperfecta.
  – *Young adults:* Osteoclastoma, bone cyst, fibrous dysplasia.
  – *Old age:* Secondaries.

Examination

Shortening, leg externally completely rotated, massive swelling of upper third of thigh and femoral triangle, bitrochanteric compression and trochanteric pressure. Painful, widening of the trochanter and shift in Bryant's triangle. Pain and bony crepitus with lack of transmitted movements.

X-ray

To know the type and the extent of the fracture and associated injuries.

Management

- **In children:** Reduction under anaesthesia and hip spica for 6–12 weeks.
- **In adults:**
  – *Stable*
    - Fixed traction in Thomas splint (Fig. 3.58a).
    - Sliding balanced skeletal traction for 6–12 weeks (Fig. 3.58b).

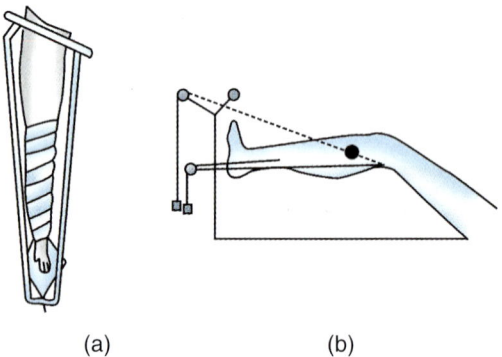

(a)   (b)

Figs 3.58a and b: (a) Fixed traction in Thomas splint (b) Sliding balanced skeletal traction

  – *Unstable (adults and also in old age)*
    - McLaughlin nail plate fixation and early mobilization (Fig. 3.59a).
    - Richard's screw and barrel plate fixation (DHS) (Fig. 3.59b).
    - 90° blade plate fixation (Fig. 3.59c).
    - Cobrahood plate fixation for comminuted fracture (Fig. 3.59d).
    - Gamma nail (Fig. 3.59e) for subtrochanteric fracture.
    - Reconstruction nail, if fracture of neck, trochanter associated with shaft femur fracture (Fig. 3.59f).

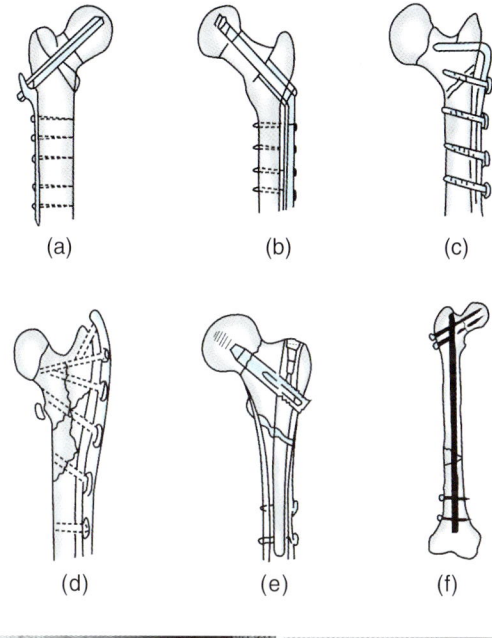

(a)   (b)   (c)

(d)   (e)   (f)

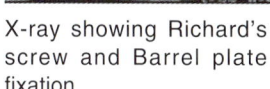

X-ray showing Richard's screw and Barrel plate fixation

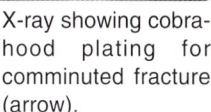

X-ray showing cobra-hood plating for comminuted fracture (arrow).

Figs 3.59a to f: Different modalities of internal fixation for unstable fracture

Complications

1. **Malunion:** Shortening, external rotation, deformity and coxa vara (reduction of neck shaft angle) causing difficulty in walking.
2. **Nonunion**

Fracture: Shaft of Femur (Fig. 3.60)

Mechanism of Injury

- In neonates, during labour of breech presentation and in children, due to the epilepsy and often fall from tree tops.
- In adults, due to the high-speed vehicular accidents and stress fracture in military recruits. In old age, due to secondaries and osteoporosis.

Clinical Features

History of trauma, thigh is painful, swollen, deformed, shortened and leg is externally rotated. Abnormal mobility of the thigh and loss of transmitted movements, bony crepitus is present. Up to one liter of the blood can be extravasated into the thigh and hence the patient may come in shock.

Always examine the distal pulsations and sensations to rule out any complications.

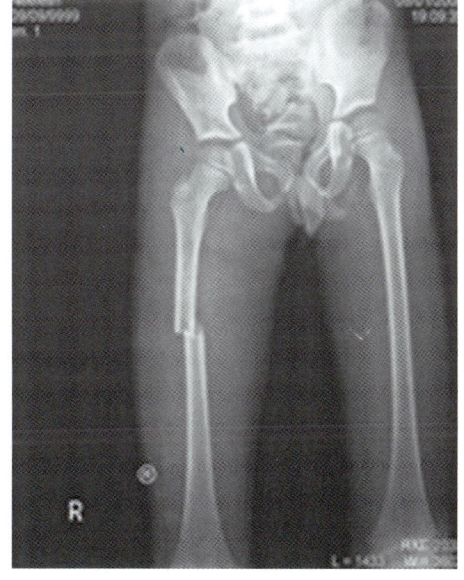

Fig. 3.60: X-ray showing mid-shaft fracture femur (R)

Management

Transportation of the patient with the injured leg bandaged to the healthy lower limb with a wooden plank or in Thomas splint (if available). Blood and fluid replacement and management of shock. Once the patient is stabilized, examine to rule out other injuries of the head, chest, abdomen and the pelvis.

Treatment

- **Children:**
  - *1 to 3 years:* Gallow's traction in wooden frame for three weeks (Fig. 3.61).
  - *3 to 10 years:* Reduction under anaesthesia and hip spica for 6 weeks. Rush nail/DCP for unstable fracture.

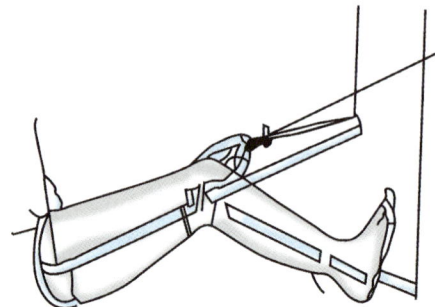

Fig. 3.62a: Skeletal traction in Thomas splint with Perkin's attachment

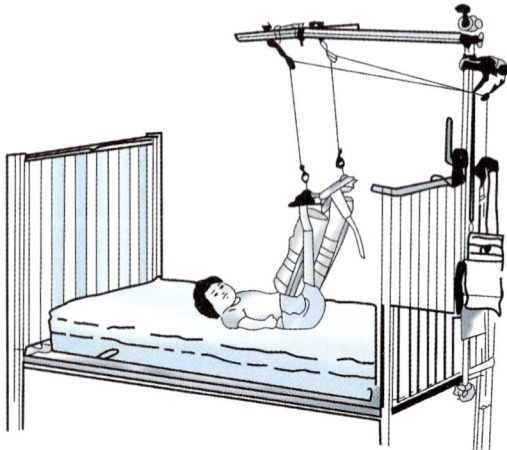

Fig. 3.61: Gallow's traction for fracture shaft femur in children

- **Adults:**
  - *Conservative*

    For soft tissue injury and compound fracture.

    External fixation or skeletal traction (Fig. 3.62a) in Thomas splint with Perkin's attachment for knee flexion.

  - *Operative:* Various operative options available are chosen depending on the fracture site and its geometry.
  - i. Intramedullary 'K' nailing, upper one-third (Fig. 3.62b) and additional bone grafting in comminuted fracture (Fig. 3.62c).
  - ii. Interlocked nail for comminuted, segmental fractures and early mobilization (Fig.3.56d).
  - iii. DC Plating for middle and lower third (Fig. 3.62e).
  - iv. Blade plate fixation for subtrochanteric fractures (Fig. 3.62f).
  - v. Illizarov fixation for difficult comminuted fractures (Fig. 3.62g).

Complications

General: The rule of 2
- Within 2 hours: Shock.
- Within 2 days: Fat embolism.
- Within 2 weeks: Thromboembolism.

Local:
- *Bone:* Delayed union, malunion, non-union, associated fractures of pelvis, neck of femur, patella especially in dash board injuries.
- *Joint:* Posterior dislocation of hip, stiffness of the knee joint due to quadricep adhesion.

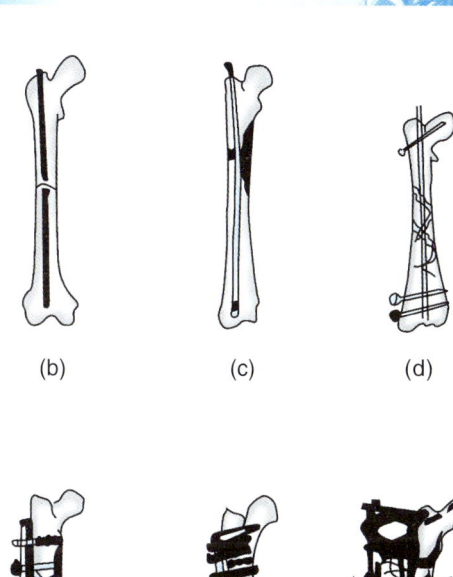

(b)   (c)   (d)

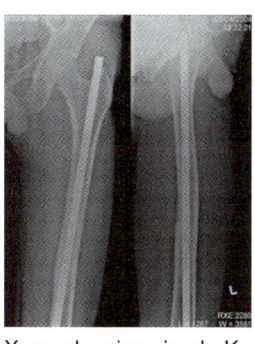
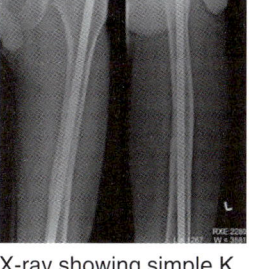
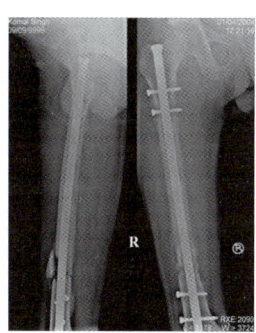

X-ray showing simple K nailing for fracture shaft femur

X-ray showing interlocking nailing for fracture shaft femur(arrow)

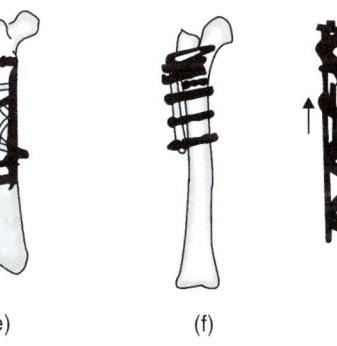
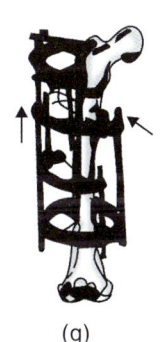

(e)   (f)   (g)

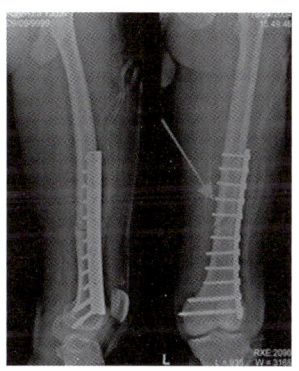

X-ray showing DC plating for middle and lower third fracture (arrow)

Figs 3.62b to g: Different modalities to stabilise femur fracture

- *Nerve:* Sciatic nerve palsy in injuries of the upper third.
- *Vessels:* Damage to the femoral artery in compound mid-shaft fracture with penetrating injuries.
- *Muscle:* Quadriceps wasting and myositis ossificans.
- *Infection:* Osteomyelitis in compound fracture and after operations at times.

Supra/Inter-Condylar Fracture

This usually presents with pain, deformity and haemarthrosis following trauma.

Management

- **First aid management:** Requires aspiration of haemarthrosis compression bandage and posterior POP slab.
- **Final**
  - 90° blade plate for lower two-thirds (Fig. 3.63a).
  - Condylar screw with plate for T-supra/inter-condylar fracture (Fig. 3.63b).
  - Cast brace for comminuted fracture (Fig. 3.63c).
  - Cancellous screws for condylar fracture (Fig. 3.63d).

Fracture

Treatment

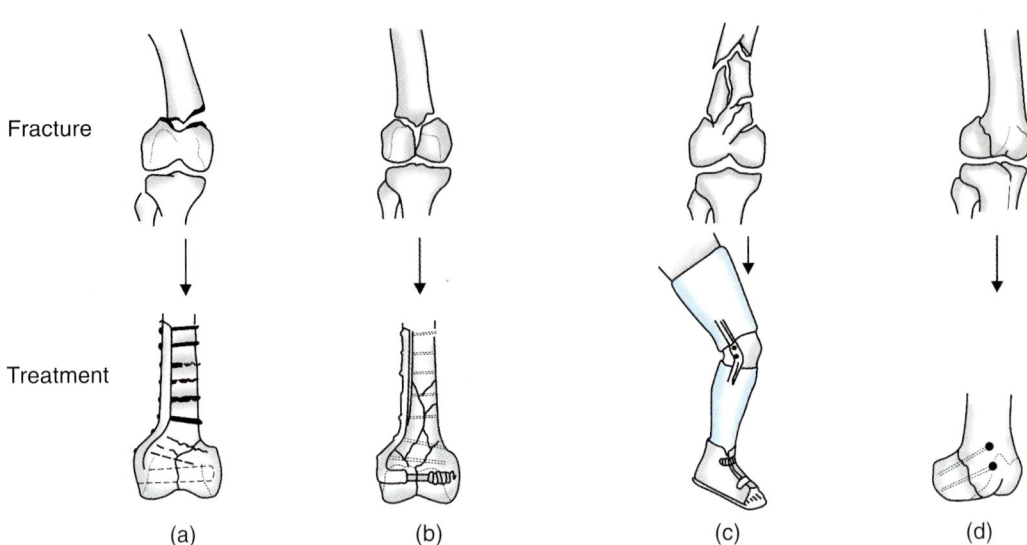

(a)　　　　　(b)　　　　　(c)　　　　　(d)

Figs 3.63a to d: Different modalities to stabilise supra/inter condylar fracture femur

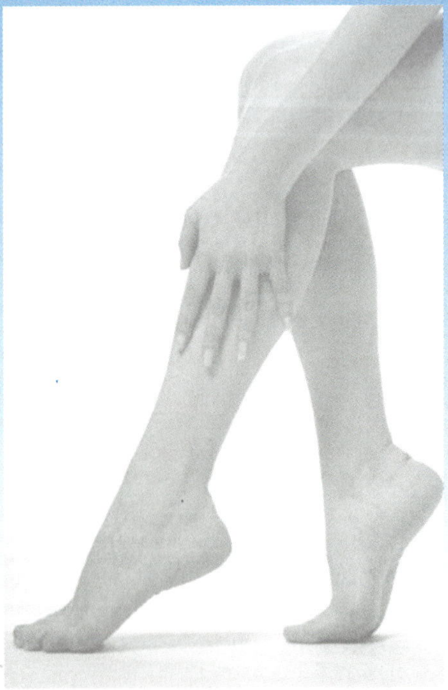

ANATOMY OF KNEE JOINT

The knee joint is made up of three bones and a variety of ligaments. The knee is formed by the femur (the thigh bone), the tibia (the shin bone), and the patella (the knee cap). Several muscles and ligaments control the motion of the knee and protect it from damage at the same time. Two ligaments on either side of the knee, called the medial and lateral collateral ligaments, stabilize the knee from side-to-side.

There are two cruciate ligaments located in the centre of the knee joint. The anterior cruciate ligament (ACL) and the posterior cruciate ligament (PCL) are the major stabilizing ligaments of the knee. In figure 3.64, on the lateral view, the posterior cruciate ligament prevents the femur from sliding forward on the tibia (or the tibia from sliding backwards on the femur). In the medial view, the anterior cruciate ligament prevents the femur from sliding backwards on the tibia (or the tibia sliding forwards on the femur). Most importantly, both of these ligaments stabilize the knee in a rotational fashion. Thus, if one of these ligaments is significantly damaged, the knee will be unstable when planting the foot of the injured extremity and pivoting, causing the knee to buckle and give way.

The weight bearing surface of knee is covered by a layer of cartilage commonly, referred as articular cartilage. There are also two shock absorbers in the knee on either side of the joint between the cartilage surfaces of the femur and the tibia. These two structures are called the medial meniscus and the lateral meniscus. The menisci are horseshoe-shaped shock absorbers that help both centre the knee joint during activity and to minimize the amount of stress on the articular cartilage. The combination of the menisci and the surface cartilage in the knee produces a nearly frictionless gliding surface.

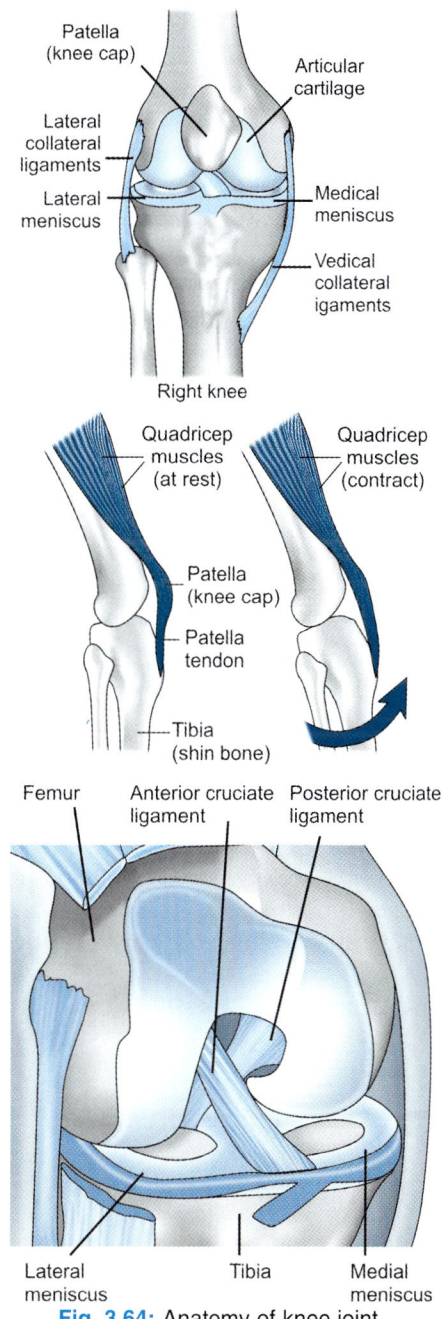

Fig. 3.64: Anatomy of knee joint

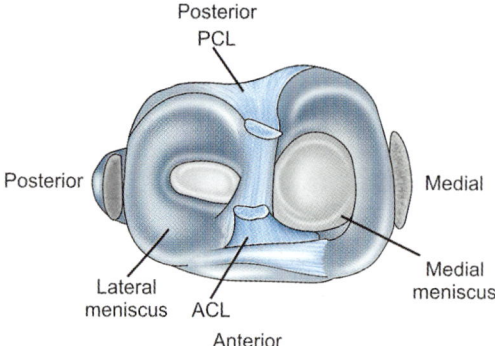

Fig. 3.65: Upper tibia showing cruciate ligaments and both meniscus

The knee is an incredible joint. It is strong, flexible, and very tough.

Movement of the Knee

The main muscles that move the knee joint are the quadriceps and hamstring muscles. The quadriceps attaches to the patella, and the patellar tendon connects this muscle to the front of the tibia. When the quadriceps muscles contract the knee extends. In contrast, when the hamstring muscles contract, they pull the knee into flexion.

INJURIES AROUND THE KNEE (INTERNAL DERANGEMENT OF KNEE)

This is a group of injuries characterized by pain, swelling, locking, muscle wasting in stability and early osteoarthritis following injury to the knee. The lesion may involve meniscus, collateral/cruciate ligaments.

Medial Meniscus (Fig. 3.65)

Types

- Anterior horn avulsion
- Posterior horn avulsion
- Bucket handle tear (most common type)

Clinical Features

It is torn more frequently than lateral because it is less mobile (being fixed to the medial

collateral ligament). The medial semilunar cartilage is more often injured being fixed to the collateral ligament whereas the lateral semicircular cartilage enjoys the advantage of being more mobile as it is not attached to the lateral collateral ligament and it gives origin to the tendon of popliteus which pulls it backwards and does not give any chance of being nipped between the two condyles of femur and the tibia. History of trauma while playing football with the knee flexed, followed by swelling, pain, recurrent effusions and locking. Tenderness at the level of medial joint line in front, behind or deep to the medial collateral ligament, depending on the site of tear. Positive McMurray's and Apley's grinding test.

Investigations

- X-ray is usually negative initially, osteoarthritis is seen in old injuries.
- Arthroscopy is very useful in precise diagnosis, and subsequent management.
- MRI is excellent non-invasive diagnostic tool.

Management

- **Acute:** Aspiration of effusion and compression bandage. Rest and quadricep exercises.
- **Chronic:** Arthroscopic repair, excision of meniscus.

Lateral Meniscus

Injuries are not very common, all the features and treatment are same, as for medial meniscus but laterally localized. **Discoid meniscus**, is at times seen, which presents as a gradually increasing swelling and needs excision.

Anterior Cruciate Ligament Tear

History of injury while playing football followed by pain, swelling (haemarthrosis), locking, muscle wasting, instability and early osteoarthritis of knee.

Clinical examination: Reveals posterior sagging knee (Fig. 3.66a), effusion, positive anterior drawer sign (anterior gliding of the tibia, knee flexed at 90° and pulled forward, Fig. 3.66b), quadriceps wasting seen in long standing cases.

Lachman test: Knee flexed at 10°, tibia pulled anteriorly, it subluxates forward and rotates medially indicating anterior cruciate and medial collateral ligament tear.

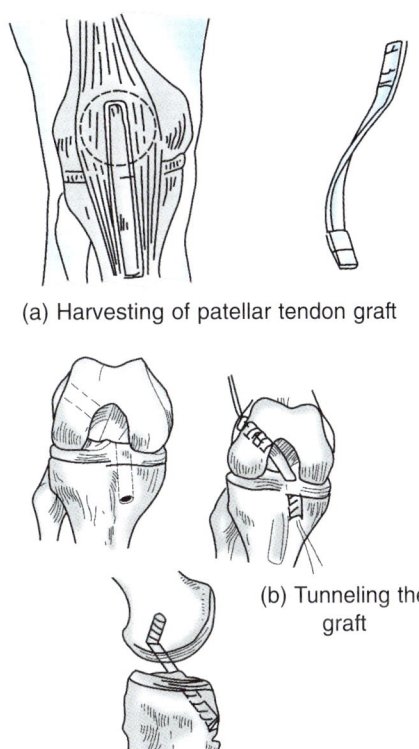

(a) Harvesting of patellar tendon graft

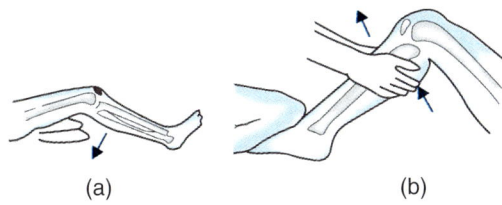

| (a) | (b) |

Figs 3.66a and b: (a) Posterior sagging knee (arrow) (b) Anterior drawer test

Investigations

- Aspiration reveals haemarthrosis.
- Arthroscopy is diagnostic as well as therapeutic.

Management

- **Acute:** Aspiration of haemarthrosis, rest and compression bandage, A/K POP cast with knee in 45° flexion for 3 weeks and subsequent repair.
- **Chronic:** Arthroscopic repair of torn ACL /replacement by patellar tendon graft or hamstrings.

A strip of ligamentum patellae along with underlying bone of the patella and tibial tuberosity is harvested and after making an appropriate tunnel in the tibia and femur the graft is passed and the two ends are then fixed to the bone with interference screws or buttons at both the ends after adequately tensioning it (Figs 3.67a to c).

(b) Tunneling the graft

(c) Fixation of graft

Figs 3.67a to c: Reconstruction with patella tendon graft

Posterior Cruciate

Clinical Features

Typical posterior sagging of the knee (Fig. 3.68a) and positive posterior drawer sign (Fig. 3.68b).

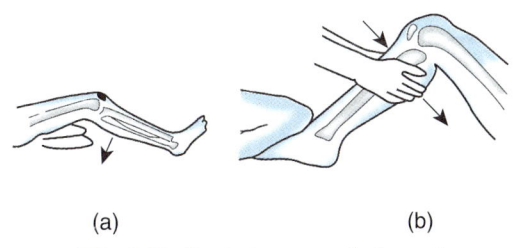

| (a) | (b) |

Fig. 3.68: Posterior sages in (arrow)

Management

- Primarily conservative.
- Repair of the torn/detached ligament (Fig. 3.69) if associated with other injuries.

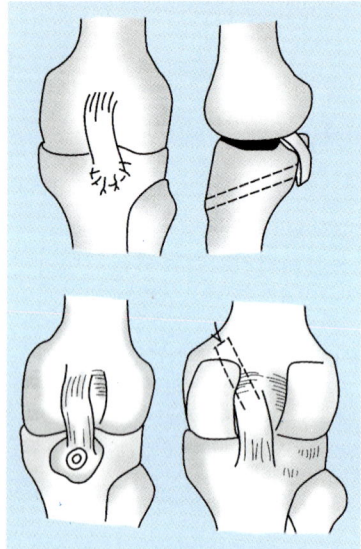

Fig. 3.69: Repair of torn/detached ligament

Medial Collateral Ligament

This is due to valgus opening of the knee joint and often associated with tear of medial meniscus.

Clinical Features

Pain, swelling, limitation of movements and tenderness at the medial joint line, exaggerated on valgus stress.

Instability

First-degree sprain: Localised joint pain and tenderness but no joint laxity (Fig. 3.70a).

Second-degree sprain: Pain and mild-joint laxity (Fig. 3.70b).

Third-degree sprain: Ligaments completely disrupted and joint is grossly unstable (Fig. 3.70c).

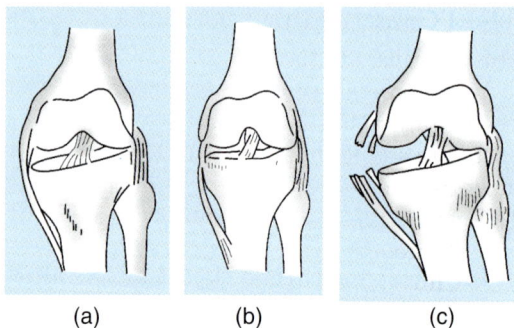

(a)   (b)   (c)

Figs 3.70a to c: (a) First-degree sprain (b) Second-degree sprain (c) Third-degree sprain

Management

- **Conservative:** Aspiration and compression bandage with A/K well moulded POP cast (for 1st and 2nd degree).
- **Surgical:** Repair of the torn ligament (for 3rd degree).

Pellegrini–Stieda disease is calcification of medial collateral ligament.

Triad of O'Donoghue: Rupture of medial collateral ligament, medial meniscus and avulsion of anterior cruciate ligament (Fig. 3.71).

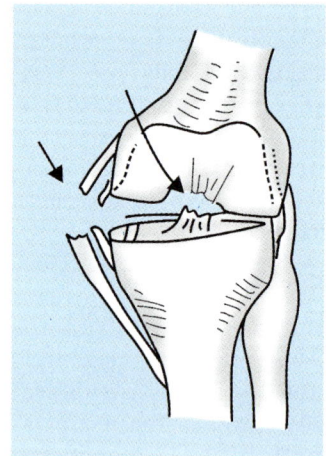

Fig. 3.71: Triad of O'Donoghue

Lateral Collateral Ligament

This is similar to medial collateral, and is due to varus strain.

Aspiration of the knee is diagnostic.

It is possible to look at the aspirate and diagnose the problem.

a. *Cruciate injury and meniscal tear*
   - **Acute:** Effusion containing blood.
   - **Chronic:** Effusion is straw coloured.
b. *Intra-articular fracture*
   Effusion containing blood and fat droplets.
c. *Ligament tear*
   Aspiration is usually negative as fluid leaks into the soft tissue.

For all injuries around the knee **quadriceps strengthening exercises is mandatory for good recovery of function.**

Fracture – Patella

Types

- Avulsion
  - Proximal pole.
  - Distal pole (Fig. 3.72a).
- Transverse
  - Undisplaced (Fig. 3.72b).
  - Displaced due to quadriceps pull.
- Comminuted (Fig. 3.73c).

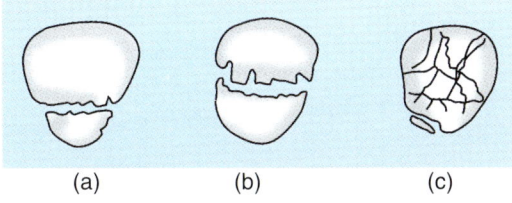

(a)   (b)   (c)

Figs 3.72a to c: Fracture patella

Mechanism of Injury

- Direct blow to the knee causing transverse, comminuted fracture.
- In tetanus and epilepsy due to violent quadriceps contraction causing avulsion fractures.

Clinical Features

- Haemarthrosis, boggy swelling in the knee joint, palpable gap between the fracture fragments.
- Pain and inability to extend the knee.
  Principle of treatment: Accurate reduction, early mobilization of the knee, good quadriceps power for the knee stabilization and movements.

Treatment

- **In undisplaced hairline fracture:** AK POP cylinder cast immobilization (Fig. 3.73a).
- **Displaced:** Open reduction and fixation with tension band wiring, or screw (Fig. 3.73b).
- **Distal pole:** Polar excision and repair of quadriceps expansion (Fig. 3.73c).
- **Comminuted fracture and old patients:** Excision of patella and repair of quadriceps tendon (Fig. 3.73d).

Complications

Quadriceps wasting, knee stiffness and early osteoarthritis.

Condylar Fractures of Tibia

These usually present with injury around the knee followed by extensive swelling in upper third of the leg, haemarthrosis, inability to stand and walk or move the knee.

Always examine for distal pulsations and sensations as incidence of compartmental syndrome is very high.

Treatment

- **Conservative:** In undisplaced fractures, aspiration of haemarthrosis followed by compression bandage and above knee POP cast for 3 –4 weeks of non-weight bearing, followed by cast brace mobilization of the knee.
- **Operative:** For displaced, depressed condylar and unstable fractures, it is always

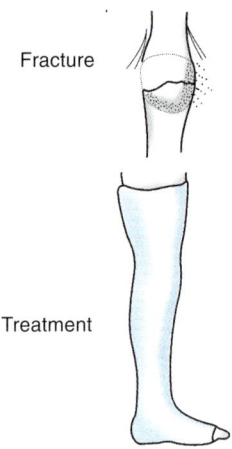

Fig. 3.73a: Fracture patella is stabilised by well padded AK pop cast

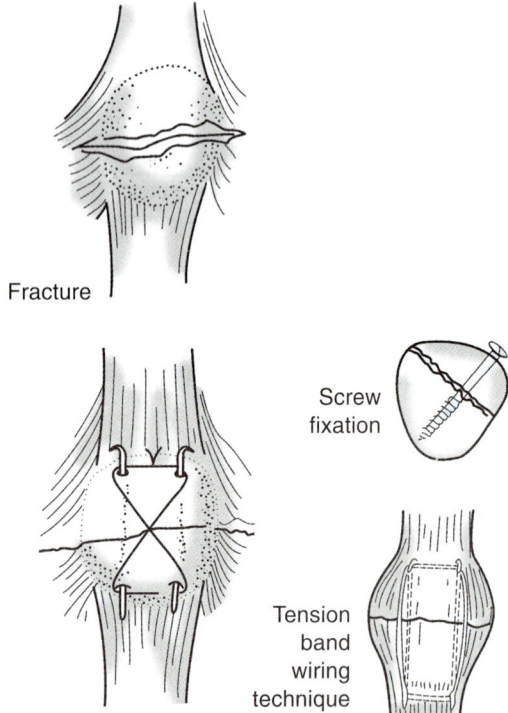

Fig. 3.73b: Displaced fracture patella is stabilised by tension band wiring technique/screw

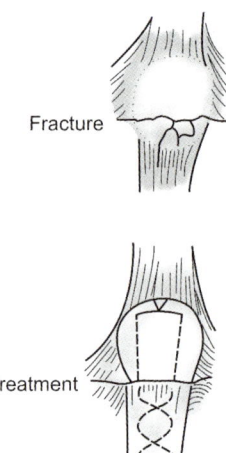

Fig. 3.73c: In comminuted distal pole fracture. Polar excision and quadricep repair

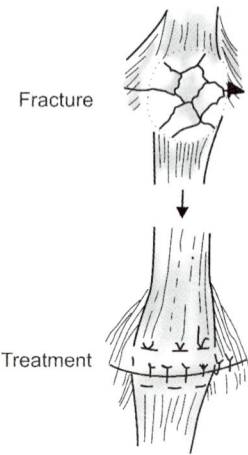

Fig. 3.73d: Total patellectomy with quadriceps repair for grossly comminuted fracture patella

preferable to accurately reduce the fracture so that the joint line is well maintained, if necessary, subcondylar bone graft packing may be done.

– Cancellous screw fixation for lateral condylar fractures (Fig. 3.74a).

– Butteress plating and subarticular bone grafting for depressed condylar fractures (Fig. 3.74b).
– T-plate for intercondylar and sub-condylar fractures (Fig. 3.74c).

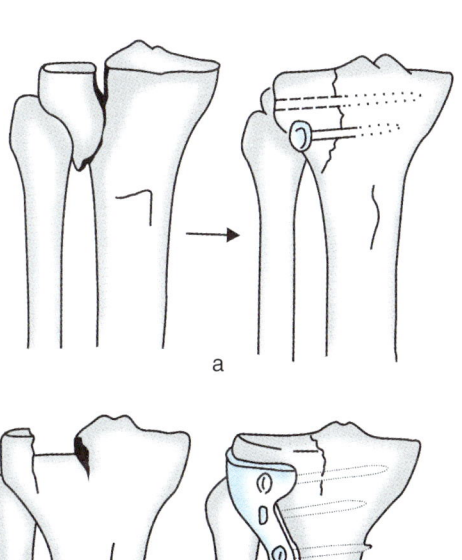

a

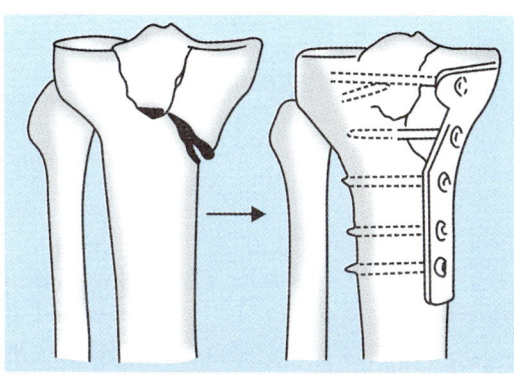

b

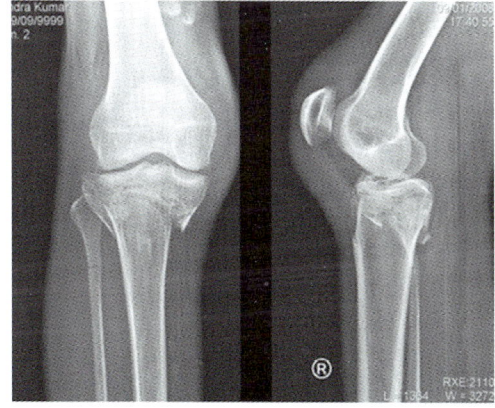

c

Complications

- Stiffness of knee and pain due to intra- and peri-articular adhesions.
- Instability due to damaged ligaments.
- Early osteoarthritis.

Fracture: Tibia/Fibula Shafts

Most common fracture in adults, often compound and gets complicated soon. Commonly due to the high speed roadside accidents.

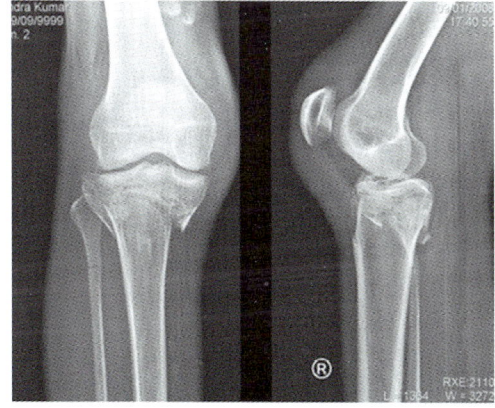

X-ray showing condylar fracture

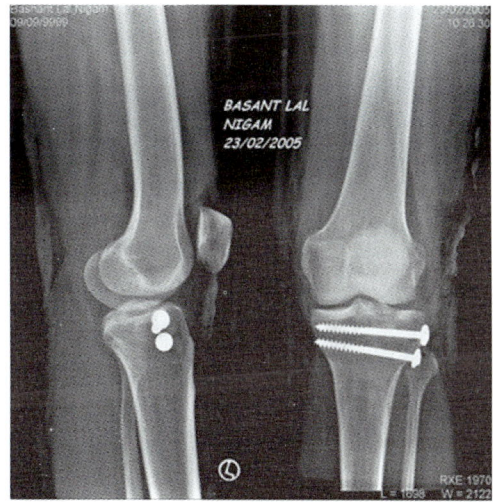

X-ray condylar fracture fixed with cancellous screw

Figs 3.74a to c: (a) Cancellous screw for lateral condylar fractures (b) Buttress plate (c) T plate

Clinical Features

Deformity, pain, swelling, blister formation, bony crepitus and abnormal movements. *Always examine the distal pulsations and sensations.*

X-ray

To see the type of the fracture and amount of the displacement.

Principle of Treatment

- **Management of simple fractures:**
  - Undisplaced and satisfactory alignment: A/K POP cast for 12 weeks.
  - Displaced: Closed reduction under anaesthesia and A/K POP cast.
  - Open reduction and internal fixation for unstable and irreducible fractures.
  - Open reduction and the internal fixation by dynamic compression plate for clean fractures (Fig. 3.75a).
  - Simple nail (Fig. 3.75b), interlocked nail for communited unstable fracture (Fig. 3.75c).
- **Management of compound fractures:**
  - If mild infection is present, allow the wound to heal, leg kept in Bohler Braun's splint with lower tibial traction.
  - External fixation for compound potentially contaminated injuries (Fig. 3.75d), Illizarov fixator for communited fractures and bone loss (Fig. 3.75e).
- **Management of complicated fractures**
  a. Management of vascular injuries followed by stabilization of bone.
  b. External fixation after fasciotomy is done, if signs of *compartmental syndrome* are obvious and final management is subsequently done for soft tissue and bony injuries.

Important Complications

- Compartmental syndrome in closed crush injuries of tibia.
- Neurovascular injuries leading to foot drop or gangrene.
- Malunion due to poor reduction of fracture fragments.
- Non-union in the lower one-third due to poor blood supply.
- Infection in compound fractures.

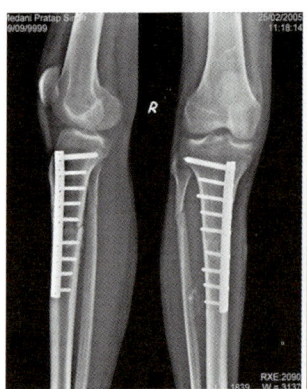 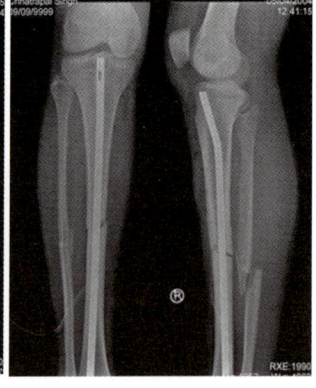 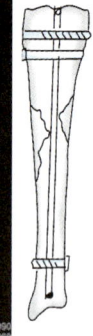 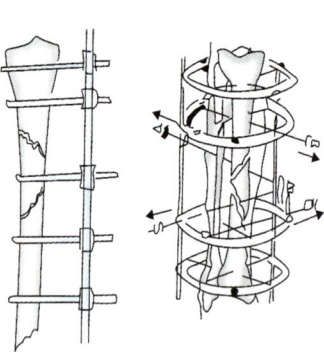

Fig. 3.75a: DC plating for fracture shaft tibia X-ray showing DC plating and cortical scews

Fig. 3.75b: Simple nailing for fracture shaft tibia. X-ray showing V nail for fracture tibia

Fig. 3.75c: Interlocked tibia nail

Fig. 3.75d

Fig. 3.75e

ANATOMY OF ANKLE JOINT

In human anatomy, the ankle joint is formed where the foot and the leg meet. The ankle, or talocrural joint, is a synovial hinge joint that connects the distal ends of the tibia and fibula in the lower limb with the proximal end of the talus bone in the foot. The articulation between the tibia and the talus bears more weight than between the smaller fibula and the talus.

Movement

The ankle joint is responsible for dorsiflexion (moving the toes up as when standing only on the heels) and plantar flexion of the foot (moving the toes down, as when standing on the toes), and allows for the greatest movement of all the joints in the foot. The ankle does not allow rotation.

In plantar flexion, the anterior ligaments of the joint become longer while the posterior ligaments become shorter. The reverse is true for dorsiflexion.

Articulation

The lateral malleolus of the fibula and the medial malleolus of the tibia along with the inferior surface of the distal tibia articulate with three facets of the talus. These surfaces are covered by cartilage.

The talus is wider in its anterior part. When the foot is dorsiflexed, the wider part of the superior talus moves into the articulating surfaces of the tibia and fibula, creating a more stable joint, than when the foot is plantar flexed.

Ligaments

The ankle joint is bound by the strong deltoid ligament and three lateral ligaments: the anterior talofibular ligament, the posterior talofibular ligament, and the calcaneofibular ligament.

- The deltoid ligament supports the medial side of the joint, and is attached at the medial malleolus of the tibia and connects in four places to the sustentaculum tali of the calcaneus, calcaneonavicular ligament, the navicular tuberosity, and to the medial surface of the talus.
- The anterior and posterior talofibular ligaments support the lateral side of the joint from the lateral malleolus of the fibula to the dorsal and ventral ends of the talus.
- The calcaneofibular ligament is attached at the lateral malleolus and to the lateral surface of the calcaneus.

The joint is most stable in dorsiflexion and a sprained ankle is more likely to occur when the foot is plantar flexed. This type of injury more frequently occurs at the anterior talofibular ligament.

ANKLE INJURIES

Pott's Fracture

It is a group of fractures around the ankle. This is due to movement of talus in the ankle mortice.

Classification: Based on mechanism of injury
- External rotation injuries.
- Abduction injuries.
- Adduction injuries.
- Vertical compression injuries.

External Rotation Injuries

First degree: Isolated spiral fracture of lateral malleolus (Fig. 3.76a).

Second degree: Avulsion fracture of medial malleolus with spiral fracture of lateral malleolus (Fig. 3.76b).

Third degree: In addition to the above injury there is associated posterior marginal fracture of tibia with subluxation of ankle joint (Fig. 3.76c).

Abduction injuries

First degree: Isolated avulsion fracture of medial malleolus (Fig. 3.77a).

Second degree: Associated communited fracture of lateral malleolus (Fig. 3.77b).

Third degree: In addition to the above posterior marginal fracture of tibia with subluxation (Fig. 3.77c).

Adduction injuries

First degree: Vertical fracture of medial malleolus (Fig. 3.78a).

Second degree: Associated transverse fracture of lateral malleolus (Fig. 3.78b).

Third degree: Associated to the above, there is fracture of posterior lip of tibia with posterior dislocation of ankle (Fig. 3.78c).

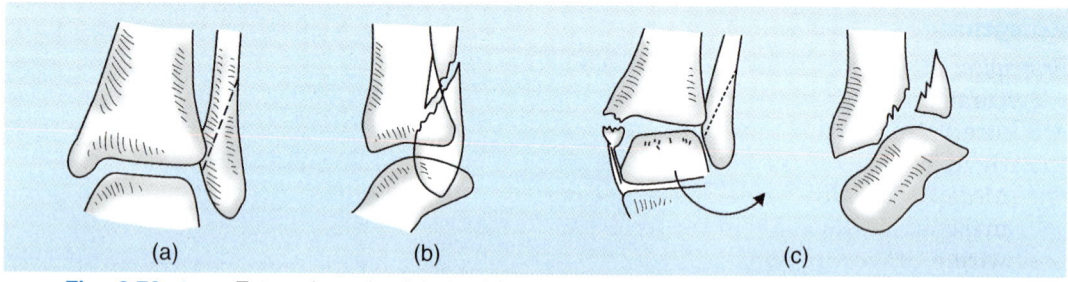

Figs 3.76a to c: External rotation injuries (a) First degree, (b) Second degree, (c) Third degree

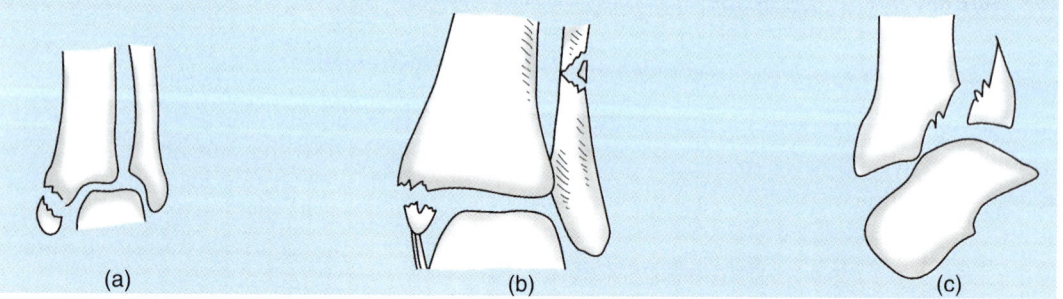

Figs 3.77a to c: Abduction fracture (a) First degree, (b) Second degree, (c) Third degree

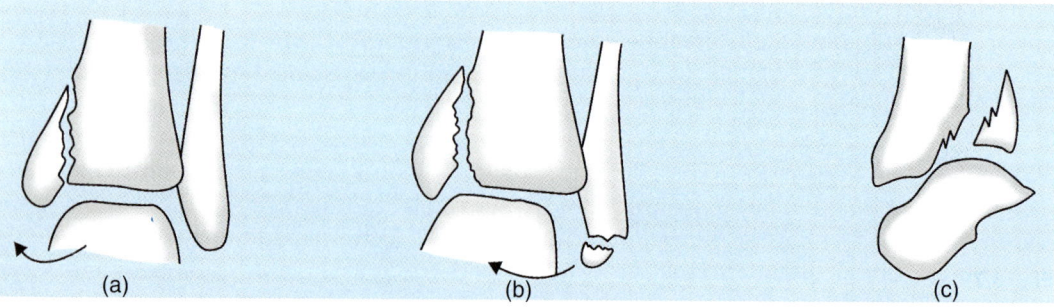

Figs 3.78a to c: Adduction fracture (a) First degree (b) Second degree (c) Third degree

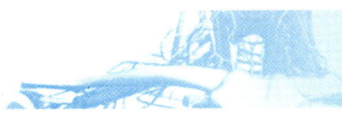

Vertical compression injuries: This results in comminuted fractures of the ankle mortise.

Clinical Features of Ankle Injuries

History of tortional injury to the foot, fall from height followed by deformity, pain, swelling and blister formation.

X-ray

X-ray of the ankle including full length of tibia and fibula to see the type of fracture.

Management

Principles:
- Accurate reduction
- Secure stabilization
- Early mobilization
  - *Medial malleolus:* Open reduction and malleolar screw fixation, or tension band wiring.
  - *Lateral malleolus:* Buttress plating, lag screw fixation (Fig. 3.79).

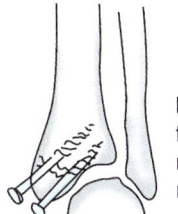

Malleolar screw fixation of medial malleolus

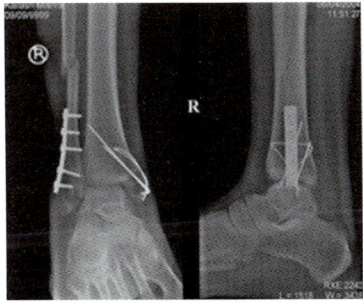

Fig. 3.79: X-ray showing tension band wiring for medial malleolus fracture and buttress plating for lateral malleolus fracture

Complications

Malunion, non-union, joint stiffness, painful swollen ankle, early osteoarthritis.

Talus Fracture

This is an important tarsal bone as it is a link between tibia, the fixed long bone of the lower extremity and the mobile part of the foot. It has no muscle attachments, and is part of the ankle and talocalcaneonavicular joint complex. Fracture of the talus is peculiar because of its precarious blood supply like that of scaphoid and head of femur. The vascular channels enter the talus from its undersurface of the neck through the vessels passing through the sinus tarsi, which ascend and then pass into the head, neck and the body; any fracture or dislocation causes damage to this vascular channel and is responsible for avascular necrosis and non-union of the fracture site.

Fractures of talus may be simple or compound. It can be classified as under :
- Fracture of the head and neck
- Fracture of the body, chipped articular cartilage
- Fracture dislocation (Fig. 3.80)
- Fracture talus associated with ankle and calcaneal injuries.

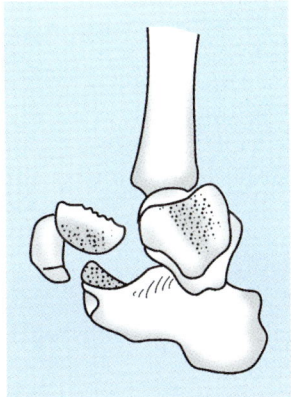

Fig. 3.80: Fracture dislocation of talus

Clinical Features

There is an obvious history of injury to the ankle, followed by immediate swelling involving the ankle and subtalar area, inability to stand and bear weight, the blood leaks into the soft tissue and all ankle movements are painful and restricted.

X-ray

Lateral view of the talus with ankle in dorsiflexion and plantar flexion, AP view and if necessary CT scan is done for a triplanar view.

Treatment

- Undisplaced fracture of the head, neck and body is initially kept in a well padded slab and subsequently converted into a non-weight bearing cast for 4–6 weeks. Non-weight bearing cast is applied with the foot fully plantar flexed (equinus) an unfamiliar and unpleasant position which is essential.
- Displaced fracture of neck and body should be treated by open reduction and fixation by K-wires or screws depending on the size of the fragment.
- Fracture dislocation in fresh cases should be reduced and fixed at the earliest.
- Old unreduced fracture, dislocations and comminuted burst fractures are best treated by Pantalar arthrodesis.

Complications

- Skin necrosis, especially in displaced fracture dislocations.
- Painful subtalar arthritis.
- Avascular necrosis of the body.

Calcaneum Fracture

History

This is usually due to the fall from the height; patient presents with pain, swelling and inability to stand following a fall and ecchymosis around the heel.

Classification

- Fracture involving subtalar joint.
- Non-articular.
  a. Anterior sustentaculum tali (Fig. 3.81a).
  b. Posterior tuberosity.
    – Vertical posterior tuberosity (Fig. 3.81b).
    – Horizontal posterior tuberosity (Fig. 3.81c).

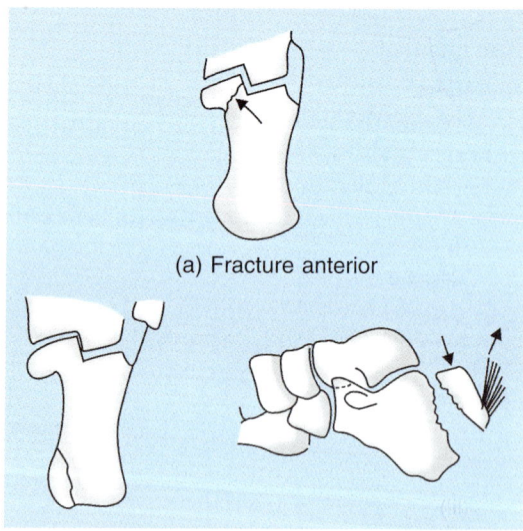

(a) Fracture anterior

(b) Fracture vertical   (c) Fracture horizontal

Figs 3.81a to c: Fracture calcaneum

X-ray

X-ray of the calcaneum is taken in AP, axial and lateral view to see the tuber angle (talocalcaneal), which is normally about 25 degrees.

Always examine dorsal lumbar spine for wedge compression fracture in a patient with a history of fall from height.

Treatment

- **Conservative:** Elevation, cold compression and POP slab/cast for 3 weeks of non-

weight bearing followed by gradual mobilization.
- **Surgery:**
  a. Open reduction and fixation for fracture of body of calcaneum and restoration of talocalcaneal joint surface.
  b. Closed pinning of posterior tuberosity (Fig. 3.82a).

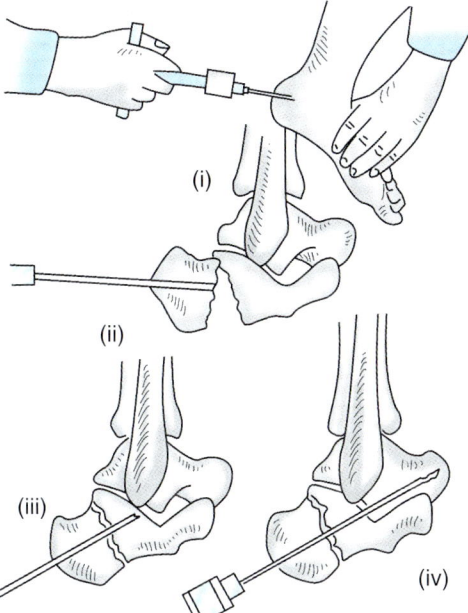

(i)

(ii)

(iii)

(iv)

Fig. 3.82a: Closed pinning of posterior tuberosity

Complications

Malunion and painful limp due to subtalar arthritis, treated by subtalar arthrodesis.

Jones Fracture

Fracture base of fifth metatarsal. This is due to inversion injury of foot due to imbalance. Usually presents with pain and swelling over base of fifth toe (Fig. 3.82b).

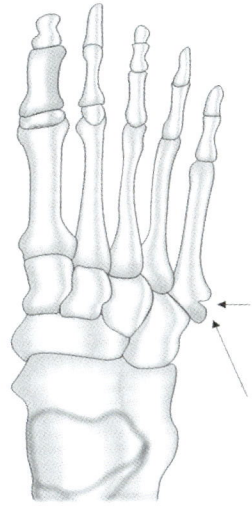

Fig. 3.82b: Jones fracture (arrow)

Treatment

- Undisplaced fracture treated by BK POP cast for 6 weeks.
- If avulsion and separation is seen, then open reduction and internal fixation with screw or tension band wiring should be done (Fig. 3.82c).

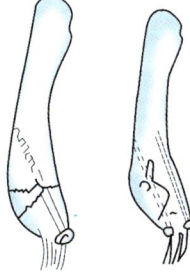

Fig. 3.82c: ORIF with a screw or tension band wire technique

March Fracture

Stress fracture of second (usually)/third metatarsal are seen on X-ray after 2 weeks of stress in army recruits. Three bones—metatarsal, fibula and tibia most common site for stress fracture in that order. It presents as painful swelling and is self-limiting, relieved by rest.

ARTHRODESIS

This is surgical ablation of movements at a joint to relieve pain, cure a disease and provide stability. This gives the joint, stability at the cost of mobility. The ideal position for the common joints are

- *Shoulder*: 60° of abduction and 30° forward flexion.
- *Elbow*: 90° of flexion for household work and straight for labourer.
- *Wrist*: 15° of dorsiflexion.
- *Hip*: 20° of flexion, 10° of abduction and 5° of external rotation.
- *Knee*: 10° of flexion.

The arthrodesis is done by excision of the articular cartilage and the fusion of the joint by intra-articular or extra-articular technique. The stability may be additionally provided by corticocancellous bone grafts, plates and screws. Charnley's compression clamp/Illizarov apparatus is used for fusion of knee/ankle.

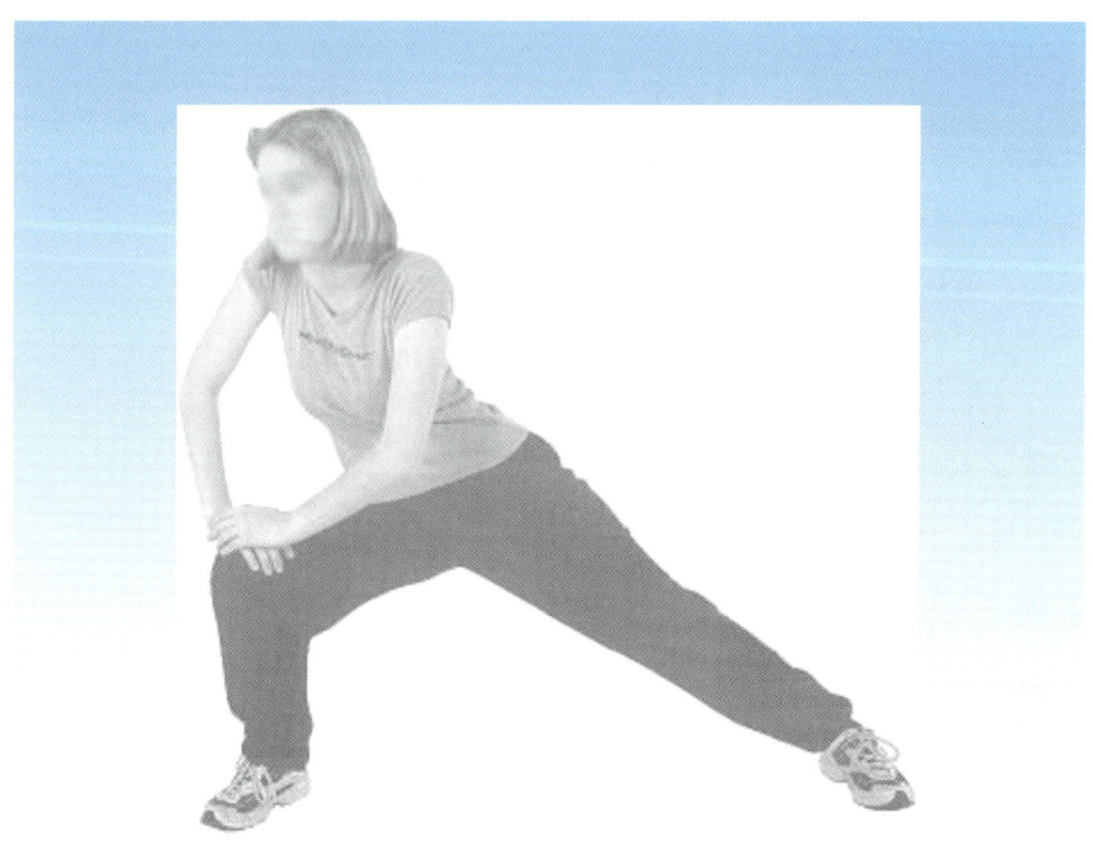

INJURIES OF PELVIS

Classification

1. Stable fracture with intact pelvic ring, an isolated fracture of ilium (Fig. 3.83a) (Duverney's), pubic rami (Fig. 3.83b), ischium (Fig. 3.83c). Duverney's, fracture of iliac wing in shown in Fig. 3.83d.

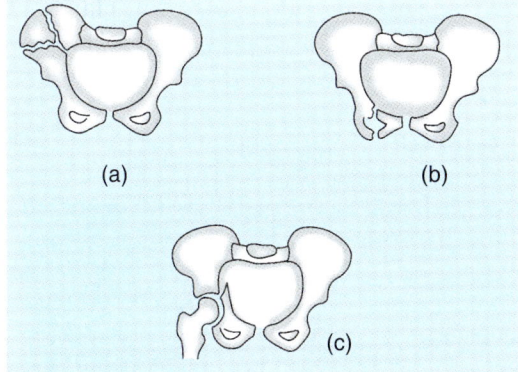

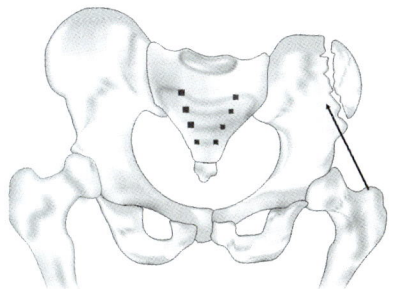

Figs 3.83a to c: Stable fracture of pelvis

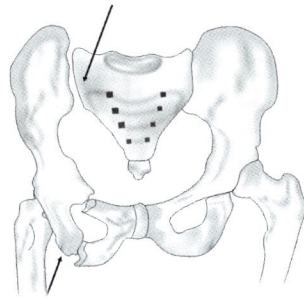

Fig. 3.83d: Duverney's fracture of illiac wing (arrow)

2. Unstable fracture (bi- and tri- planar): This involves:
   a. Double lesions like bilateral rami (Fig. 3.84a) [saddle fracture].
   b. Opening of pubic symphysis and sacroiliac joint (Fig. 3.84b).

c. Fracture of pubic rami with ala of sacrum (Fig. 3.84c). [Malgaigne's fracture]. Malgaigne's pelvic fracture is shown in Fig. 3.84d and Bucket handle fracture of pelvis is shown in Fig. 3.84e.

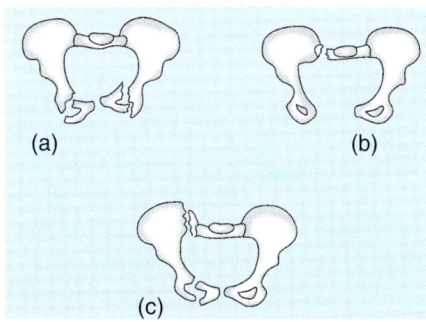

Figs 3.84a to c: Unstable fracture of pelvis

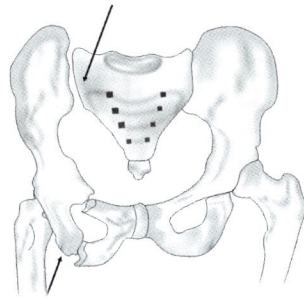

Fig. 3.84d: Malgaigne's pelvic fracture (arrow), unstable fracture of pelvis

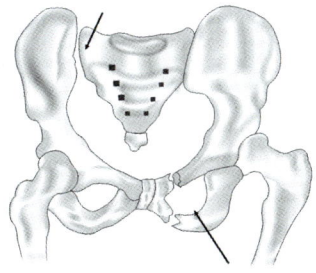

Fig. 3.84e: Unstable fracture of pelvis: Bucket handle fracture of pelvis (arrow)

3. **Complicated fracture** with visceral damage:
   - *Bladder:* Anuria with abdominal distension.
   - *Urethra:* Haematuria, anuria or incontinence of urine.
   - *Vessels:* Pelvic plexus of veins, causing shock/death.
   - *Nerve:* Posterior ring fracture, leading to sciatic nerve damage.

Clinical Features

History of major trauma due to vehicular accident, collapse of building or crush injury. The patient is usually in shock due to haemorrhage from pelvic venous plexus of veins in unstable pelvic fractures.

There is localised tenderness at fracture site and swelling. Pelvic compression and distraction is painful.

Anuria due to rupture of bladder or urethra; haematuria due to urethral injury; distension of abdomen due to bladder, visceral injury.

Investigations

- X-ray of pelvis showing AP, lateral and oblique views.
- Cystogram to evaluate bladder, urethral injury.
- Ultrasonography of abdomen to see for visceral damage.
- CT scan is at times helpful for complicated and multiplanar fractures.

Management

Principles of care are
- Management of shock by replacement of blood, fluids.
- Care of visceral damage.
- Fracture stabilization.

Treatment

- **Stable fracture:** Rest for 2–3 weeks followed by mobilization.

- **Unstable fracture:**
  - Hammock's sling with traction on both lower limbs for biplanar fractures.
  - Hip spica for children with minimal displacement.
  - ORIF for fracture of the ilium and acetabulum.
  - External fixator or plating for pelvic ring disruption.

Complications

- **Early:**
  - Shock due to haemorrhage.
  - Visceral damage consisting of urethra, bladder and bowel.
  - Damage to important vessels and sciatic nerve.
  - Associated fracture of femur, spine and hip dislocation.
- **Late:**
  - Malunion, non-union.
  - Painful gait.
  - Problems during childbirth.

Metabolic Bone Diseases

4

STRUCTURE OF BONE

Bone is a special form of connective tissue made up of microscopic crystals of phosphates of calcium (inorganic) within matrix of collagen (organic). The collagen in turn is organized in a complex three-dimensional way. The protein in bone matrix is mostly type -I, which is also the major structural protein in tendons and skin. Because of its high calcium and phosphate content, bone plays an important role in calcium homeostasis. It protects vital organs, and the rigidity that it provides, permits locomotion and the support of loads against gravity (Fig. 4.1).

Adequate amount of both protein and minerals must be available for the maintenance of normal bone structure. Bone crystals are made up of mostly hydroxyapatites. Sodium and small amounts of magnesium and carbonate are present in bone.

The cell that is concerned primarily with bone formation and resorption are osteoblasts and osteoclasts respectively. Both originate in the bone marrow.

Bone and Calcium

The adult human body contains about 1100 g (27.5 mol) of calcium (1.5% of body weight).

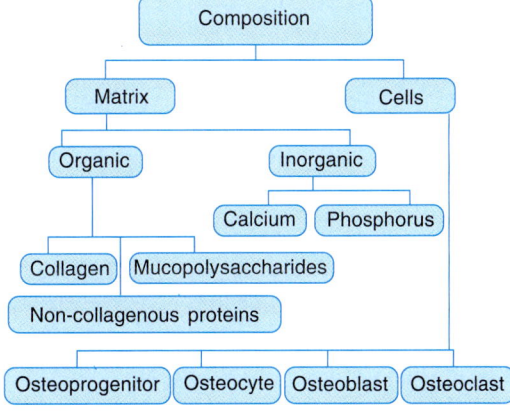

Fig. 4.1: Diagram depicting the composition of bone

Ninety nine per cent of the calcium is in the skeleton. Three hormones are primarily concerned with the regulation of calcium metabolism.

- **1, 25 dihydroxycholecalciferol** is a steroid hormone formed from vitamin D by successive hydroxylations in the liver and kidneys. Its primary action is to increase calcium absorption from the intestine.
- **Parathyroid hormone** is secreted by the parathyroid glands. Its main action is to

mobilize calcium from bone and increase urinary phosphate excretion.

- **Calcitonin** is a calcium-lowering hormone that in mammals is secreted primarily by cells in the thyroid gland inhibits bone resorption.

A fourth hormone, parathyroid hormone-related protein (PTHrP), acts on one of the PTH receptors and is important in skeletal development *in utero*. There may also be a phosphate regulating hormone, and gluco-corticoids, growth hormone, estrogens, and various growth factors also affects calcium metabolism.

RICKETS AND OSTEOMALACIA

Definition

It is the commonest metabolic disorder of childhood, characterised by abnormal minera-lization, skeletal deformities, weakness and bone pain. It affects the growth of bone and callus formation. If it occurs during the growth phase in childhood, it is called **rickets.** It is characterised by deformed bones, short stature, and increased susceptibility to fractures. In adults, such effects are termed as **osteomalacia,** first described as 'English disease' by David Whistler in 1645 due to lack of exposure to sunlight. Hess showed that prevention was possible by cod liver oil and exposure to sunlight. Some patients did not respond to cod liver oil, Albright showed that these patients had a primary renal defect.

Causes

i. **Dietary deficiency:** Vitamin D, calcium, phosphorus, exposure to sunlight.
ii. **Absorptive deficiency**
    a. *Gastric:* After gastrectomy.
    b. *Intestinal:* Chelators (antacids), phy-tates (maize), oxalates, steatorrhoeas, all of these interfere with calcium absorption.
    c. *Hepatobiliary:* Cirrhosis, pancreatitis.

iii. **Renal**
    a. *Hereditary:* Vitamin D resistant, vitamin D dependent, Fanconi's syndrome (glycosuria, phosphaturia and amino-aciduria), renal tubular acidosis.
    b. *Acquired:* Renal osteodystrophy-glomerular/tubular disease.
iv. **Miscellaneous**
    Oncogenic: Breast carcinoma, angioma. Anticonvulsant drugs (phenytoin, barbi-turates), hypophosphatemia.

Pathology

Pommer in 1885 observed changes in the growth plate and described 5 zones (Fig. 4.2):

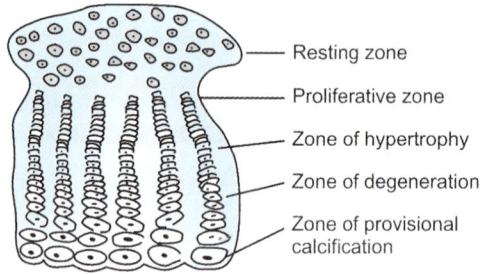

Fig. 4.2: 5 zones of an epiphyseal plate

i. In the active stage of the disease the orderly progression of endochondral ossification is interrupted. Proliferation of the cartilage cells, palisade arrangement and formation of matrix proceeds normally, but the calcification of the matrix is deficient. The cartilage cell columns proliferate 10 to 20 times the normal depth but in haphazard manner. In the metaphysis thick layers of osteoid are laid down.
ii. In the healed phase, calcium salts are deposited in the zone of provisional calci-fication. The osteoid promptly becomes calcified and is transformed to bone (Tables 4.1 and 4.2).

Table 4.1: Histological changes in rickets the 5 zones of epiphyseal plate			
S.no.	*Zones*	*Normal*	*Rickets*
1.	Resting zone	Normal	Normal
2.	Proliferation	Active cell division, cells arranged in columns	Normal
3.	Zone of hypertrophy	Ballooned cells which store glycogen arrangement	Abnormally thick and loose their columnar
4.	Provisional calcification vascular invasion	Cartilage bars calcify, chondrocytes die	Poorly calcified and vascular invasion irregular
5.	Primary spongiosa	Osteoblasts form calcified bone	Osteoid remains uncalcified

Table 4.2: Biochemical changes in different types of rickets				
Type of rickets	*Ca*	*P*	*Alkaline Phosphatase*	*PTH*
Vitamin D deficiency	Low/Normal	Low	High	High
Phosphatase Deficiency	Normal	Low	High	Normal
Gastrointestinal and enteric vitamin-D resistant	Low	Low	High	High
Hypophosphatemic (Albright)	Normal	Low	High	Normal
Type I vitamin-D dependent	Low	Low	High	High
Type II vitamin-D dependent	Low	Low	High	High
Renal tubular acidosis	Low	Low	High	High
Renal osteodystrophy	Low	High	High	High

Clinical Features

It occurs after 6 months of life up to 3 years in children, the child is restless and irritable with signs of general debility. In a classical case the findings are

i. **In rickets**
  a. **Head**
    - *Caput quadratum:* Frontal and parietal eminences with flat occiput and vertex leading to large head.
    - *Craniotabes:* Crackling cranial bone by the presence of areas of thinning and softening in the bones of the skull and widening of the sutures and fontanelles.
  b. **Chest**
    - *Rachitic rosary:* Enlarged costochondral junctions.
    - *Harrison's groove:* The soft ribs are pulled down by the attachment of diaphragm.
    - *Pigeon chest:* Chest is narrow in transverse section and elongated in AP with angled manubrium sterni.
  c. **Abdomen:** Prominent (pot-belly).
  d. **Pelvis:** Compressed transversely and decreased inlet.
  e. **Epiphysis:** The epiphyseal plate appears enlarged and deformed, the metaphysis is flared, cupped with increased height of the cartilage plate, microfractures with poor healing may be seen. Bowlegs/knock-knee, tackle deformity or wind swept (bowleg on one side and knock knee of other leg). Coxa vara with waddling gait with secondary ligamentous laxity.
  Delayed dentition, skin pale and muscle tone is poor (Fig. 4.3).
ii. **In Osteomalacia:** This is the adult for of the disease, features are mainly because of softening of bone, since the epiphysis

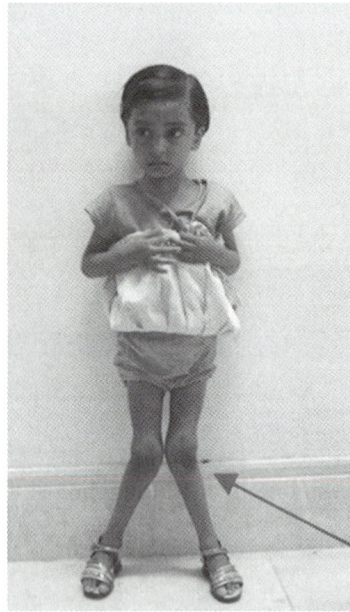

Fig. 4.3: Child with rickets is having bilateral genu valgum (arrow)

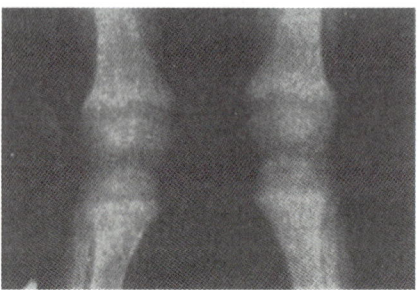

Fig. 4.4: X-ray showing rickets

has fused hence deformities are not very severe, the usual cause is dietary insufficiency or poor exposure to sunlight anorexia, bone pains, muscle weakness weight loss. Deformed femur and tibia, kyphotic spine, protrusio acetabuli, *Always look for gastric and hepatorenal causes.*

Investigations

i. **X-ray**
   a. *Rickets*
      • *Active phase:* Ossific centre of the epiphysis is small and ill-defined. Metaphysis is cup-shaped, frayed and trumpet-shaped in appearance. Epiphyseal plate is broad and thick.
      • *Healed:* A dense white line appears at epiphyseal and metaphyseal junction. Deformed metaphysis, coxa vara, bowlegs, and knock-knee (Fig. 4.4).
   b. *Osteomalacia:* Diffuse osteoporosis Pelvic deformity with protrusio acetabuli, kyphoscoliotic spine, due to wedge compression fractures, Milkman's syndrome. (multiple, symmetrical pseudo-fracture/*looser zones* (translucent zones surrounded by sclerotic bone usually running at right angle to the margin of bones) seen in upper femoral, ishiopubic rami and medial border of scapula).

ii. **Urine:** Fanconi's syndrome occurs in which renal absorption of several substances (phosphate, glucose, amino acids) is impaired.

iii. **Bone biopsy:** Decalcified specimen showing plenty of osteoid (poorly mineralized protein matrix) with increased osteoblastic activity.

iv. **Bone mineral density:** Decreased bone mass.

v. **Serum Ca × P:** <2.4 mol/l.

Treatment

i. **General:** Improve nutritional status by high protein diet, rich in milk, nuts, cheese and plenty of exposure to sunlight.

ii. **Specific**
   a. *Medical:* Vitamin D, 2000–5000 units per day which may be increased up to 3000000 units in resistant cases,

so as to elevate the serum phosphorus level up to 5 mg%. Metabolites of vitamin D like, alphacalciferol and salmon calcitonin are also available.

b. *Braces:* Prevention of progressive deformities by braces.

c. *Surgical:* Correction of coxa vara, bowleg (genu varum), knock-knee by osteotomies.

OSTEOPOROSIS

Definition

An abnormal reduction in bone tissue mass per unit volume of anatomical bone or patient whose bone mass is two standard deviations below the mean for that age and sex leading to fractures after minimal trauma. Radiologically evident as diffuse rarefaction (osteopenia) and clinically as overt fractures due to altered cellular activity either as decreased osteoblastic, increased osteoclastic or asynchrony leading to net loss of bone.

It is the single largest cause of fractures after forty, leading to morbidity and mortality in old age.

Pathophysiology

Reduction in thickness of cortex. Reduction in number of trabeculae and osteoblasts.

Types

i. **Primary**
   Type I: Postmenopausal (seen in age 45 × 65 years presenting with wrist and vertebral fractures). The main bone loss occurring in the medullary trabeculae.
   Type II: Senile (seen beyond the age of 65 years presenting with hip fractures). The main bone loss occurring in the cortical zone.

ii. **Secondary**
   a. *Endocrine:* Hypopituitarism, hypogonadism, diabetes.
   b. Chronic illness and disease, rheumatoid arthritis, liver disorder.

c. Neurological diseases
d. Alcoholism
e. Drug associated with an increased risk of generalized osteoporosis:
   • Glucocorticoids
   • Cyclosporine
   • Cytotoxic drugs
   • Anticonvulsants
   • Lithium
   • Excessive thyroxine
   • Aluminum (Present in some antacids)
   • Gonadotropin-releasing hormone agonist
   • Heparin.

Clinical Features

i. Pain
ii. Loss of height due to collapse of several vertebrae
iii. Pathological fracture, e.g. Colles' fracture, neck of femur and wedge compression fracture of the dorsolumbar spine.

Investigations

Thirty per cent of bone loss occurs before it is radiologically obvious.

i. **X-ray:** Ground glass appearance because of loss of definition of trabeculae which are coarse and cortical thinning, with fish tail shaped, wedge compression fracture of vertebra and scoliosis (Fig. 4.5).

ii. **Blood**
   Serum calcium-normal
   Serum phosphate—normal
   Serum Ca x P: > 2.4 mol/l
   Serum alkaline phosphatase may be raised.

iii. **Assessment of bone density**
   a. Dual energy X-ray absorptimetry (DEXA) determines bone density with very little radiation.
   b. Quantitative Computer tomography
   c. Ultrasonography.

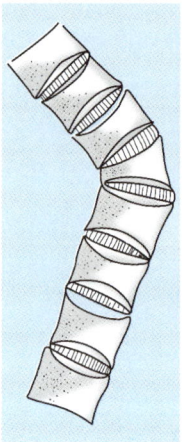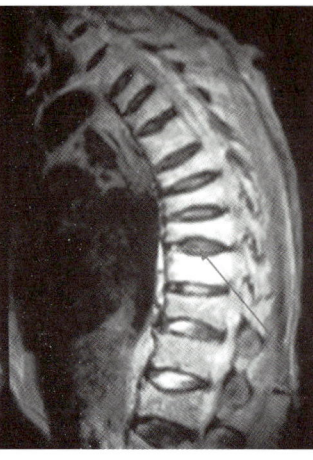

Fig. 4.5: CT scan showing disc bulges into the adjacent vertebral bodies so the disc become bi-convex in shape (cod fish appearance (arrow)). Wedging of the vertebrae are seen.

iv. Tetracycline labelled transiliac bone biopsy.
v. **Biochemical markers:**
The primary use of biochemical markers is for monitoring the response to treatment.
Biochemical markers of bone metabolism in clinical use:
Bone formation
- Serum bone specific alkaline phosphatase
- Serum osteocalcin
- Serum propeptide of type I procollagen
Bone resorption
- Urine and serum cross-linked N telopeptiide
- Urine and serum cross-linked C telopeptiide
- Urine total free deoxypyridinoline
- Urine hydroxyproline
- Serum tartrate-resistant acid phosphatase
- Serum bone sialoprotein
- Urine hydroxylysine glycosides.

The best bone markers currently available for clinical evaluation of osteoblastic activity is osteocalcin and bone specific alkaline phosphatase, pyridium cross links for bone resorbtion (others are hydroxyproline, pyridinolieoxyne).

Treatment
i. Prevention is the mainstay.
ii. Ambulation is encouraged and supports are provided to relieve pain. Proper diet and exercise are recommended.
iii. Drugs like vitamin D analogues, calcitonin, alendronate, raloxifene, biphosphonates, vitamin K, fluoride, anabolic steroids and above all high dose calcium supplementation.
iv. Oestrogen replacement: Hormone therapy in postmenopausal women.
v. Treatment of specific cause.
vi. Management of various fractures.
The drugs currently available are as follows:
- *Vitamin D:* This is the frontline drug for the management of osteoporosis given in the doses of 400 to 800 IU alongwith about 1200 mg of calcium per day. Several preparations like calcitriol (active metabolite of vitamin D), derivatives like alphacalcidol and 1-alphahydroxy cholecalciferol in doses of 0.25 mcg daily are available.
- *Calcium:* This is the frontline management of osteoporosis. The daily requirement is about 1 gm of calcium. Children absorb almost 75% of the dietary intake, whereas adults can do up to 50%. Calcium carbonate is the cheapest source of elemental calcium, calcium citrate is highly bioavailable, it can be supplemented with anabolic steroids like decadurabolin given in doses of 25 mcg weekly injections.
- *Oestrogen:* This is an integral component of hormone replacement therapy

for management of postmenopausal osteoporosis and has shown to reduce the bone loss, increase bone density both in spine and hip, thereby reducing the risk of fractures. It can be taken as a pill or patch and precautions should be taken for prescribing to the women who are at the risk of developing breast and uterus cancer. This is advisable both for prevention as well as treatment of osteoporosis.

- *Raloxifene:* This is a new class of drugs called selective oestrogen receptor modulators (SERMs) that appear to prevent bone loss at the spine, hip and total body.

- *Biphosphonates:* This group of drugs has potent anti-resorptive properties and these drugs are widely used in the treatment of osteoporosis and Paget's disease. **Alendronate** is superior to Etidronate with fewer GI side effects and is given in doses of 75 mg once a week for at least 6 months. Latest inj. zolindronic acid 300 mg i/v once a year.

- *Calcitonin:* This is a naturally occurring hormone and are responsible for maintenance of calcium balance by reducing bone loss, increasing bone density and relieving the severe bone pain associated with pathological fractures. It is available as **Salmon calcitonin,** which is 100 times more potent than natural one and is available as injection and nasal spray.

- *Vitamin K:* This is important for normal health because it is useful in calcium binding and helps in inhibition of calcium mineralization of urine. It is freely available in normal diet containing green leafy vegetables.

- *Fluoride:* This increases the life span and activity of osteoblast and helps in calcium assimilation in bones. It should always be given alongwith calcium and vitamin D.

- *Bonviva* (Idrophos) given in the dose of 150 mg once a month for 6 months or inj i.v. once in 3 months before osteolysis has shown excellent results in postmenopausal osteoporosis (Table 4.3).

Table 4.3: Clinical-pathological differences between osteoporosis and osteomalacia		
Features	*Osteoporosis*	*Osteomalacia*
Definition	Decreased amount of bone	Undermineralised bone
Symptoms	Localized to fracture sites	Generalized musculoskeletal
Radiographic features	Osteopenia, Frank fractures	Pseudo fractures with looser lines, Frank fractures
Calcium	Normal	Low or normal
Phosphate	Normal	Low or normal
Alkaline phosphatase	Normal	High
Parathyroid hormone	Normal or mildly increased	High or normal
Pathology	Thin and discontinuous bone trabeculae	Increased osteoid (the non-mineralized component of bone)
Tetracycline label	Discrete	Indistinct, smudged
Calcification rate	Normal	Decreased

OSTEOLYSIS

This is loss of bone due to rapid loss of mineralized bone which exceeds the rate of deposition, invariably due to parathyroid overactivity.

Hyperparathyroidism may be primary, secondary or tertiary.

1. Primary hyperthyroidism (von Recklinghausen's disease)/osteitis fibrosa cystica. This is due to hyperplasia of parathyroid or adenoma, characterized by Diffuse osteoporosis, cystic lesions in the long bones filled wit brown connective tissue causing, generalized bone pains, anorexia, weakness renal calculi, fractures and deformity. X-ray shows generalized osteoporosis, circumscribed bone lesions, lateral view of skull shows typical PEPPER POT appearance which is diagnostic.

   Resorption of lamina dura of the teeth. Thinning of cortex of phalanges.

   Blood: Increased serum calcium and alk PO_4, low phosphate.

   Bone biopsy from the iliac rest is often helpful.

   Treatment: It is directed to surgical excision of adenoma or removal of 2 or more parathyroid glands.

2. Secondary hyperparathyroidism is due to Renal causes, the serum calcium is usually normal or low the phosphate level varies depending upon the renal pathology.

3. Tertiary hyperparathyroidism, is due to perpetual stimulation of parathyroid glands causing irreversible over secretion and subsequent skeletal changes.

SCURVY

Barlow's Disease

This is a disease of poor children and cross country seamen due to dietary deficiency of vitamin C.

Occasionally rickets and scurvy may coexist.

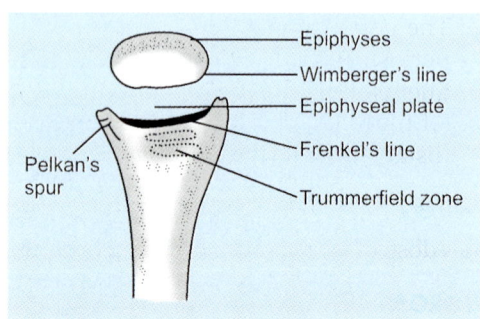

Fig. 4.6: Radiological feature is scurvy

Clinical Features

The child has poor health and low weight with bleeding gums and haemorrhages in the thigh muscle and subperiosteal zone leading to pseudoparalysis.

Radiological Features

i. The cortex is thin (Fig. 4.6 and 4.7), the metaphysis shows ground glass appearance with a prominent white line of calcification (Frenkel's line).

ii. An adjoining beak of bone (Pelkan's spur).

iii. Thin dense circle around the epiphysis (Wimberger's circle).

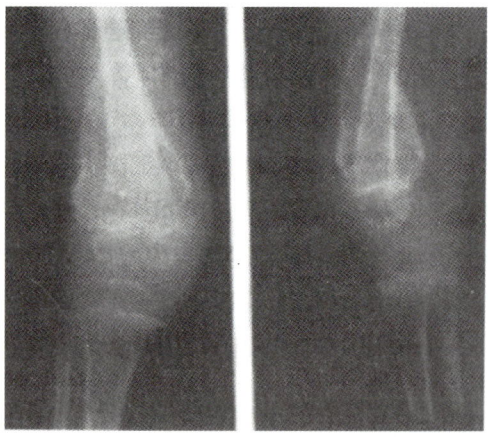

Fig. 4.7: Subperiosteal haemorrhages, which subsequently ossify in scurvy

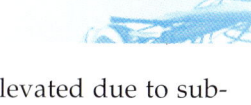

iv. The periosteum is elevated due to sub-periosteal haemorrhages, which subsequently ossify (Fig. 4.7).
v. At times there may be displacement of distal femoral epiphysis.

Treatment

High dose of vitamin C.

FLUOROSIS

Fluorine in very low concentration (≤1 ppm) has been used to reduce the incidence of dental caries. At slightly higher levels (>1.5 mg/l) it may produce mottling of the teeth (enamel of the upper incisors).

In some areas, (parts of India and Africa) where fluorine concentration in the drinking water (daily intake of 3–6 mg/l) may be above 10 ppm—Chronic fluorine intoxication (Fluorosis) is endemic and widespread skeletal abnormalities occasionally encountered in the affected population.

Fluorine directly stimulates osteoblastic activity, fluoroapatite crystals are laid down in bone and these are unusually resistant to osteoclastic resorption. The characteristic pathologic features in severe cases are subperiosteal new bone accretion and osteosclerosis which is most marked in the vertebra, ribs, pelvis and the forearm and leg bones, together with hyperostosis at the bony attachments of ligaments, tendons and fascia in these areas. Despite the apparent thickening and density of the skeleton, tensile strength is reduced and the bones fracture more easily under bending and twisting loads.

Patient complaints of backache, bone pain and joint stiffness.

Examination may show thickening of the tubular bones. Sometimes the first clinical manifestation is stress #. In the worst cases there may be deformities of the spine and lower limbs, hyperostosis can lead to vertebral canal encroachment and resultant neurological defects.

X-rays

The typical X-ray features are *osteosclerosis, osteophytosis and ossification of ligament and fascial attachments. Changes are most marked in the spine and pelvis where the bones become densely opaque, seen a bamboo spine.*

Treatment

There is no specific treatment for this condition. After exposure ceases it still takes years for bone fluoride to be excreted. If there is evidence of osteomalacia and secondary hyperparathyroidism, this can be treated with calcium and vitamin D.

Causes of Generalized Osteosclerosis

- Fluorosis
- *Osteosclerotic rim:* Growing epiphysis
- *Poisoning:* Lead, bismuth or phosphorus
- Caffey's disease
- Paget's disease of bone
- Renal osteodystrophy
- Secondaries from prostate
- Engelmann's disease
- Marble bone disease
- Melorheostosis.

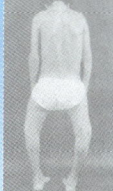

Infections

OSTEOMYELITIS

Definition

It is the inflammation of the bone involving the osteoid as well as myeloid tissue.

TYPES OF OSTEOMYELITIS

(i) Acute (ii) Sub-acute (iii) Chronic.

Acute Osteomyelitis

It is a disease of infancy and childhood, due to pyogenic infection of the metaphysis, may go for septic course and is occasionally fatal.

Aetiology

Host

Age: Below 5 years; Sex: male : female 4:1; *Site:* infection usually involves a single bone, most commonly the tibia, femur, or humerus in children and vertebral bodies in older adults and injection drug users. Trauma causes haematoma formation, which is a good culture medium for organism to grow. Antecedent focus of primary infection (boils) may be present.

Micro-organisms

More than 95% of cases of hematogenous osteomyelities are caused by a single organism.

Staphylococcus aureus accounts for 50% of isolates. Other common pathogens include group B streptococci and *E. coli* during the newborn period and group A streptococci in early childhood. Vertebral osteomyelities is due to *E. coli* and other enteric bacilli in appro. 25% of cases. *S.aureus, Pseudomonas aeuroginasa,* and *Serratia* infections are associated with intravenous drug users, and may involve the sacroiliac, sternoclavicular, or pubic joints as well as spine. *Salmonella* spp. and *S. aureus* are the major causes of long bone osteomyelities complicating sickle cell anemia and other hemoglobinopathies. Tuberculosis and brucellosis affect the spine more often than other bones. *Proteus, Pseudomonas* and *Bacteroides* seen in soft tissue damage and anaerobic areas, development of fungal infection after thorn prick injury to the foot, etc.

Pathology

Infective organisms, in neonates, are close to the joint, hence epiphyseal damage and growth disturbance is rapid and frequent (Fig. 5.1a). In a child, organisms reach the traumatized metaphyseal zone and they multiply in this zone of slow blood flow *(due to hairpin capillary flow)* and form a small medullary abscess, which soon expands, but the growth plate acts as a barrier and prevents the spread of abscess towards the joint (Fig. 5.1b).

The bone is:

- Destroyed by proteolytic enzymes.
- Necrosed by arterial thrombosis.
- Decalcified by hyperemia.
- Absorbed by activity of osteoclast.

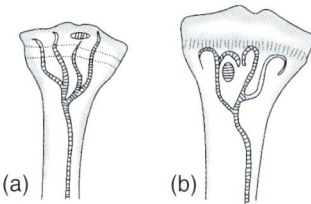

(a)   (b)

Figs 5.1a and b: (a) Epiphyseal damage and growth disturbance is rapid and frequent in neonate (b) Growth plate acts as a barrier and prevents the spread of abscess towards the joint

The medullary abscess can spread to (Fig. 5.2):

- Subperiosteal space
- Epiphysis
- Joint cavity or medullary cavity
- Through skin.

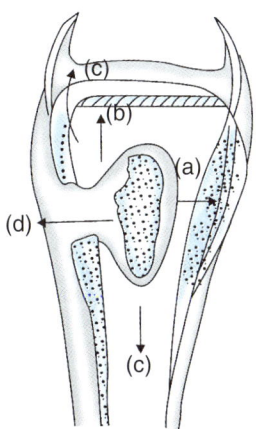

Fig. 5.2: Spreading of medullary abscess: (a) Subperiosteal space, (b) Epiphysis (c)Joint cavity or medullary cavity, and (d) Through skin

Clinical Features

The child has all the features of a febrile illness.

- **General**
  Fever, irritability, restlessness, headache, convulsions, vomiting, tachycardia and tachypnoea.
- **Local**
  Pseudoparalysis (due to severe pain, the limb is kept motionless), swelling, tenderness, redness, raised temperature around the metaphyseal area, diffuse oedema over the extremity. Sympathetic effusion of the neighbouring joints and tender regional lymphadenopathy.

Investigations

i. *For early diagnosis:* MRI, radioactive isotope uptake, CT scan to see for early signs of bone destruction.

ii. *X-ray:* Plain radiographs obtained early in the course of infection may show soft tissue swelling, but the first change in bone—*a periosteal reaction*—is not evident until at 10 days after the onset of infection. Later on, metaphyseal abscess. Periosteal lifting giving an onion peel appearance, moth eaten erosion of medulla and cortex with sequestrum formation. Lytic changes can be detected after 2 to 6 weeks, when 50 to 75% of bone density has been lost. Rarely, a well-circumscribed lytic lesion, or Brodie's abscess, is seen in a child who has been in pain for several months but has had no fever.

iii. *Blood:* Culture is invariably positive, polymorphonuclear leucocytosis, raised erythrocyte sedimentation rate (ESR).

iv. *Pus:* Aspiration of abscess and culture of organism.

Differential Diagnosis

i. *Suppurative arthritis:* All the features are the same as arthritis except that all the signs are localized to the joint. All movements are painful and restricted.

ii. *Rheumatic fever:* Fleeting arthralgia, cardiac signs, subcutaneous nodule, responds to salicylates.

iii. *Ewing's sarcoma:* A malignant primary bone tumour that arises most commonly in the first three decades of life. There is no pus, the lesion is diaphyseal in location, responds to radiotherapy. Biopsy is confirmatory. Mortality is very high.

Treatment

i. *Conservative:* Fluids, antibiotics, anti-inflammatory. Mag-sulf dressings and rest to the part with the help of a splint or traction.

ii. *Surgical:* Once pus has formed, it should be removed by aspiration, incision, drainage and if necessary drill holes in the cortex to decompress medullary abscess and irrigation of the cavity is done.

Constant Vigil should be Kept to Avoid Serious Complications

Complications

General: Anaemia, amyloidosis and septic embolization leading to septicaemia (blood poisoning).

Local

i. Acute osteomyelitis, if inadequately treated progresses to chronic osteomyelitis.

ii. Pathological fracture due to cortico-medullary erosion.

iii. Spreads to joints and causes septic arthritis especially in hip and shoulder since the metaphysis is intra-articular.

CHRONIC OSTEOMYELITIS

Definition

It is the chronic infection of the osteoid and myeloid tissue.

Types

i. **Secondary** to inadequately treated acute osteomyelitis (Fig. 5.3).

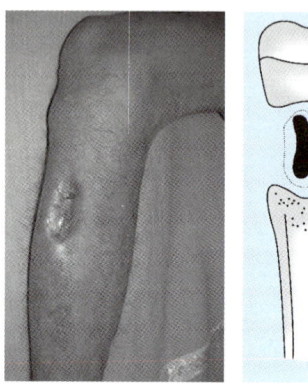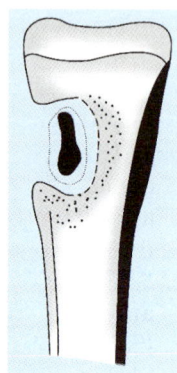

Fig. 5.3: Chronic osteomyelities: healed sinus; cavity with a sequestrum (inadequately treated acute osteomyelitis)

ii. **Insidious onset type**

a. *Brodie's abscess* (Fig. 5.4): This is sub-acute type of osteomyelities.
   • Age: 11 to 20 years

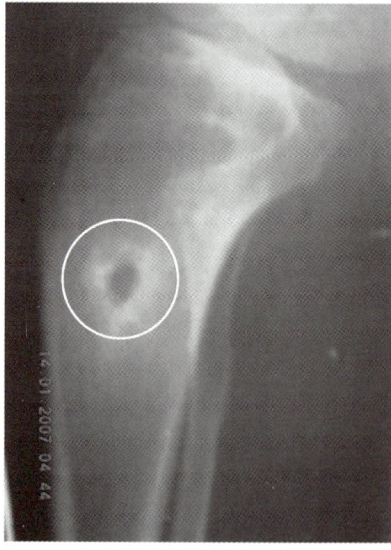

Fig. 5.4: X-rays marker showing Brodie's abscess well-defined radiolucent area surrounded by sclerotic zone

- Site: upper end of tibia and lower end of femur
- Location: metaphysis
- X-rays: it is seen as oval lytic lesion surrounded by dense fibrous tissue and sclerotic bone.
- T/t: it is best treated by curettage and bone grafting

b. *Tubercular:* This is seen in the cancellous epiphyseometaphyseal area showing a lytic lesion surrounded by an osteoporotic zone.

c. *Syphilitic:* This is seen in diaphyseal area with dense periosteal reaction (Sabre deformity of tibia).

Pathology

The avascular, dead parent bone surrounded by pus and granulation tissue is called **'sequestrum'**. Surrounding new bone formation arising from the periosteum is called **'involucrum'**. The pus and necrotic bone debris is extruded through sinuses and opening in the bone is called **'cloacae'** (Figs 5.5a and b).

Clinical Features

i. *Quiescent phase:* It shows discharging/healed sinuses, deformed and thickened bone (Fig. 5.6).

ii. *Acute flare up:* Active pus discharge with features of acute inflammation is seen.

Investigations

i. *Blood:* Haemoglobin per cent is reduced, with increase in lymphocytes and raised erythrocyte sedimentation rate.

ii. *Pus:* Culture and sensitivity test is required to decide appropriate antibiotic.

iii. *X-ray* (Fig. 5.7) to see the extent of bone involvement, sequestrum and type of infection so as to decide the line of treatment. X-ray shows corticomedullary moth eaten destruction, deformity, irregular periosteal reaction, cortical thickening, sclerosis and multiple cavities. Sequestra may be seen at several places surrounded by a zone of radiolucency (pus or granulation tissue). The sequestra may be of a wide ranging

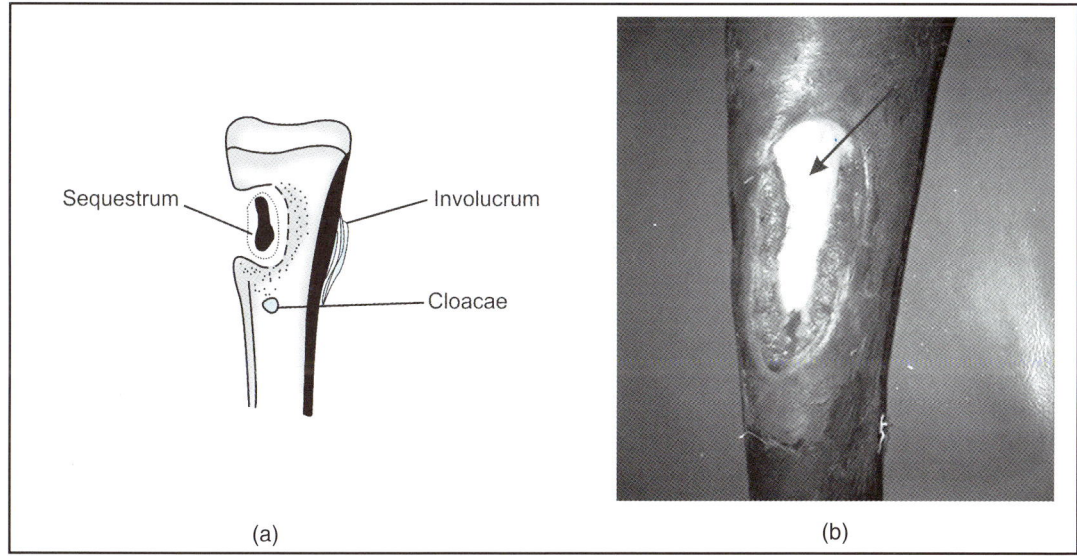

Sequestrum — Involucrum

Cloacae

(a)   (b)

Figs 5.5a and b: Sequestrum (arrow)

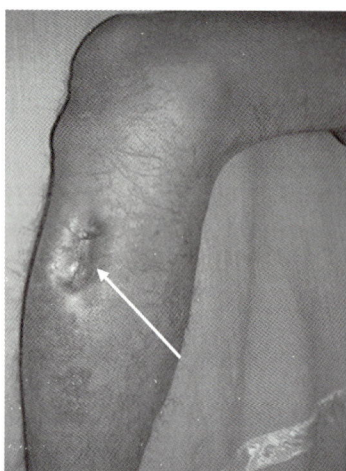

Fig. 5.6: Healed sinuses (arrow)

variety; feathery, flaky, cortical or at times extensive full length of the diaphysis often surrounded by tubular involucrum. Cloacae may be seen in the involucrum through which the sequestra may protrude. In children due to epiphyseal involvement there may be growth disturbances in the form of deformity, shortening or lengthening.

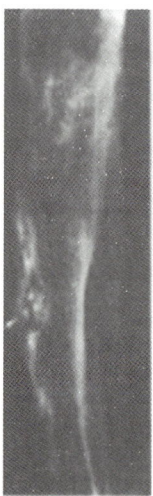

Fig. 5.7: Show corticomedullary destruction, sclerosis, cortical thickening

Treatment

General

General treatment is by building up of nutritional status and increasing the haemoglobin level.

Local

i. *Conservative:* Sterile dressings with suitable antibiotic is prescribed.

ii. *Surgical*

   a. Before surgery give broad spectrum antibiotics.

   b. Excision of sinus tract, saucerization of the cavity, sequestrectomy and filling the gap with cancellous bone/muscle pedicle graft. Gentamycin beads may be used.

   c. Closed suction irrigation to avoid collection of blood and pus.

   d. In cases of extensive osteomyelitis without obvious sequestrum continuous irrigation with suitable antibiotic, detergent and saline is done with intermittent suction till the outflow is sterile for three consecutive days.

   e. If the cause is due to an infected implant, then change over to external fixator is done or alternative mode of fixation and removal of infected implant after adequate involucrum has formed.

   f. *Soft tissue transfer:* Soft tissue transfers to fill dead space left behind after extensive debridement may range from a localized muscle flap on a vascular pedicle to microvascular free tissue transfer. The transfer of vascularized muscle tissue improves the local biological environment by bringing in a blood supply that is important in the host's defense mechanisms, as well as for antibiotic delivery and osseous and soft tissue healing

Most commonly a local muscle flap is used in the treatment of chronic osteomyelitis of the tibia. The gastrocnemius muscle is used for defects about the proximal third of the tibia, and the soleus muscle is used for defects about the middle third. A microvascular free muscle transfer is required for defects about the distal third of the tibia. A high success rate in the treatment of chronic osteomyelitis with the use of microvascular free tissue transfer. A microvascular transfer of tissue may consist of muscle that is covered with a skin graft or a myocutaneous, osseous, or osteocutaneous flap.

When a microvascular free muscle flap is used and segmental bone loss has occurred, autogenous cancellous bone grafting can be done about 6 weeks after the initial free flap transfer. A free fibular graft can be used for segmental bone loss of the tibia.

g. *Ilizarov technique:* The Ilizarov technique has been helpful in the treatment of chronic osteomyelitis and infected nonunions. This technique allows radical resection of the infected bone. A corticotomy is performed through normal bone proximal and distal to the area of disease. The bone is transported until union is achieved. Disadvantages of this technique include the time required to achieve a solid union and the high incidence of associated complications. Ilizarov procedure benefits patients who need extensive resection of bone and reconstruction.

h. *Hyperbaric oxygen therapy:* Hyperbaric oxygen therapy is another method for treating chronic osteomyelitis

Complications
Local
  i. *Bone:* Pathological fracture occurs with recurrent flare up.
 ii. *Epiphysis:*
      a. **Stimulation** causing lengthening of bone.
      b. **Destruction** causing shortening deformity.
iii. *Joint:* Septic arthritis occurs.
 iv. *Muscle:* Myositis and adhesions leading to stiffness of joint occurs.
  v. *Skin:* Chronic sinus may turn into epithelioma or fibrosarcoma or squamous cell carcinoma.

General
Anaemia, embolism, amyloidosis.

Iatrogenic or postoperative osteomyelitis: Osteomyelitis can occur after any operation on bone but especially after operating an open fracture and after procedures involving the use of foreign implants. Reported incidence of postoperative osteomyelitis varies from 0.2 to 10%. The incidence depends on the criteria for diagnosing postoperative infection. The true incidence is probably around 5% and the risk considerably greater in the elderly, obese, those with diabetes or other chronic diseases and in patients on steroids or immunosuppressive therapy.

Classification
A. *Early infection*
   1. Superficial infection
   2. Deep infection
   3. Superficial and deep infection
B. *Late infection*
   1. Following early infection
   2. Covert infection appearing later
   3. Following a long period of normality.

The organism may be introduced directly into the wound from atmosphere, the instruments, the patient or the surgeon, or indirectly by hematogenous spread from the distant focus.

The organism in postoperative osteomyelitis are usually a mixture of pathogenic bacteria (*S. aureus*, *Proteus*, *E.coli*, *Pseudomonas*) and other that are not normally pathogenic (*Staph epidermidis*) but may become so in the presence of foreign implant.

Local factors that favour bacterial invasion are:

1. Soft tissue damage.
2. Haematomas formation.
3. Bone death.

Clinical Feature

Early postoperative infection (within 1 month): The patient complaints of persistent pain and may have fever.

The skin over the implants is inflamed, and there may be a purulent discharge from the bone.

The ESR and white cell count are elevated, the blood culture may be positive. Bacteriological examination of the wound discharge will help to identify the organism and establish the antibiotic sensitivity.

Intermediate postoperative infection: (1 month – 1 year after operation)

There is a history of wound problems in the early postoperative period followed by a long quiescent period and spread when local condition favour.

Late postoperative infection: It is much more difficult to diagnose. Several years may have elapsed since the operation, during which the patient was completely asymptomatic. Pain usually starts insidiously and may never become acute. Local examination, X-ray signs of bone resorption and increased activity on radionuclide scanning may equally fail to distinguish between aseptic loosening of the implant and infection. Confirmation of the diagnosis is obtained by aspirating purulent material from the area, or by culturing the organism in washings taken after attempted aspiration.

Prevention

The risk of implant mediated infection can be reduced by

1. Avoiding operations on immunosuppressed patients
2. Eliminating any focus of infection before operation
3. Insisting on optimal operative sterility
4. Giving prophylactic antibiotics
5. Handling soft tissue gently
6. Using high quality implant material
7. Ensuring close fit and secure fixation of the implant
8. Preventing or counter acting later intercurrent infection.

Treatment

Appropriate antibiotic given intravenously and in large doses are the first line of defense.

If there is an abscess it should be drained and the wound left open until it is clean.

If these measures fail excision of infected and necrotic material followed by intermittent antibiotic irrigation and suction drainage may yet control the infection and prevent it from becoming a intractable chronic osteomyelities.

If at all possible the fixation device should be retained until the fracture has united or if the implant has to be removed in order to achieve adequate debridement, the fracture should be held securely with an external fixator.

Polymethyl Methacrylate (PMMA) Antibiotic Bead Chains

Short-term, long-term, or even permanent implantation of PMMA antibiotic beads is possible. In short-term implantation the beads are removed within 10 days, and in long-term implantation they may be left for up to 80 days, antibiotic-impregnated PMMA beads in the treatment of chronic osteomyelitis. The rationale for this treatment is to deliver levels of antibiotics locally in concentrations that exceed the minimal inhibitory concentrations.

Pharmacokinetic studies have shown that the local concentrations of antibiotic achieved are up to 200 times higher than levels achieved with systemic antibiotic administration. This has the advantage of obtaining very high local antibiotic concentrations while maintaining low serum levels and low systemic toxicity. The antibiotic is leached from the PMMA beads into the postoperative wound hematoma and secretion, which acts as a transport medium. High concentrations of the antibiotic can be achieved only with primary wound closure; if such closure cannot be performed, the wound can be covered with a water-impermeable dressing (bead pouch technique). Before the beads are implanted all infected and necrotic tissue should be adequately debrided surgically and all foreign material removed. Suction drains are not recommended because the concentration level of the antibiotic is diminished when they are used.

Biodegradable Antibiotic Delivery Systems

Various biodegradable antibiotic delivery systems have been evaluated. The main advantage of these is that a second procedure is not required to remove the implant. Furthermore, some of these biodegradable substrates contain calcium, which can be used in new bone formation. As these beads resorb they are slowly replaced by new bone and soft tissue, and this process may decrease the need for further reconstructive or coverage procedures.

MADUROMYCOSIS

This is a fungal infection involving the foot following thorn prick injury. The organism is often *Madurella mycetomi* and the tumour like mass in the foot is called **Mycetoma** or **Madura foot:** There are multiple discharging sinuses with black or yellow granules in the discharge, which is very typical. The treatment is anti-fungal, antibiotics and local debridement, often amputation has to be done to get rid of the fulminating and extensive tarsal destruction. One should keep in mind as differential diagnosis and the possibility of tubercular osteomyelitis (Fig. 5.8) of the foot.

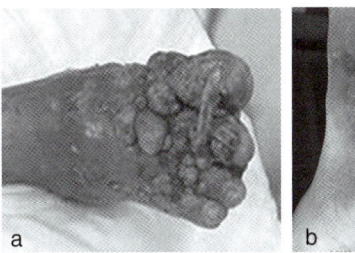 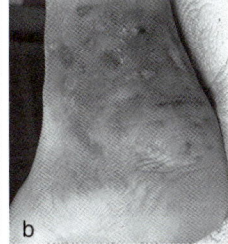

Figs 5.8a and b: (a) Madura foot; (b) Tubercular osteomyelities (multiple sinuses)

ACUTE SEPTIC ARTHRITIS

This is pyogenic infection of the joint as a result of hematogenous transmission or occasionally due to external source as in penetrating wounds.

Aetiopathology

Age is an important factor in determining the causative agent in bacterial infection. *Staphylococcus aureus* (including methicillin sodium–resistant strains) is the most common pathogen of septic arthritis in hospitalized neonates. Streptococci and gram-negative bacilli also are causative agents but to a lesser degree. In infants and toddlers younger than 2 years of age, *Haemophilus influenzae* is still recognized as the main pathogen. *S. aureus* is the leading cause in all ages followed by group A *Streptococcus* and *Enterobacter*. They also found *Klebsiella*, an organism difficult to recover by joint cultures on solid media, to be a more common cause of septic arthritis than previously recognized.

Neisseria gonorrhoeae causes approximately 75% of septic arthritis cases in healthy, sexually active young adults, although a septic joint develops in fewer than 3% of patients infected with *N. gonorrhoeae*. This infection has a slightly different presentation than other types of infectious arthritis. Often the infection is polyarticular and may be associated with a papular rash. Joint cultures often are negative, but cultures from the pharynx or urethra may be positive. Polymerase chain reaction (PCR), a DNA amplification technique that helps to identify elusive infections in tissues, blood, and bodily fluids, may help identify *N. gonorrhoeae* in culture-negative synovial fluid. Gonococcal arthritis generally has a favorable outcome if treated with appropriate antibiotics, and drainage usually is not necessary.

In older adults with nongonococcal disease, *S. aureus* infection causes about half of the cases of septic arthritis, and streptococci and gram-negative bacilli are responsible for the other half.

Polyarticular sepsis caused by *S. aureus* is extremely serious in patients with rheumatoid arthritis, hemophilia, or immunosuppression, and mortality rates have been reported to be high. Adults with systemic lupus erythematous have an increased likelihood of *Salmonella* infection, and those with a history of intravenous drug use are predisposed to gram-negative infections, including those caused by *Pseudomonas* organism

Clinical Features

There is initially synovial effusion followed by synovial proliferation, subsequent purulent collection and necrosis of articular cartilage and other joint structures.

General

Fever, pain and features of toxaemia.

Local

Joint effusion, tender, red hot swelling with diffuse oedema, muscle spasm and gross restriction of joint movements occurs.

The joint may be in the phase of:
a. Synovial effusion
b. Arthritis and joint erosion
c. Destruction and dislocation.

Investigations

i. **MRI, CT scan and Tc-99 uptake** for early diagnosis.
ii. **X-ray**
   a. *Early:* Increased joint space due to effusion.
   b. *Late:* Erosion of articular margins, diminished joint space, subluxation, subchondral cysts. In case of involvement of hip joint there may be destruction of the femoral head and pathological dislocation.
iii. **Blood:** Culture is positive and increased polymorphonuclear cells.
iv. **Pus:** Pus aspiration from the joint is positive for smear and culture.

Management

i. *Early*
   a. Broad spectrum antibiotics, analgesics are recommended.
   b. Traction to relieve the pain, spasm and deformity.
   c. Aspiration/incision and drainage of abscess, followed by continuous suction irrigation with suitable antibiotic. In acute septic arthritis, usually arthrotomy or arthroscopic drainage and antibiotic treatment are adequate.
ii. *Late*
   a. Minimal and early joint damage Wilkinson's joint clearance (synovectomy, debridement of joint),

lavage, irrigation and early mobilization.

b. Extensive joint damage
   – *For stable fixed joint:* Arthrodesis, the surgical immobilization of a joint is done.
   – *For mobile joint:* As in cases of hip and elbow involvement, excision arthroplasty and joint replacement at a later date.
   – *For deformity:* Corrective osteotomy.
   – *For shortening:* Shoe raise/limb lengthening is done.

Complications

In mild cases, with an early recovery patient may develop secondary osteoarthritis. Partial or complete damage of articular cartilage will ultimately end up with ankylosis. Deformity, shortening and instability to some extent is invariably seen in all cases.

1. *Pathological dislocation*
   Pathological dislocation occurs predominantly in children; it is rare in adults. When dislocation is recognized before severe contracture of the soft tissue has occurred, reduction is accomplished easily at the time of drainage and satisfactory function may result. However, if the femoral head has been damaged by the infection, skeletal traction should be applied through the distal femur and is continued until the femoral head is at the level of the acetabulum. After the dislocation has been reduced, the hip is immobilized in a spica cast until it is stable or until fibrous or bony ankylosis develops.

2. *Osteomyelitis*
   When the infection is confined to the joint, prompt drainage and appropriate antibiotic therapy should prevent osteomyelitis of the proximal femur. However, if osteomyelitis results in sequestration of the femoral head in children younger than 12 years of age, the head may be totally reabsorbed or it may be replaced by new bone after its circulation is restored. In older children and adults it usually remains as an infected sequestrum and requires excision.

3. *Pelvic abscess*
   Pelvic abscess complicating acute septic arthritis of the hip is caused by either suppurative infection of the iliac lymph nodes or by spread from the joint into the sheath of the iliopsoas, which may communicate with the joint. The abscess is retroperitoneal and tends to gravitate along the iliopsoas muscle beneath the inguinal ligament, eventually pointing in the medial thigh. In large abscesses the pus may track proximally along the iliopsoas and point proximal to the posterior iliac crest. Magnetic resonance imaging may help locate and determine the true extent of psoas involvement. Often this can be drained by CT-directed aspiration.

4. *Persistent infection*
   Persistent infection about the hip is difficult to treat; fortunately, it is rare. Usually, scarring is extensive, and draining sinuses have become established. Often the sinuses become blocked, causing recurring abscesses. Unless aggressive surgery is performed, chronic sepsis and its sequelae result. In addition to resecting all the infected bone, a mass of muscle also is resected to ensure drainage. This operation may result in a nearly useless pseudarthrosis or ankylosis. Marked shortening of the affected extremity results. For these reasons, this operation is a last resort. Before the operation, sinograms should be made and appropriate antibiotic therapy started. Adequate amounts of blood should be available during surgery.

TOM SMITH'S ARTHRITIS

This is septic arthritis of hip during infancy and childhood, and usually follows as a result of infected umbilical cord.

The child is usually brought late or remains undiagnosed due to the cartilaginous head of femur which is not visualized in X-ray and needs ultrasound with a 7.5 Hz probe to see the outline of the head of femur in a neonate.

The head and neck undergoes rapid destruction with resulting pathological dislocation of hip joint and this damage is irreparable and a life time of suffering, limp and shortening occurs.

On examination
- Child walks with unstable gait.
- Shortening
- Hypermobility-hip movements are increased in all directions
- Telescoping is present

For early diagnosis, help of MRI, CT scan, T-99 uptake study should be done. The delay in treatment is responsible for the destruction.

X-ray

Initially increased joint space and later destruction of head and neck of femur, with dislocation and high riding greater trochanter; the roof of acetabulum remains normal.

Management

i. **Early:** Broad spectrum antibiotics, traction and aggressive joint drainage at the earliest should take place.
ii. **Late:** Osteotomy for stabilizing the hip.

Complications

General
Septicaemia, embolism.

Local
Destruction of head and pathological dislocation, limp, shortening may occur.

BONE AND JOINT TUBERCULOSIS

Despite the attention given to tuberculosis, it remains a leading infectious cause of death worldwide. Approximately 3 million people per year die of tuberculosis and its accompanying complications. In some developing countries, more than 15% of the population is infected, and mortality is as high as 104 per 100,000.

Tuberculosis can affect virtually any organ system of the body. Extrapulmonary involvement is noted in approximately 14% of patients, with 1% to 8% having osseous disease. Approximately 50% of patients with osseous tuberculosis have pulmonary involvement, and 30% to 50% of those with osseous disease have vertebral involvement. This disease in the bone is always as a result of secondary involvement following primary lesion in lungs or intestines.

Tuberculosis is transmitted primarily through inhalation of *Mycobacterium tuberculosis* or ingestion *M. bovis*. Thereafter, lymphogenous, hematogenous, or contiguous extension to other tissues and organ systems may occur. The clinical presentation depends on the presence of either isolated musculoskeletal involvement or miliary disease. Constitutional symptoms include fever, chills, and cough, with accompanying pleuritic pain, weight loss, and fatigue. The patient may have acute or chronic symptoms. A high index of suspicion is in order for previously described high-risk populations, children younger than 5 years of age, and elderly individuals.

Pathology

The organism is usually
- *Typical: Mycobacterium tuberculosis* in human (lungs), in bovine (intestines).
- *Atypical:* This causes resistant type of lesion, seen in patients suffering from multidrug resistance (MDR) and AIDS.

The organisms enter into the blood stream from the primary foci, i.e. the lungs and the intestines as a phase of transient bacteraemia and settle in various parts of the skeleton. In 90% of the cases the lesion heals, unfortunately in 10% of the patients the organisms lie dormant in the metaphyseal area for a long time, waiting for a suitable environment for multiplication.

Trauma to the metaphyseal area causes haematoma formation, which is a good culture medium for the organisms to start multiplying.

A typical tubercle consists of:

Central area of caseation, surrounded by epithelioid cells and Langhan's giant cells, lymphocytes, surrounded by a fibrous capsule.

The tubercle takes one of the following courses depending upon the virulence of the organism and host resistance.

- If virulence is low and host resistance is good:
  - Complete resolution.
  - Fibrous encapsulation.
  - Calcification.
- If virulence is high and host resistance is poor:
  - Granuloma formation.
  - Cold abscess.

Lecithin, a fatty acid in the cell wall of *Mycobacterium tuberculosis* inhibits activity of osteoblasts and hence in tubercular involvement of bone, no new bone formation is seen.

Clinically, the disease may start in the synovium or in the bone (metaphyseal area). The common sites of osteoarticular tuberculosis are

- Arthritis involving knee, hip, wrist, elbow and PIP joints.
- Osteomyelitis involving upper tibia, ribs, trochanter, calcaneum, olecranon.

- Spondylitis (Pott's spine) involving inter-vertebral, body, posterior facet joints.

Whatever be the site, the basic presentation is pain, deformity and cold abscess. Management principles are usually the same.

The disease is usually **monofocal** with **insidious** onset.

Clinical Features

Local

Pain, deformity, cold abscess.

i. *Pain:* Limp, stiffness, spasm, restricted movements, muscle wasting and night cries.
ii. *Deformity:* Deformity depending on muscle spasm and stage of disease.
iii. *Cold abscess:* Swelling, cord compression, multiple discharging sinuses.

General

Tubercular toxaemia causing fever, anorexia, weight loss, malaise, evening rise of temperature, night sweats, tachycardia, tachypnea.

Additional

Depending on features of

i. *Primary focus:* Lungs and intestines.
ii. *Secondary focus:*
   a. Brain and meninges: Meningitis.
   b. Spine: Paraplegia.
   c. Kidney: Haematuria, albuminuria.

Investigations

i. **Blood**
   - **Haemoglobin** for anaemia.
   - **ESR** for prognosis and status of the disease.
   - **TLC** for immune status and host reaction.
   - **Lymphocyte:** Monocyte ratio, if less than 5, then immune status is poor and so patient should avoid surgery.
ii. **ELISA**
   - **IgG** for chronic tubercular infection.
   - **IgA, IgM** for recent tubercular infection.

iii. **Urine**
- *RBC:* Indicates tubercular nephritis.
- *Albumin:* Indicates nephrotic syndrome.
- *Pus cells:* Indicates UTI.
- *Sugar:* To rule out diabetes.

iv. **X-ray** (Fig. 5.9)
- *Changes in the joint*
  - Initially increased joint space due to effusion.
  - Later reduction in joint space due to erosion.
  - Wandering acetabulum due to subluxation.
  - Pathological dislocation seen as break in Shenton's line.
  - Parafocal osteoporosis is obvious due to increased vascularity.
  - Focal trabecular destruction.
- *Extra-articular lesions:* Osteomyelitic cavities may be seen in the hip joint (roof of acetabulum, head of femur, Babcock's triangle), trochanter, calcaneum, olecranon and vertebral body.

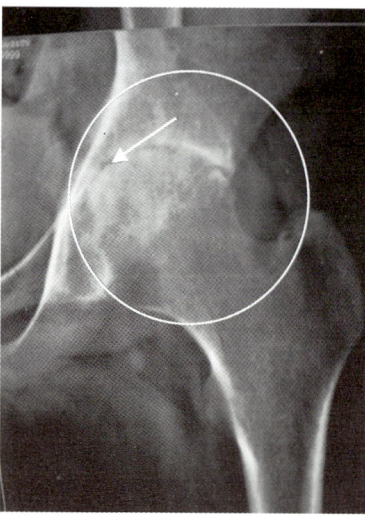

Fig.5.9: TB Hip:Erosion of articular margins, decreased joint space (arrow), Periarticular osteoporosis

There is tubercular destruction of bone without new bone formation due to inhibition of osteoblastic activity.

v. **Pus:** Pus from cold abscess for AFB by ZN stain, newer fluorescent technique by auramine, rhodamine staining microscopy. Culture and guinea pig inoculation.

vi. **Culture:** By LJ media (new Middle Brook TH10, Bactac 460 culture media gives results in 2–3 weeks).

vii. **Biopsy:** From synovium/joint for histopathological examination.

viii. **CT scan and MRI:** For early diagnosis and assessment of the extent of the lesion, especially in children where X-ray is not very helpful.

ix. **Tc 99 uptake:** For disseminated lesions in body scanning.

x. Molecular diagnosis is latest, using polymerase chain reaction (PCR), detects viable TB and MDR strain within 2 hrs.

Treatment

i. **Anti-tubercular drugs**
  a. For first line management of osteoarticular tuberculosis (4 drugs for 3 months followed by 3 drugs for 9 months, as in the table 5.1).
  b. Second line drugs for resistant cases: Aminoglycoside, kanamycin, ethionamide, ofloxacin, cycloserine.

ii. **Local management**
  a. *Conservative:* Traction, splintage, rest.
  b. *Changes in the joint:* Surgery
    - *Early:* Aspiration of joint effusion, drainage of cold abscess, synovectomy, arthrotomy, joint lavage.
    - *Late*
      - *For joint involvement:* Arthrodesis, excision arthroplasty, joint replacement.
      - *For deformities:* Corrective osteotomy.

Table 5.1: "The Rule of 5"			
Drug	*Dose*	*Side effects*	*Management*
INH	5 to 10 mg/kg	Anaemia, peripheral neuropathy	Add 50 mg of B_6
Rifampicin	10 mg/kg	Cloestatic jaundice	Stop drug
Streptomycin	20 mg/kg	Oto/Nephrotoxic	Do. S. test
Ethambutol	25 mg/kg	Optic neuritis	Avoid in child
Pyrazinamide	20 to 30 mg/kg	Hyperuricemia	Avoid in gout and pregnancy

TUBERCULOSIS OF HIP

Usually mono-articular infection by *Mycobacterium tuberculosis bacilli* as a secondary lesion with an insidious onset.

Clinical Features

Pain (probably the first symptom), limp (earliest sign), deformity, multiple discharging sinuses, the course stretched over months and years, ultimately leading to fibrous ankylosis of the joint, associated with shortening and deformity of the concerned lower limb. It starts in childhood and adolescence and drags onto middle age.

Age: 5 to 35 years, commonest before 10 years of age.

Sex: Males are more prone to this disease than females due to greater exposure to trauma.

Signs and Symptoms

i. **Constitutional symptoms** as fever (evening rise of temperature), anorexia, weight loss, lethargy, irritable.

ii. **Local features**
   a. *Pain:* Initially mild, later constant dull ache, aggravation during evening hours after exertion, night cries, limp.
   b. *Deformity:* Depending on the stage of the disease which are as follows :
   - *Stage of synovitis:* Flexion, abduction, external rotation and apparent lengthening of the limb is observed (Fig. 5.10a).
   - *Stage of arthritis:* Flexion, adduction, internal rotation and apparent shortening of the bone is observed (Fig. 5.10b).
   - *Pathological dislocation:* Flexion, adduction, internal rotation and real shortening of the bone is observed (Fig. 5.10c).
   c. *Abscess:* It could be mid-inguinal, trochanteric, gluteal with active/healed multiple discharging sinuses.
   d. Bitrochanteric compression test is positive with local tenderness below mid-inguinal point. *Gauvian's sign* positive (rotation of lower limb causes abdominal spasm).
   e. Proximal shift of trochanter as measured by Bryant's triangle.
   f. Disproportionate/gross wasting of gluteii.
   g. Antalgic gait with positive Trendelenburg test, positive pump handle test in old cases.
   h. Always examine the spine and other sites for primary lesion.

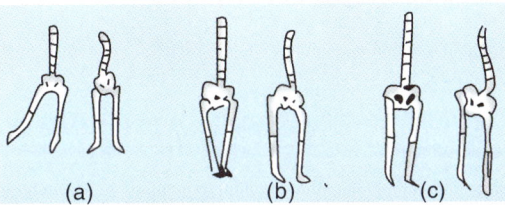

Figs 5.10a to c: Deformity: Depending on the stage of the disease. (a) Stage of synovitis; (b) Stage of arthritis; (c) Pathological dislocation

Investigations

i. **Blood:** Low Hb, high ESR, high TLC, increased lymphocytes, L/M ratio should be 5, if less, it shows poor immune status (avoid surgery).

ii. **Urine:** RBC in urine shows silent haematuria and nephritic TB. RBC+ albuminuria shows UTI. Sugar indicates diabetes mellitus.

iii. **Biopsy:** Lymph node, synovial biopsy from the hip joint.

iv. **Mantoux test:** Positive result shows prior sensitisation to tuberculous bacilli.

v. **Pus:** AFB staining.

vi. **Culture:** LJ media.

vii. **Inoculation:** Guinea pig.

viii. **X-ray of the hip joint**
 a. *Early:* Increased joint space with paraarticular osteoporosis.
 b. *Late:* Decreased joint space, erosion of articular margins, osteoporosis, break in Shenton's line, wandering acetabulum.
 c. *Occasional extraarticular focus:* Head, neck, roof of acetabulum, trochanteric osteomyelitis.

ix. **X-ray of chest:** For pulmonary Koch's.

x. **MRI/CT** scan for early diagnosis especially in children.

xi. **Ultrasonography** for neonates to see the cartilaginous head.

Differential Diagnosis

Septic arthritis, Perthes' disease, irritable hip, regional lymphadenitis.

Management

General

Improve haemoglobin, protein status, drugs: ATT for 15 months.

Local

i. *Conservative:* Skin traction to the patient, to correct deformity, decreases muscle spasm and distracts inflamed joint surface.

ii. *Surgery*
 a. Active lesions
1st stage	– Synovectomy.
2nd stage	– Wilkinson's joint clearance
3rd stage	– Excision, arthroplasty for a mobile joint, and arthrodesis for a stable fixed joint
b. Healed lesions
Shortening	– Lengthening of bone.
Deformity	– Corrective osteotomy
Ankylosis	– Total hip replacement

TUBERCULOSIS OF KNEE

Clinical Features

i. **Age:** 15 to 30 years.

ii. **History:** Trauma to the knee followed by pain and swelling.

iii. **Examination:** Synovial bulge, wasting of quadriceps and triple deformity (flexion, external rotation, posterior subluxation), tender joint line and painful movements.

X-ray

i. **Initially:** Increased joint space and synovial bulge, enlarged ossification centre (due to paraarticular hyperemia).

ii. **Later:** Reduced joint space, erosion of joint margins, triple deformity, extra articular focus of infection may be seen in the tibial condyles ends as ankylosis.

Progression of Tubercular Disease Process
(Fig. 5.11)

Treatment

i. Anti-tubercular drugs.

ii. Conservative
 – 90°–90° traction to correct triple deformity.
 – Aspiration of effusion and compression bandage with POP cast immobilization for 3 to 6 weeks.

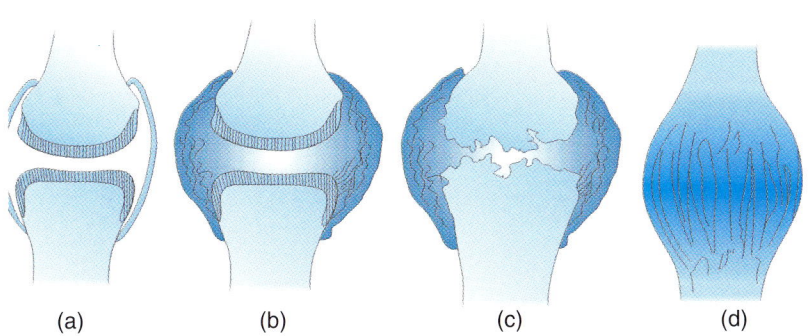

Figs 5.11a to d: (a) Synovial effusion, (b) synovial proliferation, (c) arthritis, (d) ankylosis

iii. Surgical
    a. **Early:** Synovial excision. Wilkinson's joint clearance.
    b. **Late:** Arthrodesis (in position of 15° of flexion), for damaged and deformed joint. Total Knee replacement for ankylosing joint.

TUBERCULOSIS OF SPINE

(Pott's Spine) Osteitis or caries of the vertebrae, usually occurring as a complication of tuberculosis of the lungs. First described by Sir John Percivall Pott as the most crippling lesion characterised by pain, spinal deformity, cold abscess and paralysis. This is a disease which, if diagnosed early, can avoid a lot of complications and morbidity.

The spine is the most common (30 to 50%) site of osseous involvement, especially in elderly individuals; however, it is also common in children and in young adults from developing countries. A primary accompanying lesion may be discovered from the pulmonary or urogenital system or from an unknown source. Lymphogenous and hematogenous spread has been implicated in thoracolumbar lesions, but less often in cervical or sacral lesions. Usually, active spinal lesions involve a particular segment: two vertebral bodies and the corresponding disc. Some have speculated that these areas are affected most often because of the generous arterial and venous supply and the high O_2 pressure requirement of the tuberculosis bacilli. A peridiscal presentation occurs in approximately 80% of patients, with the anterior vertebral body affected and contiguous progression through subligamentous burrowing (anterior longitudinal ligament) and eventual extension to the adjacent vertebrae. Less frequently, lesions occur centrally in the vertebral body. These lesions are more difficult to diagnose and may mimic a tumor or contribute to significant spinal deformities. Patients may have intramedullary granulomas, arachnoiditis, segmental collapse with anterior wedging, and gibbus formation (Pott's disease). Rarely are the posterior elements of the spine the only sites affected. Perispinal abscesses with sinus extension to the skin also may arise and extend through tissue planes to reach intraperitoneal structures. They have been reported to occur as far distally as the popliteal fossa. Patients present with pain, weakness, and, in the late stages, paralysis.

Age: 5 to 35 years.

Sex: Males are more prone to this disease than females due to activities.

Site: The commonest site is thoracolumbar junction, followed by cervical. 1 0% have double lesion, 40% have extra-articular lesion.

Types

i. Intervertebral or Paradiscal (most common): 95% (tubercular spondylitis).
ii. Body (tubercular osteomyelitis).
iii. Posterior facet joint involvement (this has presentation like spinal cord tumour syndrome).

Clinical Features

i. **Pain:** Usually in the evening after day's activity, night cries.
ii. **Radicular pains:** This is due to posterior facet tubercular lesion.
iii. **Muscle spasm**
   a. *Cervical zone:* Rust sign (chin supporting).
   b. *Thoracic:* Military man attitude.
   c. *Lumbar:* Alderman's gait (pregnant type).
iv. **Deformity**
   a. Kyphosis, scoliosis, lumbar lordosis.
   b. Knuckle deformity (due to collapse of one intervertebral disc space).
   c. Gibbus deformity (due to collapse of more than 2 vertebrae).
   d. Scoliosis (due to collapse of several vertebrae).
v. **Abscess:** Travels along sheath of vessels, nerves, muscles and facial tracts.
   a. *Cervical:* Retropharyngeal and paravertebral, post border of sternomastoid, back of the neck and may travel along the brachial plexus into axilla and paravertebral fascia into mediastinum.
   b. *Thoracic:* Intercostal nerves, paraspinal (postspinal nerves), along the rectus sheath, along paravertebral zones.
   c. *Lumbar:* Psoas muscle—Iliac fossa, mid-inguinal point and femoral triangle.
   Obturator nerve: Popliteal fossa.

Aorta, pudendal artery: Ischiorectal fossa.

vi. **Paraplegia:** This is the most dreaded complication of Pott's spine, occurs in 15% of the patients.

This is classified into following four grades:

Grade I : Patient is unaware of his problem and is diagnosed by the physician. Examination reveals extensor plantar and ankle clonus.

Grade II : Patient walks with support and has spastic gait.

Grade III : Patient is bedridden with paralysis in extension and sensory deficit less than 50%.

Grade IV : Flaccid paralysis with extensive sensory deficit and bladder/bowel involvement.

Paraplegia of early onset is usually due to inflammatory oedema, granulation tissue or cold abscess and prognosis is good.

Paraplegia of late onset is usually due to mechanical factors and cord damage, the recovery is poor.

Investigations

i. **X-ray**
   a. *Spine*
      – *AP view:* To see paravertebral abscess (Fig. 5.12a).
      – *Lateral:* Reduced intervertebral joint space (earliest sign). Erosion of adjoining surface. Collapse of vertebra (kyphosis). Parafocal osteoporosis. To see skip lesions in the vertebra above/below (Fig. 5.12c).
   b. *Chest:* To rule out pulmonary tuberculosis.
   i. *CT scan:* Destruction of intervertebra disc and adjoining vertebra (Figs 5.12b and 5.13).
ii. *MRI:* For early diagnosis, to see the extent of osseous destruction as well as cold

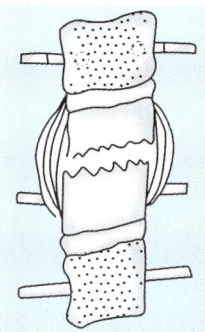

Fig. 5.12a: Paravertebral abscess

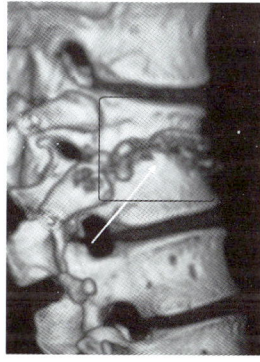

Fig. 5.12b: CT scan showing erosion of adjoining surface of vertebrae, obliteration of disc space, collapse of vertebrae with anterior wedge compression (arrow)

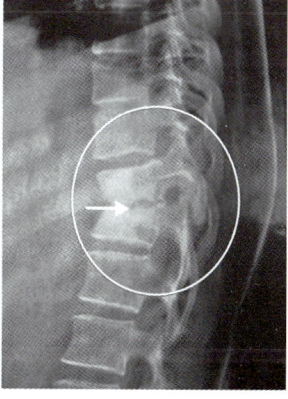

Fig. 5.12c: X-ray lateral view showing reduced intervertebral joint space (arrow). Collapse of the vertebrae (kyphosis). Para focal osteopenia. (marker)

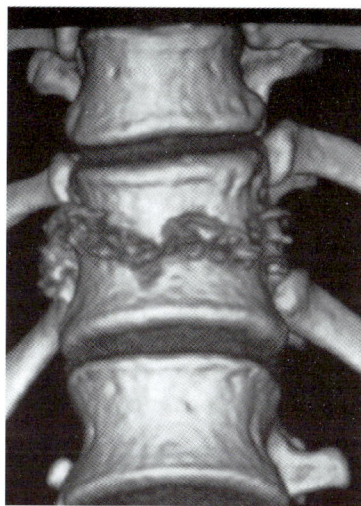

Fig. 5.13: AP view of spine showing tubercular spine D_{11}–D_{12}

abscess. Other investigations are as mentioned in the general management.

Treatment

i. *Conservative:* Patient should rest on hard bed, antitubercular drugs and spinal braces are prescribed.

ii. *Surgery:* Drainage of cold abscess, spinal decompression and spinal fusion.

iii. *Management of paraplegia:* Care of back, bowel and bladder. Rehabilitation.

SPINA VENTOSA (Fig. 5.14)

This is tubercular involvement of proximal phalanx, presenting as 'spindle' shaped deformity of the finger which is tender, swollen and may show cold abscess or multiple discharging sinuses.

PONCET'S DISEASE

This is a type of tubercular presentation characterised by polyarticular pains, swelling as seen in rheumatoid arthritis, responding to antitubercular drugs.

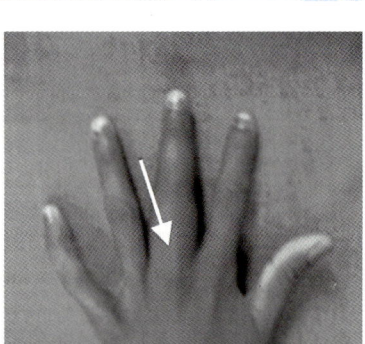

Fig. 5.14: Spina ventosa: spindle-shaped deformity of the finger, swollen (arrow)

TUBERCULAR OSTEOMYELITIS OF FOOT

Tubercular involvement of the small bones of the foot swelling, multiple discharging sinuses and tarsal destruction as seen in **Madura foot** (Fig. 5.8). When it involves the calcaneum or cuboid, it presents as pain, swelling and cold abscess. X-ray shows a lytic lesion in the bone with parafocal osteoporosis. This needs a course of ATT followed by drainage of the cold abscess.

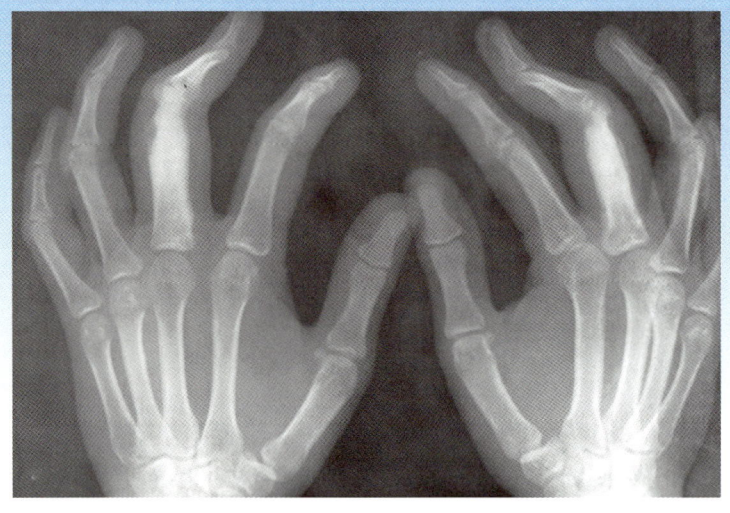

Developmental Disorders

6

DWARF

- *Short limbs* as in achondroplasia.
- *Short trunk* as in chondro-osteodystrophy, vertebral anomalies.
- *Deformity with short stature* as in osteogenesis imperfecta.

Achondroplasia (Dwarfism) (Fig. 6.1)

This disorders is among the more common types of dwarfism. It is inherited as autosomal dominant trait, although most cases are sporadic and due to new fibroblast growth factor receptor 3 (FGFR 3) which inhibits chondrocytes proliferation in the growth plate. The abnormal proliferation at the growth plate leaving other areas relatively unaffected in the tubular bones, causes production of short bones that are proportionately thick (these children are often seen as jokers in the circus).

Clinical Features

- The appearance of short limb, particularly the proximal portions, with normal trunk is characteristically accompanied by a large head, a saddle nose and an exaggerated lumber lordosis.
- The fingers appear stubby and somewhat splayed *(trident hand).*
- The length of spine is almost always normal.
- Those who survive infancy usually have normal sexual and mental development and lifespan may be normal.
- Spinal deformity nevertheless may lead to a cord compression and nerve root encroachment.

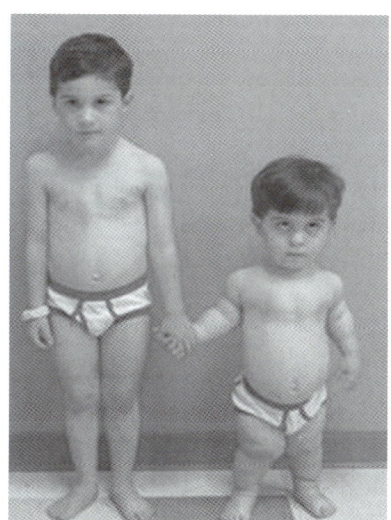

Fig. 6.1: Achondroplasic dwarfism (second child)

Chondro-osteodystrophy

This is also known as **Morquio–Brailsford disease** and is a hereditary dysplasia of growing bones due to excessive storage of mucopolysaccharides in which there is a defect in degradation of glycosaminoglycans, is inherited as an autosomal recessive trait. There is defective maturation of chondroblast of the epiphyseal plate leading to broadening and fragmentation of the epiphyseal zone of the spine and limbs leading to **dwarfism**. The child is characterized by severe skeletal defects with short stature, large head, sunken eyes (with corneal opacities) and angulated chest (a marked manubriosternal angle almost 90° is pathgnomonic) and spine with ligament laxity. Knock-knee, flat feet and obvious kyphosis.

X-ray

The vertebral bodies are flattened, tongue shaped, best seen in the midthoracic area. The femoral epiphyseal shows flattening and fragmentation with deformed acetabulum. X-ray of the hand shows short metacarpals.

Urine

Urine examination shows excessive excretion of keratan sulfate.

Hurler's Disease

This is also known as **Gargoylism**. This is due to defect in the mucopolysaccharide metabolism and is characterized by dwarfism, multiple skeletal deformities with mental retardation, corneal opacity and hepatosplenomegaly. The child has a frog-like look due to large head, wide set eyes, broad nose bridge, and low set ears.

Osteogenesis Imperfecta

This is also known as **'Fragilitas ossium'**. This is a familial disease characterized by fragile bones due to defective osteoid and failure of maturation of collagen leading to poor, thin cortex, which easily bends and breaks.

Types

i. **Congenita:** The child develops multiple fractures *in utero* or soon after birth causing death.

ii. **Tarda:** In this, fractures during childhood causes bent, broken, and deformed limbs (Figs 6.2a and b). In a dwarf child the exuberant callus during healing of fracture may mimic a sarcoma. The limbs are thin and long with hyper-mobile joints. The teeth are of poor quality and translucent due to imperfect dentine. *The classical features are blue sclera,*

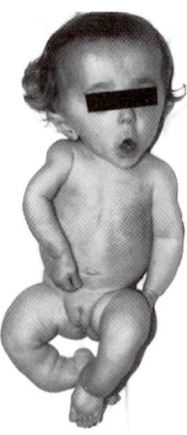

Fig. 6.2a: Osteogenesis imperfecta

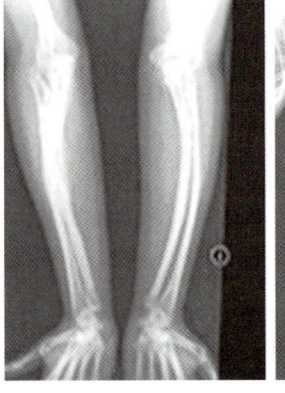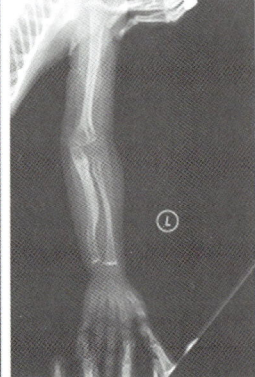

Fig. 6.2b: X-ray of the bones of child of osteogenesis imperfecta showing multiple fractures and deformity

deafness due to otosclerosis and deformities.

Treatment

This is aimed at prevention of fractures and correction of deformities. Correction of gross deformities of long bones is done by multiple osteotomies and fixation by expanding **Sofield's rods** (Figs 6.3a and b).

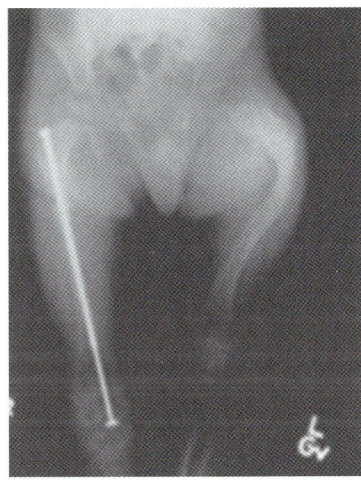

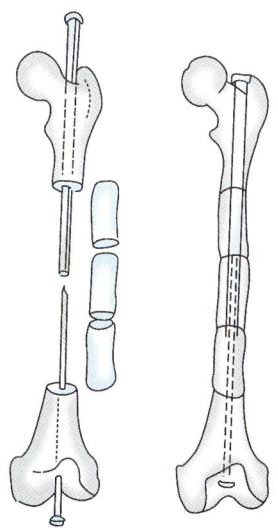

Figs 6.3a and b: Expanding intramedullary rods (Sofield's rods) for correction of deformity

Osteopetrosis

This is also known as **'Marble bone disease'** or **'Albers-Schönberg disease'**. This is characterized by hereditary increase in generalized bone density. The bone appears hard, chalky, and brittle. The medulla is also obliterated leading to aplastic anaemia with hepatosplenomegaly.

The child is brought with pathological fracture of brittle bones or neuropathy due to osteosclerosis of optic and cranial nerve foramina leading to blindness and deafness.

X-ray picture shows dense sclerotic bones without corticomedullary differentiation (Fig. 6.4). If periosteal reaction appears as flowing down of molten wax from a candle then it is known as **melorheostosis.**

Fibrous Dysplasia

In this disorder, bone is replaced by fibroosseous tissue instead of normal healthy bone during the process of bone turnover. This mass gradually proliferates leading to erosion of surrounding cortical bone, which becomes thin and expanded. It may be localized or generalized, the latter often associated

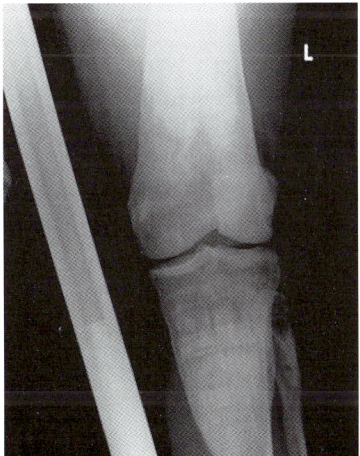

Fig. 6.4: X-ray shows dense sclerotic bones without corticomedullary destruction

with hormonal disorder and cutaneous pigmentation in young girls, better known as **Albright's disease**.

X-ray

It shows a corticomedullary destruction, which is ground glass in appearance and causes thinning and expansion of the cortex with a multilocular appearance. It may produce bending of the bone (the weight bearing bone may be bent; and one of the classic feature is the *'shepherd's crook' deformity of proximal femur)* and pathogical fracture (Fig. 6.5).

Blood test

It shows normal serum calcium which differentiates it from hyperparathyroidism.

Treatment

Treatment is usually required when patients present with pain and pathological fractures. Surgical treatment is directed towards curettage of the cavity and cancellous bone grafting.

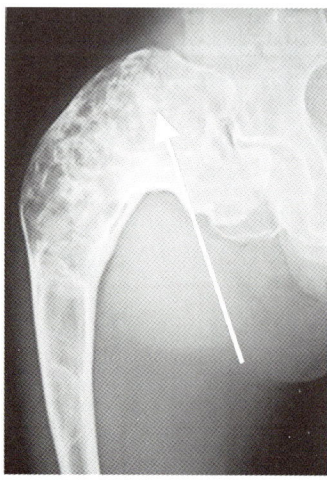

Fig. 6.5: Fibrous dysplasia of femur. X-ray showing corticomedullary destruction, which is ground glass in appearance. Classic feature is the "Shepherd crook" deformity of proximal femur (arrow)

Multiple Neurofibromatosis (von Recklinghausen's Disease)

This is a rare genetic disorder characterised by multiple fibromatosis along the cutaneous nerves with scoliosis, café-au-lait spots with skin nodules and occasional hypertrophy of one limb with strange skeletal disturbances of growth, and pseudoarthrosis of tibia. (*Rule out other causes like congenital defect, fibrous dysplasia, and acquired tibia defects following fracture.*)

X-ray shows kyphoscoliotic deformity of tibia and non-union following fracture (pseudoarthrosis of tibia Fig. 6.6a). Pressure erosion of bone, and sometimes one of the tumours may undergo malignant change.

Treatment

Types

Type I: Complete defect of the bone.
Type II: Congenital bony cyst resembling fibrous dysplasia.
Type III: Congenital bowing, complicated.
  i. Excision of painful nodules in the limbs and vertebrae with spinal decompression and fusion for scoliosis.
  ii. Pseudoarthrosis (Fig. 6.6a) of tibia requires excision of fibrous defect and bone grafting as given below
     a. Boyd's Dual onlay bone graft (Fig. 6.6b).

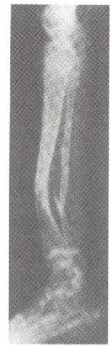
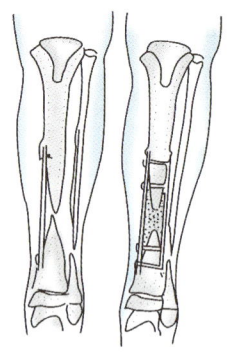

Fig. 6.6a: Pseudoarthrosis of tibia

Fig. 6.6b: Boyd's Dual onlay bone graft

b. Mac Farland's by-pass bone grafting.

c. Sofield's osteotomy and rotation of the fibrous defect.

d. Excision of the non-union, acute docking of the refreshed site and proximal osteotomy lengthening by Illizarov apparatus.

iii. Elephantiasis requires soft tissue dissection.

These patients are prone to fatal haemor-rhage during surgery.

NAIL-PATELLA SYNDROME
(Onycho-osteodysplasia)

It is inherited as an autosomal dominant trait. The nails are hypoplastic and the patella unusually small or absent. The radial head is subluxated laterally and the elbow may lack full extension.

X-ray

The characteristic X-ray features are hypoplastic or absent patella

The presence of *bony protuberances (iliac wings) on the lateral aspect of the iliac blades*

MARFAN'S SYNDROME (Arachnodactyly)

This is a generalized disorder affecting the skeletal, joint ligaments, eyes and cardio-vascular structures. There is a defect of crosslinkage in collagen and elastin. The genetic abnormality has been mapped to the fibrilin gene on chromosome 15. It is transmitted as autosomal dominant but sporadic cases also occur. Males and females are equally affected.

Clinical Features

Patients are tall, with disproportionately long legs and arms and often with flattening or hollowing of the chest (pectus excavatum). Upper body segment is shorter than the lower (ratio < 0.8 is suggestive) and arm span exceeds height by 5 cm or more. The digits are

unusually long (spider finger), scoliosis, spondylolisthesis, slipped upper femoral epiphysis, generalised joint laxity, flat feet, dislocation of patella or shoulder, high arched

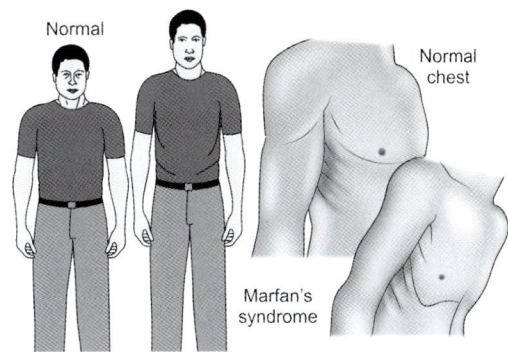

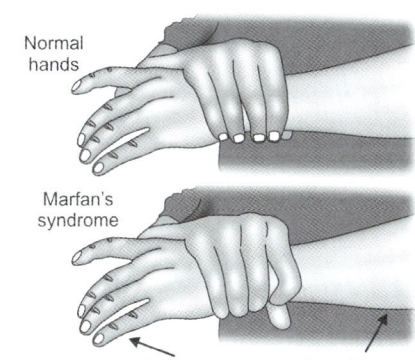

Elongated finger and arm bones

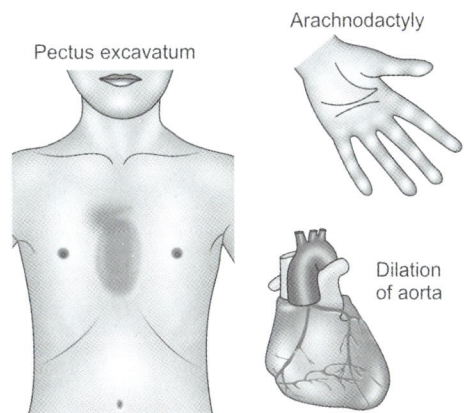

Fig.6.7: Showing features (arrow) of Marfan's syndrome

palate, hernias, lens dislocation, retinal detachment, aortic aneurism and mitral or aortic incompetence can occur (Fig. 6.7).

X-rays

Bone structure appears normal but may reveal scoliosis, spondylolisthesis or slipped epiphysis.

Diagnosis

Marfanoid features along with ophthalmic and cardiovascular defects are diagnostic.

Management

Patients occasionally need treatment for progressive scoliosis or flat feet. The heart should be carefully checked before operation.

DOWN SYNDROME (TRISOMY 21)

This condition results from having an extra copy of chromosome 21. It is much more common than any of the skeletal dysplasia. Characteristic features at birth includes head is foreshortened eyes slant upward, prominent epicanthal fold, nose is flattened, lips are parted, tongue protrudes, abnormal palmar creases, clinodactyly, spreading of first and second toes, hypotonicity and delayed skeletal development. Children are short with varying degrees of mental retardation and joint laxity. Adults have atlanto-axial

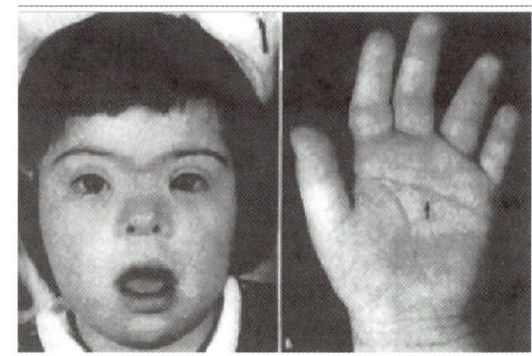

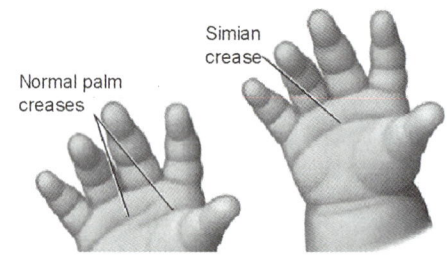

Fig. 6.8: Features of Down syndrome (mongoloid fascies; arrow)

instability, cardiac defects, and decreased resistance to infection (Fig. 6.8).

Treatment

There is no specific treatment but surgery can offer considerable cosmetic improvement. Atlanto-axial fusion is occasionally needed for patients with neurological symptoms.

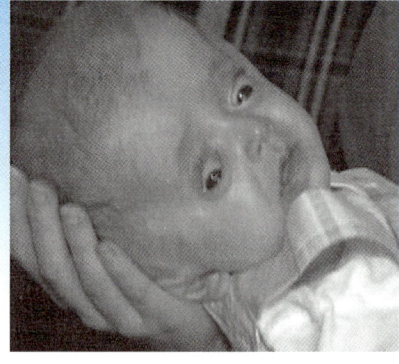

Diseases of Joints

ARTHRITIS

Synovial Fluid

- **Normal (knee):** Synovial fluid of normal knee is 3–5 ml in volume. It is clear, viscous, transparent, with WBC count of less than 200, with 25% of it formed by neutrophils. Firm mucin clot and glucose level same as that of blood.

- **Non-inflammatory synovial effusion:** Volume of synovial fluid more than 5 ml transparent, straw coloured and viscous. WBC count is 200–2000. Rest same.

- **Septic arthritis:** Plenty of synovial fluid which is opaque, purulent, yellow to green coloured. WBC count is more than 1 lac; of it 75% is neutrophils. Mucin clot is friable and culture is positive. Glucose level drops.

- **If RBC are seen in plenty:** Possibilities are trauma, haemophilia or bleeding disorders, neuropathic arthropathy, pigmented villonodular synovitis, haemangioma.

- **Crystals**
  - *Gout:* Monosodium urate crystals, are long needle shaped, negatively birefringent and usually intracellular.
  - *Pseudogout and chondrocalcinosis:* Calcium pyrophosphate dihydrate crystals are usually short, rhomboid shaped and positively birefringent.

Always remember when you are sending samples of synovial fluid for:
  a. *Cells:* Send it in a heparinized bottles.
  b. *Mucin clot:* Add a few drops in 5 ml 5% acetic acid.
  c. *Sugar:* Send in fluoride tube and the patient should be fasting.

HAEMARTHROSIS

This is collection of blood in the joint.

Causes

  i. Traumatic (iatrogenic or accidental)
  ii. Bleeding disorders like haemophilia
  iii. Neuropathic arthropathy
  iv. Pigmented villonodular synovitis
  v. Tumours: Synovioma, haemangioma
  vi. Traumatic injury while passing the needle into the knee joint for aspiration.

If aspirated, blood contains fat globules, it indicates intra-articular fracture.

Clinical Features

Warm, boggy, post-traumatic swelling limited to the joint capsule due to injury or bleeding disorder. Must be aspirated and controlled, otherwise, it can lead to ankylosis.

Treatment

i. Treat primary cause.
ii. Aspirate with 16-guage needle and apply Robert–Jones 3 layer compression bandage.
iii. Plaster immobilization in cases of fractures.

Sites of Arthritis

In general:
Sites of hand or wrist involvement and their potential disease besides knee, shoulder and hip joint.
- *DIP:* Osteoarthritis (Heberden's nodes); psoriatic; Reiter's
- *PIP:* Osteoarthritis (Bouchard's nodes); SLE; RA; psoriatic
- *MCP:* RA Pseudogout; hemochromatosis
- *1st CMC:* Osteoarthritis (characteristic)
- *Wrist:* RA: Pseudogout; gonococcal arthritis; juvenile arthritis; carpel tunnel syndrome
- *Focal wrist pain localized to radial aspect:* de Quervain's tenosynovitis.

OSTEOARTHRITIS OF KNEE

It may be primary or secondary due to overweight, diabetes or post-traumatic.

Clinical Features

Progressive pain, swelling and limitation of knee movements while squatting, going up and down a stair. Pain is mild in the morning but increases with activity and is relieved by rest. Instability gradually limits mobility of the patient in due course of time and formation of the genu varum (bowleg) as seen in Fig.7.1. Rule out a secondary cause.

Management

Aims
i. *Relief of pain:* Rest, analgesics, chondroprotective drugs.
ii. *Increase mobility:* Exercises and physiotherapy.
iii. *Reduce instability:* Braces.
iv. *Surgery:* Synovectomy, HTO, arthrodesis, joint replacement.
   a. High tibial osteotomy (Figs 7.2 to 7.4). In this a lateral wedge of the tibia is excised to correct the varus and realign the knee weight bearing axis. It is advisable for early osteoarthritis which is monocompartmental, especially in a young patient.
   b. If ligament laxity leads to genu varum and subluxation (Fig. 7.1) and severe damage of all the three compartments of the knee joint with gross disability **takes place then total knee replacement** (Fig. 7.3) is the treatment of choice

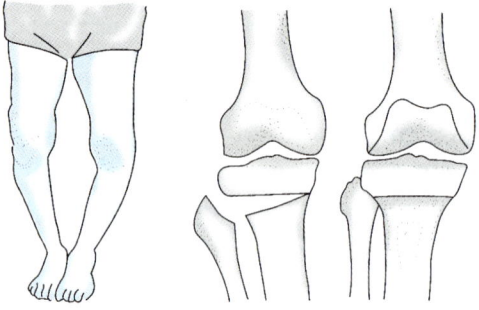

Fig. 7.1: Genu valgum

Fig. 7.2: High tibial osteotomy (HTO)

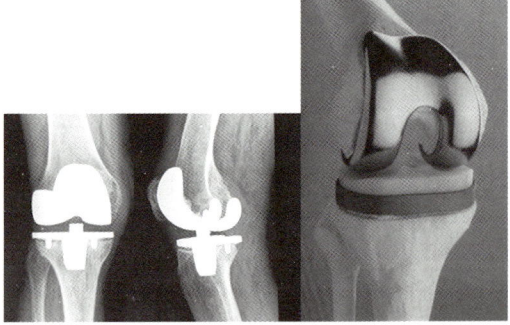

Fig. 7.3: Total knee replacement

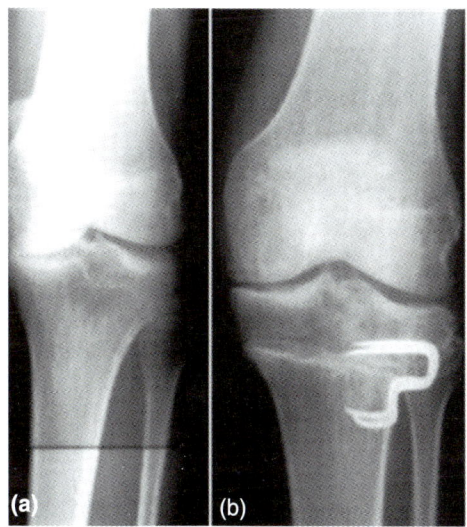

Figs 7.4a and b: (a) X-ray OA knee before and (b) after HTO fixed with staple

provided the patient accepts new and limited lifestyle.

CHARCOT'S JOINT
(Neuropathic Arthropathy)

This is a degenerated painless joint due to loss of pain, temperature and proprioceptive sensation to the joint.

It was first described by Jean Mortin Charcot in 1868 in patients with tabes dorsalis.

Disorder Associated with Neuropathic Joint Disease

- Tabes dorsalis
- Diabetes mellitus (DM)
- Meningomyelocele
- Syringomyelia
- Amyloidosis
- Leprosy
- Peroneal muscular atrophy
- Spinal cord injuries
- Pernicious anaemia
- Repeated hydrocortisone injection in the joints

Joint involvements

- *Tabes dorsalis:* knee, hips and ankles are most commonly affected
- *Syringomyelia:* glenohumeral joint, elbow and wrist
- *Diabetes mellitus:* tarsal and tarsometatarsal

Usually involves large joints like knee, ankles, etc. Enlarged, boggy, deformed joints, painless abnormal mobility, eroded cartilage with osteophytes and multiple loose bodies (Fig. 7.5).

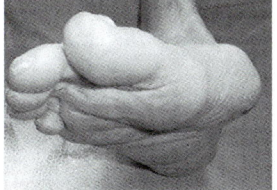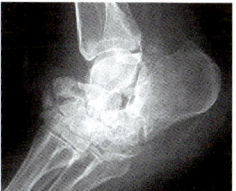

Fig. 7.5: Charcot's joint; X-ray showing neuropathic arthropathy of ankle joint

Management

i. Treat primary cause.
ii. Arthrodesis/amputation.
iii. Braces.

HAEMOPHILIA

Clinical Features

i. Family history.
ii. Exclusively in males (X-linked recessive inheritance).
iii. Haemophillia A is by far the more common type, constituting 85% of cases.
iv. In order of frequency, the joint most commonly involved/affected are the *knees, ankles, elbows, shoulders, and hips.* Small joints of the hands and feet are occasionally involved.
v. Pseudotumour (haemophilic cyst) due to intramuscular bleeding causing involvement of associated nerves and paralysis example bleeding into the iliacus sheath

may cause Femoral nerve paralysis, or into the forearm compartment leading to Median and ulnar nerve damage or periosteal haemorrhage.

vi. History of repeated episodes of bleeding from gums, after any cut.

vii. Bleeding into joints causing damage to articular cartilage, deformity and later ankylosis of joint.

viii. Clotting time increased due to lack of antihaemophilic factor—Haemophilia A (factor VIII) or Haemophilia B (Christmas factor).

ix. X-ray: Distended joint, articular surfaces intact but thinned out. In late cases, genu valgum and genu varum deformities may be associated due to epiphyseal asymmetric overgrowth.

x. Squaring of patella, widening of intercondylar notch of femur is typical finding seen in late cases.

Treatment

i. Replacement therapy of factor VIII: whole blood, fresh frozen plasma, cryoprecipitate.

ii. Acute case: Aspiration of joints and cold compression.

iii. For chronic cases
   a. Bracing/orthotic appliances.
   b. Dynamic splintage.
   c. Synovectomy for early cases with synovial proliferation.
   d. Arthrodesis in painful disorganized joints.

RHEUMATOID ARTHRITIS

It is the commonest inflammatory disease of middle age characterized by progressive, chronic, symmetric inflammation and deformity involving small joints of the hand, fingers, large joints, soft tissue and always associated with constitutional symptoms.

Clinical Features

Rheumatoid arthritis involves 1–3% of the population (usually between 30–50 years), with a male and female ratio of 1:3, symmetric, insidious onset with preferential involvement of knee, ankle and PIP joints of the fingers associated with general symptoms as fever, malaise, fatigue, anorexia and weight loss. Morning stiffness is an integral symptom, which subsides by the day. Joints show pain, swelling and warmth with synovial effusion and then progressive deformities develop.

It may occur in children less than 15 years (polyarticular juvenile rheumatoid arthritis). This is called **Still's disease** if it is associated with high fever, rash, lymphadenopathy, splenomegaly and involvement of one or few joints, leukocytosis, absence of RA factor and chronic iridocyclitis leading to blindness.

Deformities

i. *Wrist:* **Bent fork deformity** due to collapse of carpal bones and subluxation of intercarpal joints (Fig. 7.6a).

ii. *MCP joints:* Ulnar deviation and swollen knuckles.

iii. *IP joints:* **Swan neck deformity** (Fig. 7.6b), i.e. hyperextension of PIP and flexion of MP and DIP; **Boutonniere deformity** (Fig. 7.6c), i.e. flexion of PIP and hyperextension of DIP joints).

iv. *Feet:* Hallux valgus deformity of great toe.

v. *Knee:* Swelling, flexion contracture and later ankylosis.

vi. Tenosynovitis involving the extensor tendons of the hand, tendon Achilles at the heel, etc.

vii. *Elbow and shoulder:* Effusion and later contractures.

Other features are:

Palmer erythema, subcutaneous nodules along ulnar border in 30% of the patients.

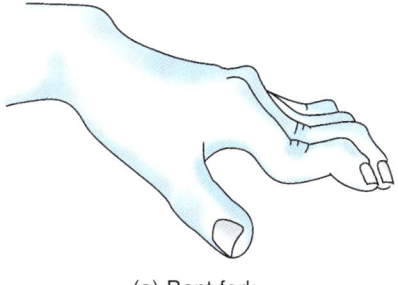

(a) Bent fork

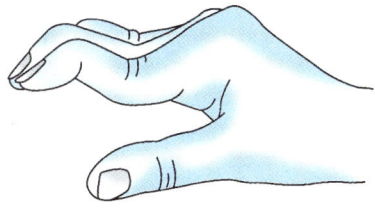

(b) Swan neck

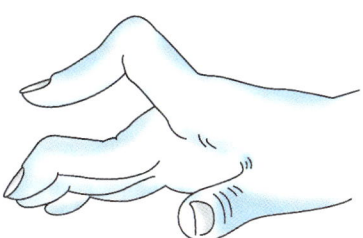

(c) Boutonniere

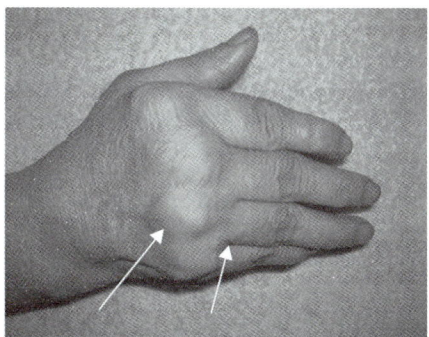

(d) Ulnar deviation, swollen knuckles (arrow) and deformed fingers

Figs 7.6a to d: Various deformities in rheumatoid arthritis

Enlarged spleen in 10% and lymph nodes in 30%, subungual haemorrhage.

Atrophy of skin over the hand, knee, and feet.

Sjögren's syndrome: *Dryness of eyes, keratoconjunctivitis, episcleritis, dry mouth and parotid swelling.*

Felty's syndrome: *Triad of seropositive RA associated with splenomegaly, neutropenia and cutaneous ulcers.*

Additional features of systemic involvement

a. *Pulmonary:* Pleuritis, pleural effusion, fibrosis.
b. *Cardiac:* Pericarditis, effusion and fibrosis.
c. *Ocular:* Xerophthalmia, scleritis, episcleritis.
d. Peripheral neuropathy, lymphadenitis and anaemia.

Diagnosis

It is based on history, clinical features, and investigations.

The criteria of **American Rheumatism Association** (ARA) requires at least four features to be present out of the following:

i. Progressive stiffness lasting more than one hour.
ii. Arthritis involving more than 3 joints simultaneously.
iii. Arthritis of PIP joints, MCP or wrist joints.
iv. Symmetric arthritis.
v. Rheumatoid nodules.
vi. Positive rheumatoid factor test.
vii. Radiographic changes of RA (Para-articular osteopenia, erosion).

- *Classic* case should have seven criteria for atleast six months.
- *Definite* case should have five criteria for six months.
- *Probable* case should have atleast

three criteria for a minimum of 4 weeks.

Investigations

i. **Blood**
   a. *RA factor:* It is an auto-antibody that binds to IgG, positive in 75–85% of patients, false positive in Sjögren's syndrome, macro-globulinemia, leishmaniasis, hepatitis.
   b. Increased ESR, CRP, anaemia, thrombocytosis, increased gamma-globulins, leukopenia associated with splenomegaly.
ii. **Synovial fluid:** Yellowish, cloudy, low viscosity, poor stringing effect. Leukocyte count more than 25000 cells/mm^3; mainly neutrophils (more than 70%).
iii. **X-ray**
   a. *Early stage:* Increased joint space (due to effusion and synovial proliferation) and osteopenia.
   b. *Late stage:* Decreased joint space, articular erosion, subchondral cyst and deformed, ankylosed joints.

Differential Diagnosis

i. *Acute:* Rheumatic fever, viral arthritis, SLE.
ii. *Chronic:* Osteoarthritis, gout, psoriatic arthropathy, Reiter's syndrome.

Management

i. **Conservative**
   a. *Rest:* Physical, emotional, articular.
   b. *Physiotherapy:* Fomentation, exercise.
   c. *Drugs*
      • For slowly progressive RA: Indomethacin, Brufen, Diclofenac sodium, Celecoxib, Aspirin, Ketoprofen, Naproxen, etc.
      • For aggressive RA:
        – DMARD (Disease modifying anti-rheumatoid drugs). Methotrexate, Hydroxy-chloroquine, Sulfasalazine, Gold and Cyclosporine, Leflunomide.
   – Corticosteroids.
   – New drugs
      a. TFN inhibitors like Infliximab, Etanercept
      b. Beta cell targeting—Rituximab
      c. T cell targeting—Abacept
      d. Osteoclcast inhibitors—Zolindronic acid

ii. **Surgery**
   a. *Early*
      • Aspiration of synovial fluid and compression.
      • Subtotal synovectomy (arthroscopic).
      • Tenosynovectomy.
      • Ligament reconstruction, tendon transfer.
   b. *Late*
      • Joint replacement indications are as follows:
        – Intractable daily pain even at rest.
        – Gross functional limitations.
        – Advanced radiological changes of degeneration and instability.
      • Arthrodesis: Grossly deranged, unstable progressive disease. Sites of arthrodesis are knee, IP joints of fingers, wrist (this corrects deformity, improves other joint functions).
      • Corrective osteotomy: For deformities in arm, hip and knee.

GOUT

It is a familial disease of adult males (95%) characterized by acute onset, monoarticular inflammation (podagra, MP joint of great toe in more than 50%), the involvement of knee and heel pad.

It is associated with hyperuricemia (serum uric acid more than 7 mg/100 ml). This presents as acute inflammatory response due to deposits of *monosodium urate crystals* in the synovial fluid, urate deposits in the soft tissues like tendons, pinna and kidney with dramatic response to colchicine and asymptomatic periods in between.

Pathophysiology

There is an increase in uric acid levels leading to deposits of monosodium urate monohydrate crystals in the synovial fluid, capsule, ligaments, kidney, pinna, etc. either because of

i. **Primary causes**
   a. *Increased production of uric acid:*
   - *Exogenous:* Intake of purine rich diet like liver, kidney, bone, soups.
   - Endogenous production of purine.
   - Lesch–Nyhan syndrome, Kelly-Seegmiller syndrome.
   b. *Decreased excretion of uric acid:* Diabetic ketoacidosis, salicylates, thiazide diuretics and chronic alcoholism.
   c. *Both (a) and (b) mentioned above* i.e. increased production coupled with decreased excretion, e.g. chronic alcoholism, G6PD deficiency and fructose intolerance.

ii. **Secondary causes**
   Acquired hyperuricemia with myeloproliferative disorder, multiple myeloma, haemoglobinopathies, malignancies and increased breakdown of nucleic acid as in leukaemia and lymphomas.

Clinical Features

i. First described by Hippocrates in fifth century BC. The patient has a nice party with lot of drinks and non-veg diet, gets up at midnight or morning with acute excruciating pain, redness, swelling involving the great toe (50%) (Fig. 7.7)

(tendon Achilles), knee, ankle, or hand. The inflammation gradually subsides and the overlying skin desquamates subsequently, there is always associated fever, malaise, headache, tachycardia.

ii. Chronic alcoholism, thiazide diuretics may cause precipitation of gout.

iii. Chronic/recurrent pain with secondary degenerative arthritis with hallux valgus. Renal stones (20%), tophaceous deposits in the joint cartilage, capsule, ear and tendons.

iv. Chronic renal damage may lead to hypertension and renal failure.

Investigations

i. **Blood**
   a. Increased uric acid level more than 7 mg/100 ml.
   b. Increased WBC and ESR.
   c. Increased urea and serum creatinine in patient with decreased renal function.

ii. **Synovial fluid:** Examination under polarised microscopy shows negatively birefringent crystals of monosodium urate.

iii. **X-ray:** Punched out subchondral, para-articular cystic lesion and later changes of OA.

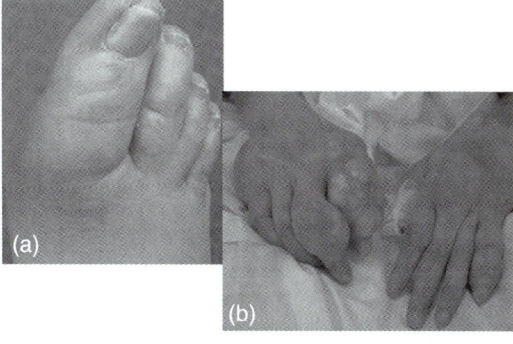

Figs 7.7a and b: Acute gout (a) with erythema (redness) of the great toe joint gout (b) showing Tophi in the hand (fingers)

Differential Diagnosis

i. **Secondary osteoarthritis** due to tubercular, pyogenic arthritis, osteoarthritis, rheumatoid arthritis.

ii. **Crystal synovitis (psuedogout)**

a. *Ca pyrophosphate:* The crystals are rod shaped, weakly positive birefringent, symmetric arthritis (usually polyarticular). Calcification of ligament/IV disc, cartilage and menisci (alkaptonuria), associated hyperparathyroidism, haemochromatosis, ochronosis, decreased PO_4, decreased Mg (Fig. 7.8).

b. *Ca hydroxyapatite:* This primary mineral of bone and teeth can get deposited over damaged tissue, as in hypercalcemia, hyperparathyroidism.

c. *Ca oxalate/renal type:* The crystals are bipyramidal strongly positive birefringent on polarized microscopy. Seen in patients with nephro-calcinosis/chronic renal failure, ascorbic acid is metabolized to oxalic acid, this is poorly excreted by the kidney in CRF and gets deposited in the kidney, joints and soft tissues.

Management

i. **Prevention**

a. Increased urine output by increased water intake.

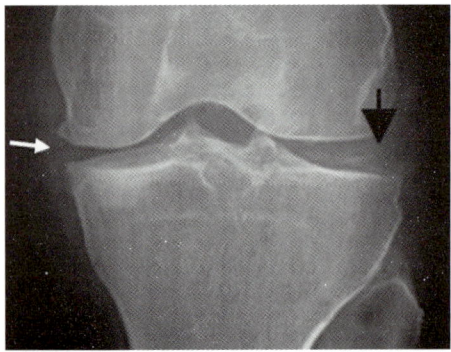

Fig. 7.8: Alkaptonuria showing calcification of meniscus

b. Alkalinize the urine with sodabicarbonate.

c. Decrease purine rich food intake, alcohol, avoid thiazide diuretics, vitamin C in CRF, fasting and dehydration.

ii. **Acute**

a. Bedrest, cold compression for inflamed joints.

b. Drugs

Colchicine: 0.5 mg hourly till the pain decreases or diarrhoea.

Indomethacin: 50 mg 6 hourly.

Voveran/Brufen/Naproxen/Steroids: Oral/local.

iii. **Chronic**

a. **Uricosuric drugs**, *used for increasing uric acid clearance.*

• Probenicid 500 mg daily.

• Sulfinpyrazone 100–200 mg/day.

Care while using uricosuric drugs:

• Urine 2 litres of output per day and the pH > 4.

• Avoid using salicylates (antagonistic).

• Contraindicated in patient with kidney stones.

b. Drugs used for *reduction of urate production.*

Allopurinol (zyloric) in the dose of 200–400 mg/day decreases urate and urinary uric acid concentration, mobilizes tophaseous deposits. Good for endogenous type of gout.

Sometimes causes precipitation of gout, hence avoid in acute stage and in patients with poor renal function.

Note: Some patients of gout have normal serum uric acid levels.

SERONEGATIVE ARTHROPATHY

This is a group of clinical conditions presenting with spondyloarthropathy, oligoarticular peripheral arthritis, enthesis, genetically predisposed individuals with HLA-B27 *positive* and are negative for RA factor test in the blood.

- Ankylosing spondylitis.
- Psoriatic arthritis.
- Reiter's disease (urethritis, conjunctivitis and arthritis).
- Ulcerative colitis.
- Crohn's disease.

Ankylosing Spondylitis

Seronegative spondyloarthropathy affecting males in the 18–30 age group. Pain and stiffness in dorsolumbar and sacroiliac regions more in the morning and after exertion. Progressive limitation of chest expansion, if < 2.5 cm then it is highly suggestive (Fig. 7.9a).

- The most common extraarticular manifestation is acute anterior uveitis, which occurs in 40% of patients and can antedate the spondylitis. Attacks are typically unilateral, causing pain, photophobia, and increased lacrimation. Up to 60% of patients have inflammation in the colon or ileum. This is usually asymptomatic, but fran inflammatory bowel disease (IBD) occurs in 5–10% of patients with AS. 10% of patients

meeting criteria for AS have psoriasis Aortic insufficiency, sometimes producing symptoms of congestive heart failure, occur in a few per cent of patients. Prostatitis has been reported to have an increased prevalence. Amyloidosis is rare

- Rest aggravates and activity relieves pain and stiffness. Poker back in advanced cases.
- Restricted spinal movements, especially in flexion and large joints become stiff.
- There may be history of urethritis and ulcerative colitis.
- There is predilection in HLA B27 positive individuals (85%).

Schober's test is positive.

- It is used to measure the ability of a patient to flex his/her lower back. The examiner makes a mark approximately at the level of L5 (fifth lumbar vertebra). The examiner then places one finger ~5 cm below this mark, and another, second, finger, ~10 cm above this mark. The patient is asked to touch his/her toes. By doing so, the distance between the two fingers of the examiner increases. However, a restriction in the lumbar flexion of the patient reduces this increase; if the

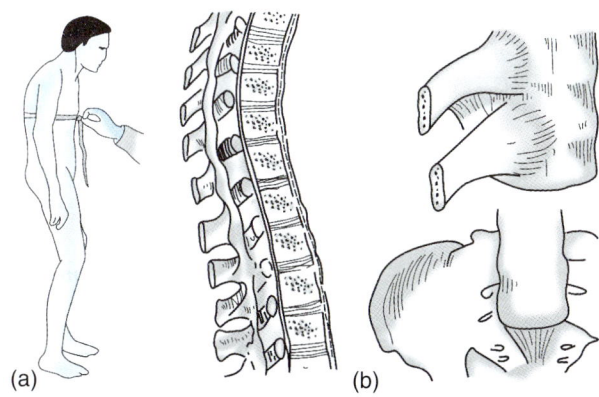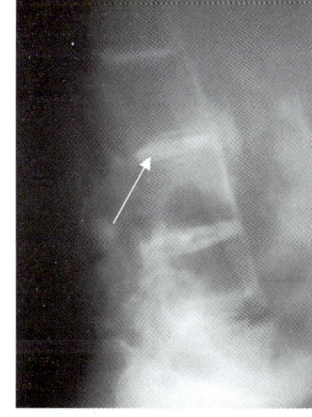

Figs 7.9a to c: (a) Progressive limitation of chest expansion; (b) Calcification of the collateral ligaments and sacroiliac joint fusion; (c) Bamboo spine due to calcification of the collateral ligament and paradiscal calcification

distance increases less than 5 cm, then there is an indication that the flexion of the lower back is limited.

Investigations

X-ray

Bamboo spine due to calcification of collateral ligaments (Fig. 7.9b), sacroiliac joints fusion, paradiscal calcification (Fig. 7.9c), *rule out fluorosis /diabetes*.

Treatment

i. **Conservative:**
   a. Proper posture maintenance.
   b. Exercises
   c. Drug therapy:
      - Anti-inflammatory drugs (NSAIDs) have been the mainstay of pharmacologic therapy for AS like Indomethacin 250 mg thrice a day, Naproxn 500 mg twice a day. These agents reduce pain and tenderness and increase mobility in many patients with AS
      - Sulfasalazine, in doses of 2–3 g/d, has been shown to be of modest benefit, primarily for peripheral arthritis.
      - Methotrexate, although widely used, has not been shown to be of benefit in AS, nor has any therapeutic role for gold or oral glucocorticoids been documented.
      - Attacks of uveitis are usually managed effectively with local glucocorticoid administration in conjunction with mydriatic agents
      - *Recent therapy:* There is now accumulating evidence that anti-TNF therapy is highly effective in AS. The anti-TNF α agents currently available, infliximab, Etanercept and adalimumab
   d. Radiotherapy to relieve stiffness.

ii. **Surgery:**
   a. Osteotomy of spine, for severe kyphosis.
   b. Total hip replacement, if hip ankylosed.

Differential Diagnosis
(of diffuse osteosclerosis)

Mnemonic (FROM)

Fluorosis, increased vitamin D.

Renal osteodystrophy.

Osteopetrosis, sickle cell anaemia.

Myelosclerosis, mastocytosis, metastatic (prostrate).

Ochronotic Arthritis

Ochronotic arthritis (alkaptonuric arthritis)
Homogentisic acid is formed due to incomplete breakdown of amino acid tyrosine and phenylalanine, its a rare congenital disorder.

Homogentisic acid is a strong reducing agent, which on oxidation turns to a dark pigment with an affinity to cartilage, sclera ligaments, tendon, intervertebral disc and joints, leading to early degenerative changes.

The urine changes to black on standing. The sclera and ear cartilage is pigmented black. Thoracic spine is kyphotic. The urine turns black on standing and this change may be accelerated by heating or alkalising the urine. A few drops of ferric chloride solution turns the urine bluish green. There is no treatment other than high dose of vit. C.

OSTEOARTHRITIS
(DEGENERATIVE JOINT DISEASE)

This is the commonest cause of morbidity after the age of 45, involving 60% of the population, characterized by joint pains, reduced mobility, instability and crippling deformity. The basic cause is due to progressive articular degeneration accompanied by poor repair, remodelling of subchondral bone and osteophyte formation.

Aetiopathology

Primary Osteoarthritis

This is age-related and gradually progressive.

Secondary Osteoarthritis

This is due to:
- Damage to the articular cartilage due to trauma, infection, irradiation, gout, steroids and alcohol.
- Alteration in the vascular supply to the cartilage as in storage diseases, haemoglobinopathy, Paget's disease, Caisson sickness (disease caused by nitrogen bubbles in deep sea divers), osteoporosis and osteomalacia.
- Alteration in joint alignment/bio-mechanics following injury, deformity or limb shortening.

Diagnosis

This is based on history, clinical examination and corroborative findings on X-ray.

History

Pain in relation to the joint activity and relief by rest, grinding and joint crepitus, gradually progressive loss of joint movements, recurrent swellings and crippling deformities.

Examination

The patient shows obvious signs of ageing, wrinkles on the face and arcus senilis.

Examination of joints in general reveals joint line tenderness, palpable crepitus osteophytic, reduced mobility, joint instability, deformity and muscle atrophy. There may be associated neurological signs depending on root involvement especially the cervical and lumbar zone.

- **Hand:** Osteoarthritis here occurs more common in females with classical signs of **Heberden's nodes** on the distal interphalangeal joints or **Bouchard's nodes** over proximal interphalangeal joints (Fig. 7.10).
- **Knee:** This causes pain during routine activities of life, stiffness, instability and progressive varus deformity leading to bowlegs.
- **Hip:** This presents as groin pain and progressive antalgic gait.
- **Spine:** The degeneration may involve intervertebral disc, facet joints or exiting nerves and presents as radicular pains as well as local stiffness (Fig. 7.11).

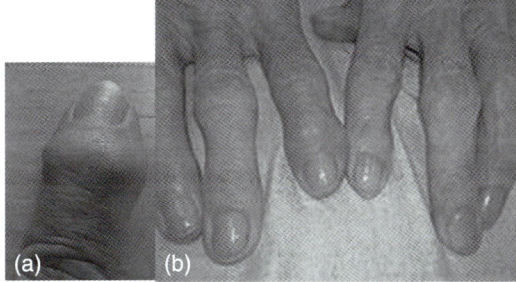

Figs 7.10a and b: (a) Heberden's nodes (b) Bouchard's nodes

Investigations

- **X-ray** of knee shows reduction of joint space, increased density of subchondral bone, osteophytes/loose bodies, joint subluxation, deformity and malalignment of joint (Fig. 7.12).
- Synovial fluid, blood and urine examination is necessary to rule out secondary causes.

Treatment

This is based on the severity of the disease and demands of the patients.

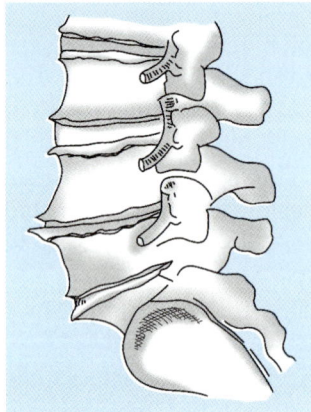

Fig. 7.11: Degenerative spine (loss of lumbar lardosis, decrease in disc space, osteopenia and lipping of the vertebrae)

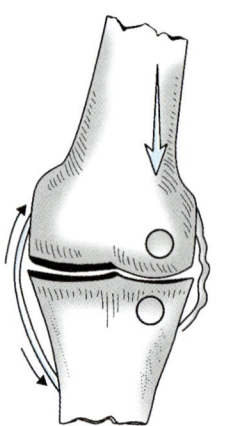 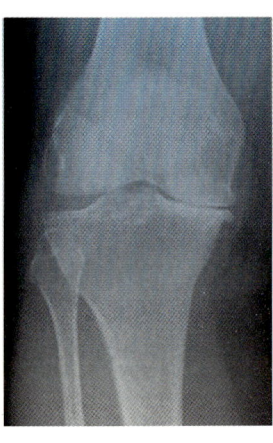

Fig. 7.12: X-ray showing osteoarthritis of a knee joint (decrease in joint space)

- **Conservative**
  - Exercises to improve the joint movements and muscle power.
  - Reduce weight so as to cut down the load on the major weight bearing joints.
  - Local therapy by hot fomentation, massage and anti-inflammatory liniments.
  - Supportive aids like splints, braces, canes, and crutches.
  - Change in lifestyle and joint demands.

  - Drugs: Analgesic/anti-inflammatory drugs, cartilage rejuvenators like glucosamine.
- **Surgery**
  - Joint realignment by osteotomies around hip and knee
  - Stability of joint by arthrodesis in the hand and knee
  - Joint replacement especially hip, knee, elbow, shoulder, and small joints of the fingers.

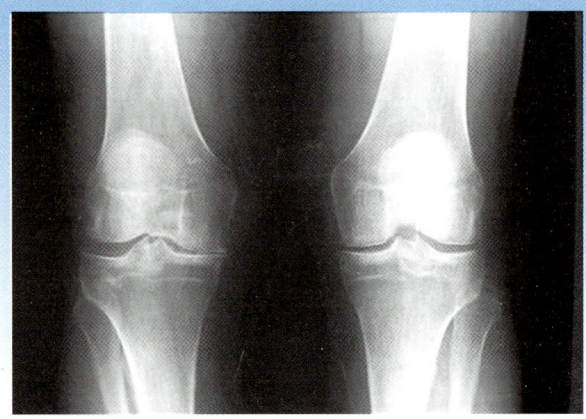

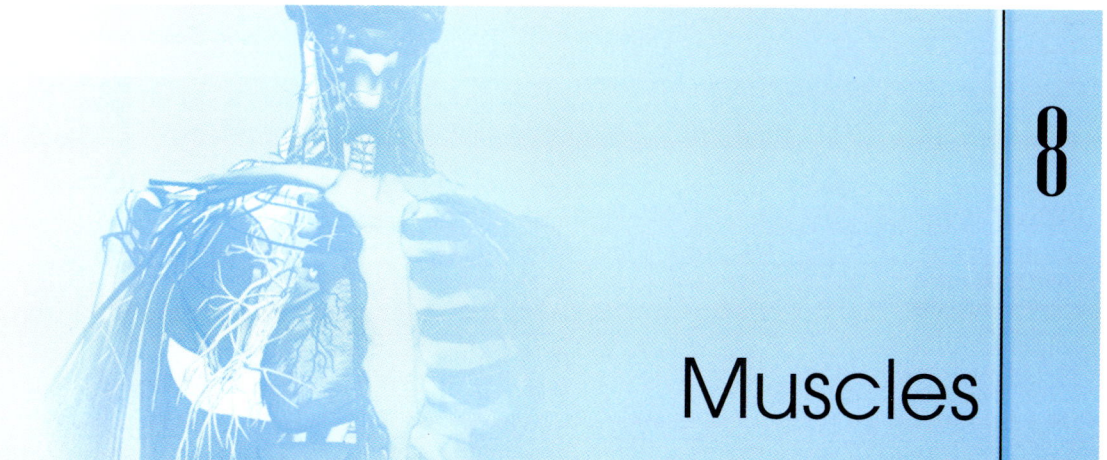

Muscles

8

Muscle is a contractile tissue, which brings about movements. Muscles are motors of the body.

Types of Muscles

Basically the muscles are of three types smooth, skeletal, and cardiac.

Cardiac

Cardiac muscle tissue forms the bulk of the wall of the heart. Like skeletal muscle tissue, these are striated. Unlike skeletal muscle tissue their contraction is usually not under conscious control (involuntary).

Smooth

Smooth muscles tissues are located in the walls of hollow internal structures such as blood vessels, the stomach, intestines, and urinary bladder. Smooth muscle fibres are usually involuntary, and they are nonstriated and therefore called as smooth muscles. Smooth muscle tissue, like skeletal and cardiac muscle tissue, can undergo hypertrophy and in addition, certain smooth muscle fibres, such as those in the uterus, retain their capacity for division and can grow by hyperplasia.

Skeletal

Skeletal muscle tissue is named for its location —attached to bones. It is striated; that is, the fibres (cells) contain alternating light and dark bands (striations) that are perpendicular to the long axes of the fibres. Skeletal muscle tissue can be made to contract or relax by voluntary control.

All skeletal muscle fibres are not alike in structure or function. For example, skeletal muscle fibres vary in colour depending on their content of myoglobin (myoglobin stores oxygen until needed by mitochondria). Skeletal muscle fibres contract with different velocities, depending on their ability to split adenosine triphosphate (ATP). Faster contracting fibres have greater ability to split ATP. In addition, skeletal muscle fibres vary with respect to the metabolic processes they use to generate ATP. They also differ in terms of the onset of fatigue. On the basis of various structural and functional characteristics, skeletal muscle fibres are classified into three types: Type I fibres, Type II B fibres, and Type II A fibres (Table 8.1).

Nerve Supply of Skeletal Muscle

Motor nerve is the nerve that supplies a muscle. In fact it is a mixed nerve, and consists of the following type of fibres.

Table 8.1: Characteristics of muscle types			
Fibre Type	*Type I fibres*	*Type II A fibres*	*Type II B fibres*
Contraction time	Slow	Fast	Very fast
Size of motor neuron	Small	Large	Very large
Resistance to fatigue	High	Intermediate	Low
Activity used for	Aerobic	Long-term anaerobic	Short-term anaerobic
Force production	Low	High	Very high
Mitochondrial density	High	High	Low
Capillary density	High	Intermediate	Low
Oxidative capacity	High	High	Low
Glycolytic capacity	Low	High	High
Major storage fuel	Triglycerides	CP, glycogen	CP, glycogen

1. **Motor fibres (60%)** comprise of: (a) large myelinated α efferent which supply extrafusal muscle fibres; (b) smaller myelinated γ efferent which supply intrafusal fibres of the muscle spindles; and (c) the fine non-myelinated autonomic efferent which supply smooth muscle fibres of the blood vessels.
2. **Sensory fibres (40%)** comprises of: (a) myelinated fibres distributed to muscle spindles, tendons, and local fascia; and (b) non-myelinated fibres carrying pain sensations of uncertain origin.

   • **Motor point** is the site where the motor nerve enters the muscle. It may be one or more than one.
   • **Motor unit** (myone) is defined as a single α motor neuron (Figs 8.1a and b).

Neuromuscular junctions are cholinergic in nature. On approaching the muscle the axons of motor nerve lose their myelin sheath and break up into a number of branches to

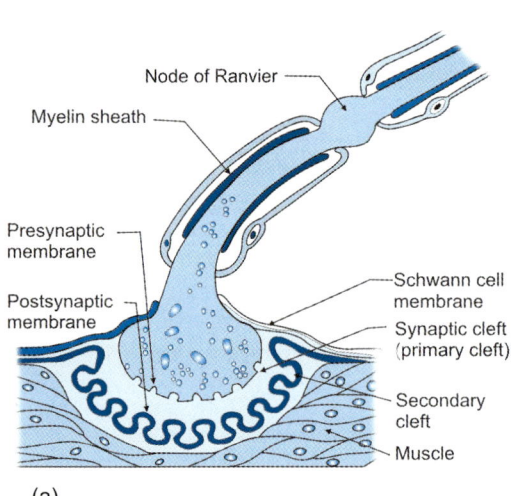

(a)

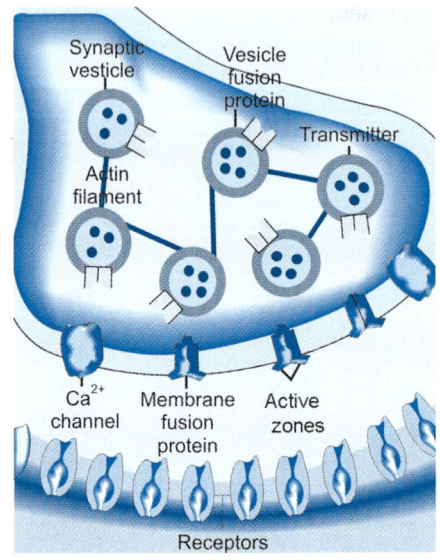

(b)

Figs 8.1a and b: Neuromuscular junctions

supply the individual muscle fibres specialised motor nerve endings, rich in acetylcholine. At the neuromuscular junction, the muscle fibre also is specialised into a sole plate, which is a localised collection of granular sarcoplasm containing many nuclei and mitochondria, and presenting synaptic gutters for the end plate. The sacrolemmal folds in the synaptic gutter are rich in acetyl cholinesterase which destroys the liberated acetylcholine after each neuromuscular transmission of impulse.

Muscle spindles (Neuromuscular spindles) are spindle-shaped sensory end organs of the skeletal muscle. Each spindle contains 6–14 intrafusal muscle fibres which are of two types, the larger nuclear bag fibres, and the smaller nuclear chain fibres. The spindle is innervated by both the sensory and motor nerves. Muscles spindles act as stretch receptors. They record and help regulate the degree and rate of contraction of the extrafusal fibres by influencing the neurons. Recent evidence shows that the spindle activity is represented in the sensory cortex, which plays a part in conscious appreciation of the position and movements of the joints (Fig. 8.2).

Some Definitions

- *Isotonic or concentric contraction* occurs if the length of muscles is reduced by one-third or more.
- During *isometric contraction* the tension is same as load and length of the muscles does not change, e.g. holding the arm outstretched.
- During *eccentric contraction*, tension is less than the load, i.e. muscle fibres are lengthening to bring about a particular movement, example lowering the arm to the side.
- *Active insufficiency:* A particular tendon crossing number of joints cannot work with efficiency at all the joints of the same time, e.g. flexor digitorum profundus muscles on the wrist, metacarpophalangeal and interphalangeal joints.
- *Passive insufficiency:* The extensors cannot extend all the joints at the same time, e.g. extensor digitorum on the wrist and joints of metacarpals and phalanges.

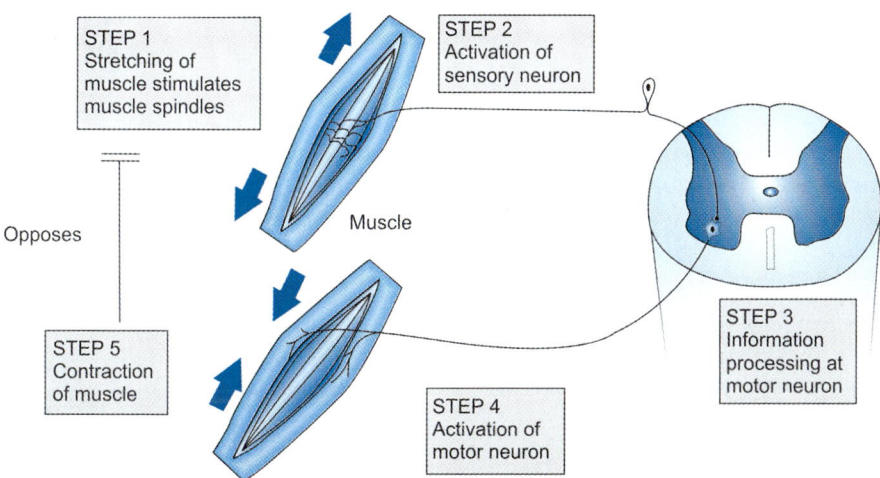

Fig. 8.2: Nerve supply of the muscle spindle

MECHANICS OF MUSCLES

When a muscle contracts the force of contraction is said to have three main components example

Swing which is transaxial

- This component is maximum during the contraction of branchialis muscle while flexing the elbow joint. Shunt, which is transarticular:
- Shunt component is maximum when the origin of the muscle is close to a joint while insertion is at a distance example: branchioradialis muscle.

Spin, which is rotary along its axis

- Spin component is predominant in the pronator quadratus muscle, wrapped on the anterior surfaces of lower ends of radius and ulna bones.

Applied Anatomy

Paralysis

- Loss of motor power (power of movement) is called paralysis.
- This is due to inability of the muscles to contract caused either by damage to the motor neural pathways (upper or lower motor neuron), or by the inherent disease of muscles (myopathy).
- Damage to the upper motor neuron causes spastic paralysis with exaggerated tendon jerks.
- Damage to the lower motor neuron causes flaccid paralysis with loss of tendon jerks.

Muscular Spasm

- These are quite painful.
- Localised muscle spasm is commonly caused by a 'muscle pull'.
- In order to relieve its pain the muscle should be relaxed by appropriate treatment (relaxant and other).
- Generalised muscle spasms occur in tetanus and epilepsy.

Disused Atrophy and Hypertrophy

- The muscles which are not used for long times become weak and thin.
- This is called disused atrophy conversely; adequate or excessive use of particular muscles causes their better development, or even hypertrophy.
- Muscular wasting is a feature of lower motor neuron paralysis and generalised debility.

Regeneration of Skeletal Muscle

- Skeletal muscle is capable of limited regeneration.
- If large regions are damaged, regeneration does not occur and the missing muscle is replaced by connective tissue.

ELECTROMYOGRAPHY

Introduction

Electromyography is a technique used to diagnose the neuromuscular disease or trauma. In electromyography, the study of the electrical activity of contracting muscle gives information regarding the structure and function of the motor units. This may make it possible not only to localize the site of pathology affecting either muscle or its innervation but also it frequently provides evidence regarding the nature of the pathological process. It is also helpful in studying muscle function from kinesiologic point of view and also to study the integrity of different portion of motor unit. There are two types of electromyography.

Clinical Electromyography

- The electrical potentials are detected and recorded from skeletal muscle fibres
- Usually clinical electromyography deals in terms of instrumentation requirements and data analysis techniques.
- This procedure, give information regarding the myopathy or extent of nerve injury.

Kinesiologic Electromyography

- This type of electromyography is used for studying muscle activity
- This procedure helps in establishing the role of different muscles for specific activity.

Physiology of the Muscle in Relation to Electromyography

Under electromyography in the true sense, we study the motor unit activity; the motor unit is composed of:

- One axon.
- Neuromuscular junctions.
- One anterior horn cell.
- All the muscle fibres innervated by that axon.

The impulse is conducted by single axon to all its muscle fibres and at the same time the depolarization occurs in the muscle fibres. The depolarization thus results in the electrical activity that is known as *motor unit action potential (MUAP)* and this is graphically recorded as electromyogram (Fig. 8.3).

Motor Unit Action Potential

The *motor unit action potential (MUAP)* means when the depolarization results in the electrical activity and graphically recorded by electromyogram it represents potential derived from group of muscle fibres that are contracting nearly synchronously and frequently activated by a single neuron.

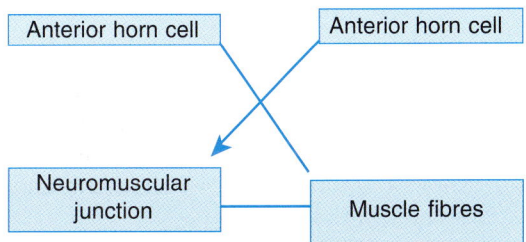

Fig. 8.3: Motor unit

Components of Electromyography

The electromyography instrument needs:

Amplifies

- This is used in the *processor phase* for amplifying small electrical signals which is thousand times amplified.

Electrodes

- They are used in *input phase* for picking up electric potential from muscle contracting.

Display

- This is used in *output phase* in which a device is used which converts the electrical signal to visual or audible signal.
- This is used for analysing the data.

Normal Motor Unit Action Potential

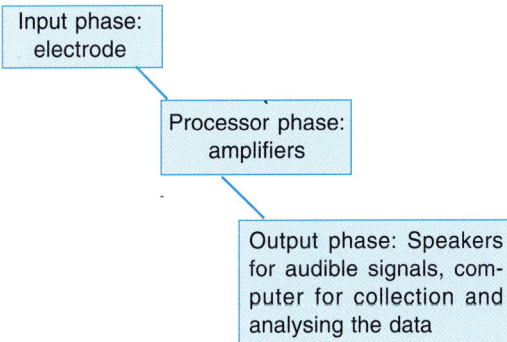

The normal motor unit action potential is the sum of electrical potential of the muscle fibres present in the single motor unit, having the capability of being recorded by the electrodes. The normal MUAP depends on the given five factors that is amplitude, duration, shape, sound and frequency.

In normal muscle, the amplitude of single motor unit action potential may range from 300 mV to 5 mV from peak to peak. The total duration measured from initial baseline will normally range from 3 to 16 msec.

There are four classification of the spontaneous activity:
1. Fibrillation activity (a).
2. Positive sharp waves (b).
3. Fasciculation potentials (c).
4. Repetitive discharges (Fig. 8.4).

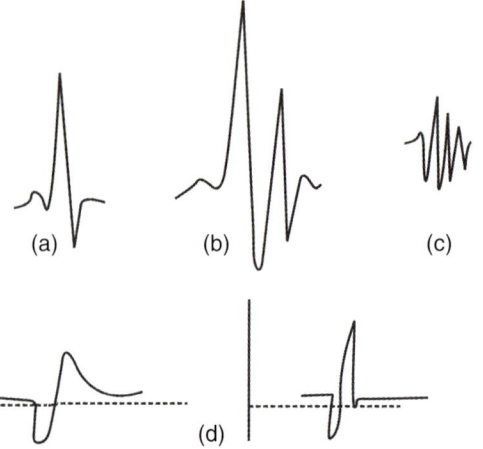

Figs 8.4a to d: (a) Normal wave pattern; (b) Positive sharp waves (1–2 wks); (c) Denervation fibrillation (3–4 wks); (d) Repetitive discharge

Fibrillation Potential

Fibrillation potential is seen in the denervated muscle as they give spontaneous discharges because they are hypersensitive to circulating acetylcholine. Classically, it is seen in lower motor neuron disorders such as:
• Anterior horn lesions.
• Radiculopathies.
• Peripheral nerve lesions
• Polyneuropathies with axonal degeneration, it is seen in myopathic disease.
  a. Dermatomyositis
  b. Polymyositis
  c. Muscular dystrophy
  d. Myasthenia gravis.

Positive Sharp Waves

It is a form of *electrical potential associated with fibrillating muscle* fibres which are recorded as

a biphasic, positive negative action potential initiated by needle movement and recurring in uniform patterns.

Positive sharp wave is *seen in primary muscle disease* like muscular dystrophy, polymyositis but some times it is also seen in upper motor neuron lesions. These waves are characteristic features of denervated muscle.

Fasciculations

A *random spontaneous twitching of muscle fibres* or a group may be visible through skin. This is seen in irritation or degeneration of anterior horn cell.
• *Muscle spasm or cramps*
• *Motor neuron disease*
• *Nerve root compression*
• *Pathology of spinal cord*
• *Pathology of root level.*

Repetitive Discharges

These are also known as bizarre *high frequency discharge.* The potential of repetitive discharge represents various forms. The characteristic features of the repetitive discharges are,

    Amplitude   – 50 mV to 1 mV
    Frequency   – 5 to 100 per sec

Indication of Clinical Electromyography Test

1. *Disorders of peripheral nerve:* In peripheral nerve disorders the lesions are of three types.
   • Neuropraxia
   • Axonotmesis
   • Neurotmesis.
2. *Polyneuropathies*
3. *Motor neuron disease*

   This includes degenerative disease of the anterior horn cells. They include:
   • neurotmesis
   • poliomyelitis
   • syringomyelia.

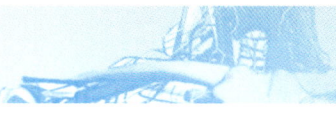

Some disease characterised by degeneration of both upper lower motor neurons such as

- amylotrophic lateral sclerosis
- progressive bulbar palsy
- progressive muscular atrophy
- spinal muscular atrophies.

4. Radiculopathy
5. Myasthenia gravis
6. Myotonia
7. Myopathies

8. Spinal cord compression
   - cord tumours
   - cervical spondylosis
   - syringomyelia
   - lumbar disc lesions.
9. Facial nerve palsy
10. Movement disorders
    - rigidity
    - spasticity
    - tremor.

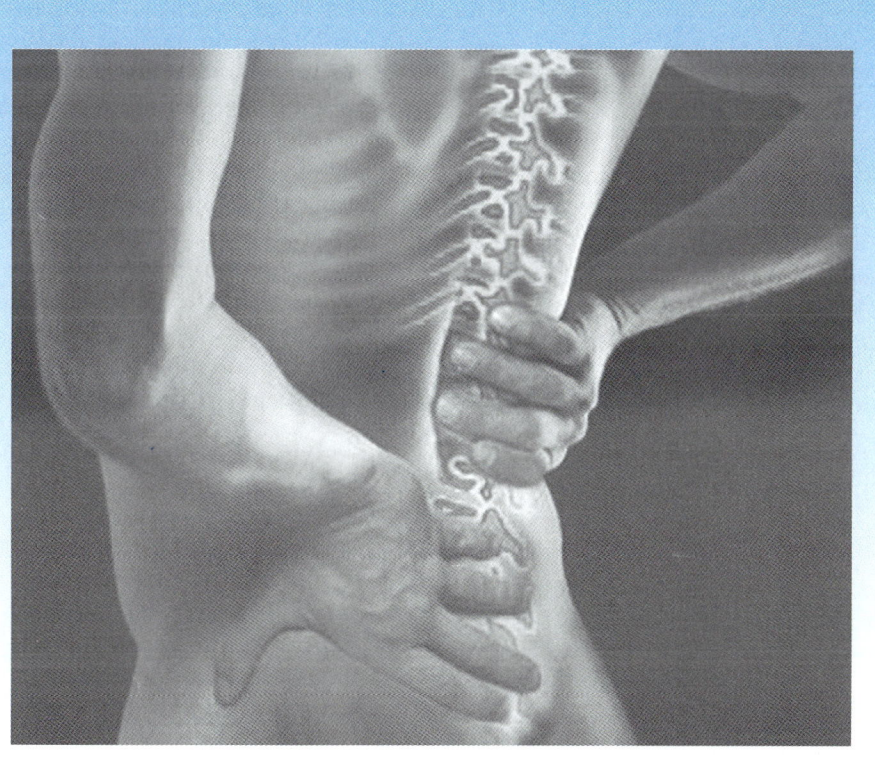

9

Diseases of Muscles

MUSCULAR ATROPHY

This is due to degeneration of nerve cell or axon of LMN. Non-familial, generally occurs late in life, affects **distal muscles** especially of hands. Fasciculations may be seen, spastic, exaggerated, deep tendon reflex (DTR), extensor plantar reflex, e.g. amyotrophic lateral sclerosis, Charcot–Marie–Tooth disease, myelopathic muscular atrophy.

MUSCULAR DYSTROPHY

This is familial, occurs in childhood, involves **proximal muscles, no spasticity or fasciculations**, e.g. progressive muscular dystrophy. Characterized by onset in childhood, weakness of shoulder, hip and calf. Waddling gait, climbing up on a body in an attempt to stand up (Gowers' sign). Contractures, scoliosis, lordosis. Absent or decreased deep tendon reflex.

Investigations

Positive muscle biopsy, EMG, increased levels of serum creatinine phosphokinase (CPK) and aldolase.

Treatment

Physiotherapy and general supportive measures.

Types of Dystrophy

i. **Duchenne dystrophy** (pseudohyper-trophic muscular dystrophy): The most common childhood muscular dystrophy. Enlarged calf and gluteal muscles (due to infiltration of muscle by fat and fibrous tissue), common in males, caused by a mutation of the gene that encodes **dystrophin**. It is localized to the short arm of the *'X'-chromosome at Xp21*. Dystrophin is a part of a large complex of sarcolemal proteins and glycoproteins. It starts in first 3 years of life, rapid progression, child is unable to stand and walk by 10 years of age. There is cardio-myopathy, mental impairment.

ii. **Landouzy–Dejerine dystrophy** (fascio-scapulohumeral muscular dystrophy): Childhood to adult onset, both sexes involved, muscular pseudohypertrophy, contracture and skeletal deformities. It has the characteristic cartoon 'Popeye' look, drooping eyelids, facial atrophy (myopathic face), thickened over-hanging upper lip (tapier lip), weak shoulder and arm (winging of scapula), no involvement of forearm muscles.

130

iii. **Erb's** (limb girdle): It involves shoulder and pelvic girdle muscle. Face is not affected, both sexes affected (2nd to 3rd decade), pseudohypertrophy is uncommon.

CONGENITA MYOTONIA (Thomsen's Disease)

This is a heridofamilial disease characterized by delayed muscular relaxation after a strong voluntary contraction. Difficulty in activities of the child can be seen in early childhood. There is a surprising generalized muscular hypertrophy giving it a Herculean appearance. Characteristically, the first few attempts at movement are associated with painless stiffening contractions with slow relaxation, but subsequently the movements become easier. Affected patients have a typical *hatchet faced appearance* due to temporalis, masseter, and facial muscle atrophy and weakness.

Cardiac disturbance occurs; other features associated include intellectual impairment, hypersomnia, posterior subcapsular cataracts, frontal baldness, gonadal atrophy, insulin resistance and decreased esophageal and colonic motility.

It is diagnosed by a simple percussion test, which produces spasm followed by slow relaxation. An electrical stimulation of brief duration initiates a prolonged contraction and repeated electrical stimuli will abolish the phenomenon. Electromyography is diagnostic. The hypertrophic muscle has a greater ability to store creatine, with high urinary excretion of creatinine.

Treatment

Quinine is specific and has to be continued indefinitely. Calcium is a useful adjunct. Newer drugs like procainamide in doses of 250 mg, thrice a day give excellent results.

MYASTHENIA GRAVIS

A disorder of neuromuscular transmission marked by fluctuating weakness and fatigue of certain voluntary muscles.

This is due to rapid depletion of acetylcholine receptors at the neuromuscular junction, characterized by involvement of bulbar innervated muscles, i.e. face, lips, eyes, tongue, throat, and neck.

Clinical Features

Common in females, 20–30 years of age, pronounced fatigue of following muscles:
- **Eyes:** Causing ptosis and diplopia.
- **Oral:** Causing dysarthria (speech) and difficulty in swallowing.
  - The **limb weakness** in myasthenia gravis is often proximal and may be asymmetric. Despite the muscle weakness deep tendon reflexes are preserved.
  - In about 65% the **thymus is 'hyperplastic'**, with the presence of active germinal centres, while 10% of patients have **thymic tumours (thymomas)**.

Treatment

Prompt response with edrophonium chloride and neostigmine.
- **Medical:** Neostigmine, pyridostigmine, edrophonium chloride, high dose of steroids/corticotropin/ACTH.
- **Surgical:** Beneficial results have been shown after thymectomy or irradiation of thymus (3000 R over 3–6 weeks).

FAMILIAL PERIODIC PARALYSIS

This is a rare heridofamilial type of intermittent paralysis. Periodic attacks of flaccid paralysis occur, with loss of reflexes affecting the trunk and limbs lasting for a few hours to several days with gradual recovery. It usually starts in the back and travels up and down, but does not involve muscles supplied by radial nerves and respiration. It is usually preceded by excessive thirst and perspiration. It is usually precipitated by excessive cold, heavy carbohydrate ingestion or vigorous exercise. Serum potassium is invariably low. It is treated by potassium chloride 5 to 10 gm orally and in severe conditions intravenously.

ARTHROGRYPOSIS MULTIPLEX CONGENITAL

This is failure of development of skeletal muscles congenitally, resulting in deforming contracture of joints. The child is usually born with involvement of one or all limbs with fixed deformities. The knee and elbow are straight with club foot, club hand and scoliosis. The head muscles are usually spared.

Treatment

It is basically aimed at stretching out the contractures and surgical treatment of various joint deformities.

MYOSITIS

It is inflammation of the muscle following bacterial, parasitic virus or even traumatic injury.

TRAUMATIC MYOSITIS

This is myositis ossificans traumatica invariably following an injury or massage around the joint (for details see complications of fracture).

MYOSITIS OSSIFICANS PROGRESSIVA

It is a congenital condition (autosomal dominant) characterized by ossification of muscles, fascia and tendons, often starting in the paraspinal muscles and then subsequently all over. Blood shows elevated eosinophil count. Radiologically sheets of ossified zones may be seen in the neck and cervicodorsal region, often obviously visible. Associated anomalies are shortening of the big toe and thumb. Treatment with diphosphonates may prevent progression. In the worst cases movements are restricted and the patient is severely disabled.

There is no known effective treatment.

PRUSSIAN DISEASE

This is usually seen in soldiers doing a lot of horse riding and develop ossification in the adductor muscle of the thigh which are constantly damaged by the saddle, and the deltoids by carrying rifles hanging around the shoulders.

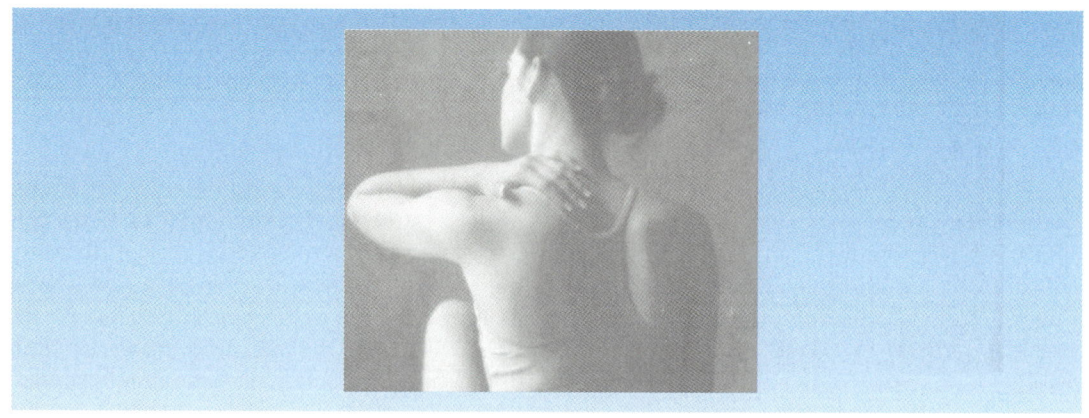

Orthopaedic Neurology

10

ANATOMY OF THE SPINE

- Discs (shown as arrow)
- Vertebrae
  - Body
    - Front section, shaped like drum
    - Supports weight
  - Lamina
    - Towards the back
    - Bony arch surrounds spinal canal
  - Spinous process
    - Bony process from arch
    - Points of attachment for muscles and ligaments
    - Cushions between vertebrae.

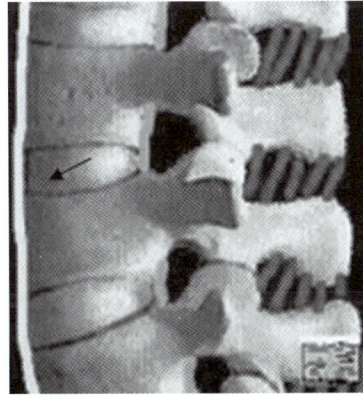

Fig. 10.1: Intervertebral disc (arrow)

Spinal column can be divided into three parts (Denis)

1. *Anterior column:* Anterior longitudinal ligament, anterior portion of disc, and anterior half of body of vertebra.
2. *Middle column*: Posterior longitudinal ligament, posterior portion of disc, and posterior half of body of vertebra.
3. *Posterior column:* Posterior bony arch comprises of pedicle, facets, posterior ligamentous complex of supraspinous, interspinous, ligametum flava and facet joint capsules.

The vertebral column is made up of:
- 7 Cervical
  - Flexion, extension, bending and turning of head
- 12 Thoracic
  - Chest region, allows mostly for rotation
- 5 Lumbar
  - Larger boney structures to support added wgt
- 5 sacral fused together
- Coccyx.

CLASSIFICATION OF SPINAL CORD INJURY

1. **ASIA impairment scale:**

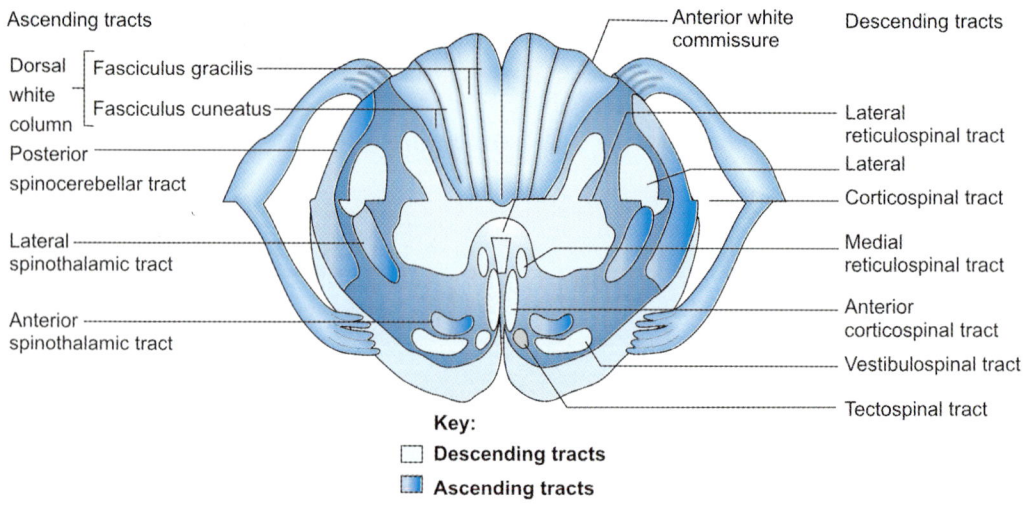

Ascending tracts

Dorsal white column — Fasciculus gracilis

Fasciculus cuneatus

Posterior spinocerebellar tract

Lateral spinothalamic tract

Anterior spinothalamic tract

Anterior white commissure

Descending tracts

Lateral reticulospinal tract

Lateral Corticospinal tract

Medial reticulospinal tract

Anterior corticospinal tract

Vestibulospinal tract

Tectospinal tract

Key:
☐ **Descending tracts**
▨ **Ascending tracts**

Fig. 10.2: Cross-section of the spinal cord to show the different tracts

- A = *Complete:* No motor or sensory function preserved in the sacral segments S4–5 (i.e. NO perianal sensation, deep anal sensation, or voluntary anal contraction)
- B = *Incomplete:* Sensory but no motor function preserved in the sacral segments (may not be normal, but is present!)
- C = *Incomplete:* Motor function is preserved below the neurologic level, and > ½ of the key muscles below the NLI have a muscle grade of < 3
- D = *Incomplete:* Motor function is preserved below the neurologic level, and ≥ ½ of the key muscles below the NLI have a muscle grade of ≥ 3

2. **Frankel classification:**
   - Grade A Absent motor and sensory function
   - Grade B Absent motor function, sensory function present
   - Grade C Motor function present but not useful (2/5 or 3/5), sensation present

- Grade D Motor function present and useful (4/5), sensation present
- Grade E motor and sensory function normal

SPINAL INJURIES

Types of Spinal Injuries

Definition

Stability: The ability of the spine under physiologic loads to prevent displacements which would injure or irritate neural tissue.
Instability: It is the loss of the ability of spine to tolerate physiological loading, without incurring neurological deficit, pain or progressive structural deficit.
   i. Stable
   ii. Unstable.

Mechanism of injury
   i. *Flexion:* Wedge compression fracture-usually stable.
   ii. *Flex/rotation:* It causes fracture dislocation, which is unstable injury, and paraplegia is often seen.

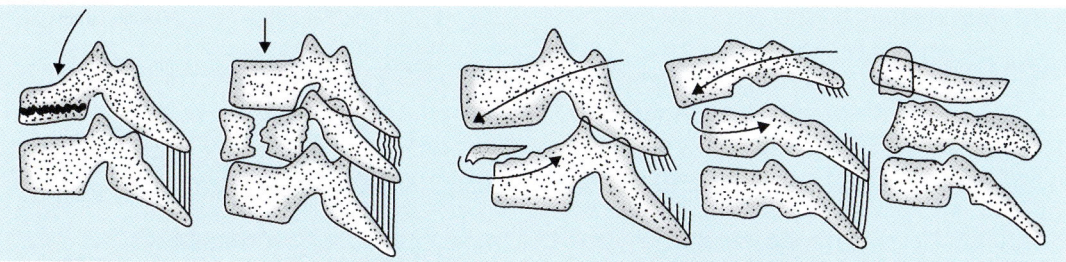

a. Stable: Intact posterior, ligament complex   b. Unstable: Tear of posterior ligaments, subluxation and dislocation, fracture of odontoid

Figs 10.3a and b

iii. **Extension:** There is rupture of anterior ligaments and is called whiplash injury. It is a stable type of injury.
iv. **Compression:** This causes burst fracture and is stable but the bone fragments may cause cord damage which is a serious complication.
v. **Penetrating:** This is due to bullet or stab injuries that damage the cord directly or as a result of high frequency waves.

Clinical Features

Sixty per cent fractures occur between T12 and L2.

EXAMINATION

History of injury, due to fall, vehicular accident or war injuries. Local tenderness, deformity, spasm and bruising occurs.
- There are two key objectives of the clinical assessment of the patient who has suffered an injury to the spine.
- *The first* is to ascertain the presence of concomitant injuries. One study found 47% of patients with spine trauma had associated injuries; 26% with head injuries; 24% with chest injuries; and 23% long bone injuries.
- Abdominal injuries and lumbar spine fractures often coexist and are overlooked. There is a common association b/w flexion-distraction (Chance type) lumbar injuries

and hollow viscus injuries in seat-belt injuries.
- *The second* objective is to ascertain the presence of a neurological deficit.
- The initial neurological assessment must be meticulous and well documented including rectal examination as this provides a reference baseline with which to assess further worsening or improving neurology and consequently decide on the urgency and type of management.

Neurological Examination

i. *Cervical:* Quadriplegia, root damage.
ii. *Thoracic:* Paraplegia.
iii. *Lumbar:* Cauda equina syndrome.

One must always look for bladder and bowel function.

Examine the patient from head to toe to rule out other important associated injuries, as this is usually a high velocity trauma.

Key indicators of damage of the level of cord are

- **Sensory level**
  - *Dermatome*: (Patch of skin innervated by a given spinal cord level)

    | C7 | – Middle finger. |
    | T4 | – Nipple. |
    | T10 | – Navel. |
    | L5 | – Dorsum of foot. |
    | S2 | – Posterior aspect of thigh. |

- **Motor level**
  - The term *"myotome"* is also used to describe the muscles served by a single nerve.

C4	– Respiration (diaphragm)
C5/6	– Elbow flexor
C8/T1	– Hand muscles (intrinsic)
L3/4	– Knee extensor
L5	– Great toe extensor
S1	– Great toe flexor
S2/3	– Anal sphincter

Root Pain Occurs if there is Injury to the Nerve Roots

- *Investigations*
  1. Most important initial study is a complete plain film series of the spine. 5–20% of fractures are multiple.

2. CT is used to define the bony anatomy in the injured area.
3. MRI essential to define spinal cord anatomy and also for assessing ligamentous injury.
4. Myelography and EMG.

SOME COMMON FRACTURES

Burst Fracture

- Compression fracture of body with superior and inferior end plate fractures, posterior arch fracture with laterally displaced pedicles (Fig. 10.5).
- Very unstable
- Over 2/3 have cord injury from retropulsed fragments.

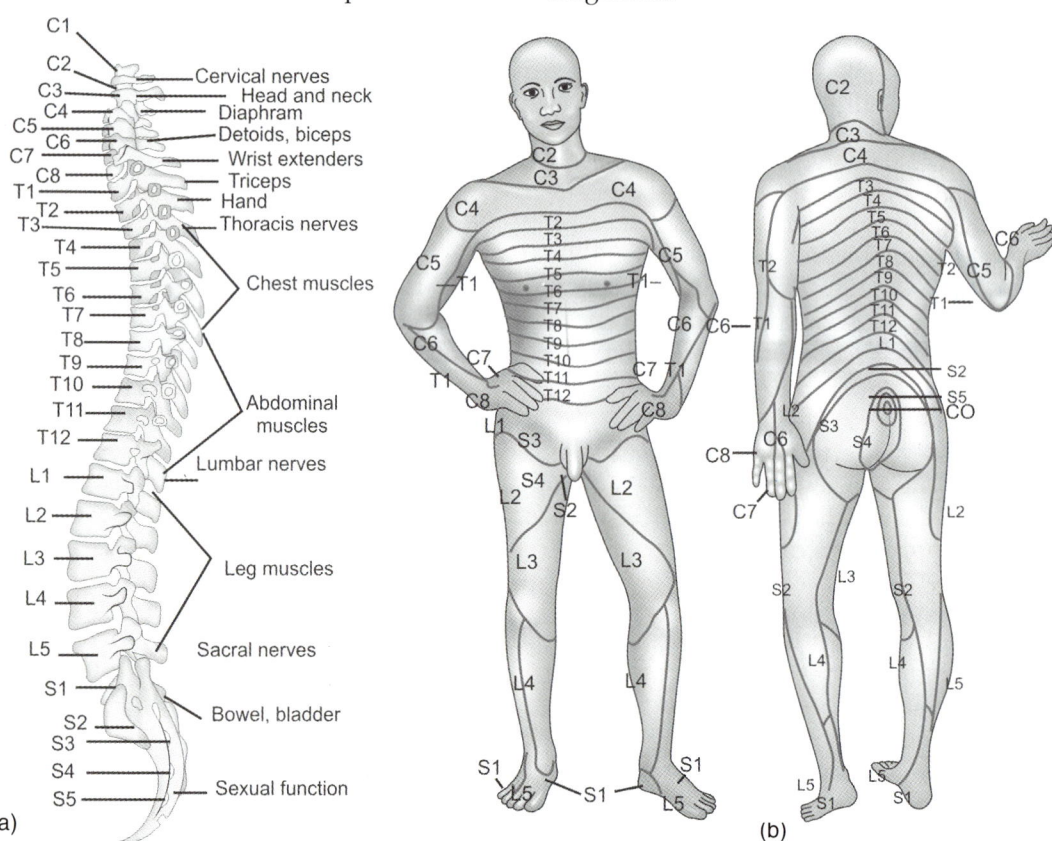

(a)   (b)

Figs 10.4a and b: (a) Myotomes (b) Dermatomes

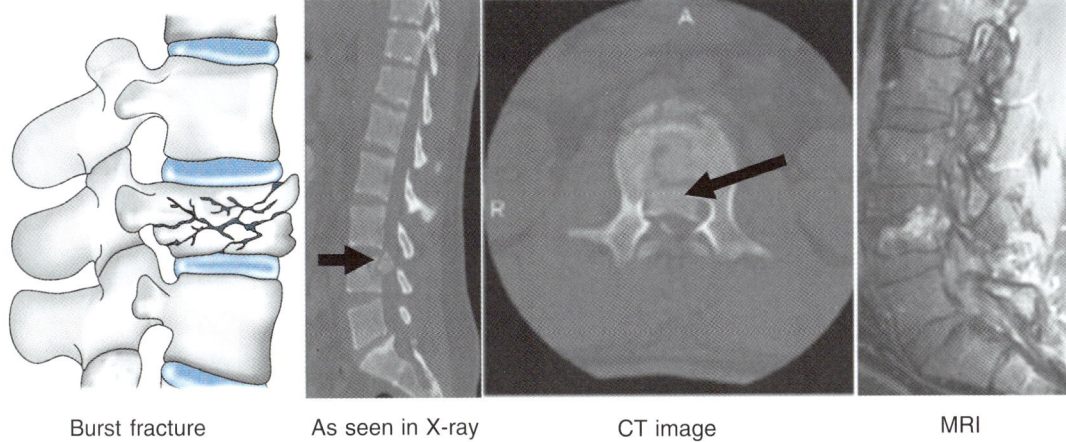

| Burst fracture | As seen in X-ray | CT image | MRI |

Fig. 10.5

- Axial load/flexion combined mechanism
  Stable: Isolated to body, less than 50% loss of height, 1 or 2 levels only
  Unstable: Posterior arch involved, or more than 50% loss of height, or more than 2 levels
  - Look for loss of height, loss of straight or anterior concave surface of body
  - *Mechanism:* FLEXION very common
  - *Neurologic injury:* Uncommon

Compression Fractures

- **Stable:** Isolated to body, less than 50% loss of height, 1 or 2 levels only
- **Unstable:** Posterior arch involved, or more than 50% loss of height, or more than 2 levels
- Look for loss of height, loss of straight or anterior concave surface of body
- **Mechanism:** FLEXION. Very common
- **Neurologic injury:** Uncommon (Fig. 10.6).

Chance Fracture

- Most common at T10–L2
- Unstable
- Neurologic injury in 15%, abdominal injury in 50% (tear of mesentery, bowel injury): always CT spine and abdomen

- Compression fracture of body and transverse posterior arch fracture
- Mechanism: FLEXION over a lap seat belt (Fig. 10.7).

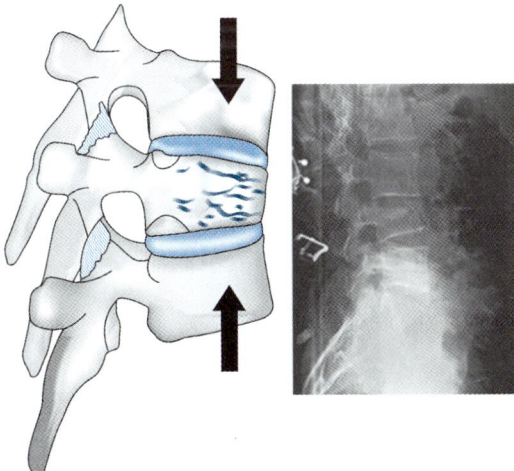

Figs 10.6a and b: (a) Compression forces (b) Compression fracture in X-ray

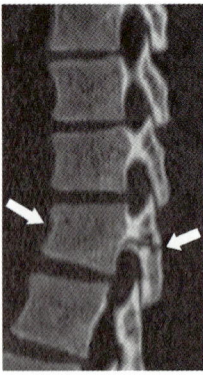 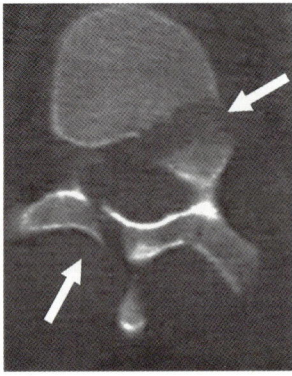

Figs 10.7a and b: (a) Chance fracture in X-ray (b) Chance fracture in CT

SEAT BELT INJURIES (Fig. 10.8)

This type of injury accounts for 6% of major spinal injuries. Caused by hyperflexion and Distraction of the posterior elements. During vehicular accidents.

COMMON SYNDROMES ASSOCIATED WITH SPINE INJURY

1. *Central cord syndrome:* Greater weakness in the upper limbs than in the lower limbs, occurs in cervical region
   • The *most common* of the incomplete syndromes

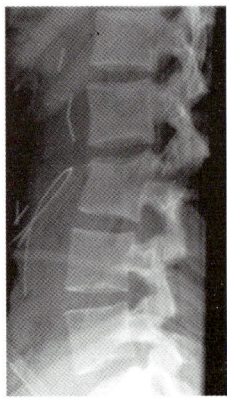

Fig. 10.8: Seat belt injuries

• Frequently seen in elderly patients with cervical stenosis
• Good prognosis for recovery but age a predictor

	<50 yr	>50 yr
• Ambulation	97%	41%
• ADLs	77%	12%
• Bowel	63%	24%
• Bladder	83%	29%

2. *Brown-Séquard's syndrome*
   • 2–4 % of all traumatic SCI (spinal cord injury)
   • Hemi-section injury of the spinal cord producing greater ipsilateral proprioceptive and motor loss with contralateral loss of pain and temperature sensation
   • Overall best prognosis for recovery
     Ambulation   75% (40% if >50 yr)
     ADLs   70%
     Bowel   82%
     Bladder   89%
3. *Anterior cord syndrome*
   • Injury involving anterior 2/3 of spinal cord with variable loss of motor function, pain and temperature, with preserved proprioception and light touch
   • Poor prognosis for recovery only 10–20% have any motor recovery and it's almost always non-functional
4. *Posterior cord syndrome*
   • *Least frequent*
   • Preserves pain, temperature, and light touch with varying degrees of motor preservation and loss of proprioception
   • Prognosis for ambulation is poor

CAUDA EQUINA SYNDROME

• Patients with lesions affecting only the cauda equina can present with polyradiculopathy in the lumbosacral area, with pain, radicular sensory changes, asymmetric LMN type leg weakness and sphincter dysfunction.

- This may be difficult to differentiate from plexus or nerve involvement.
- Lesions affecting only the CONUS MEDULLARIS cause early disturbance of bowel and bladder.

RADICULOPATHY SYNDROME

Patients with radicular involvement present with dermatomal sensory changes and with myotomal weakness. Radicular pain increases with increased intra-spinal pressure, e.g. coughing, sneezing, and valsalva manoeuvre.

Management

The management of traumatic paraplegia is prolonged and needs dedicated care givers, which includes a team of paramedical staff, physicians, orthopaedic surgeons, physiotherapists, nursing staff, and most importantly caring attendants and family members.

First aid care at the site of injury is most crucial. It is mandatory to put a cervical collar to a victim of polytrauma and the patient should be shifted with utmost care to avoid further injuries to the cord. The various stages of management roughly coincide with the natural progression of the disease:

1. Initial BLS and critical care for immediate injury.
2. Management of spinal shock.
3. Management of the bony and neurological injury as determined after detailed assessment, which can be operative or conservative.
4. Postoperative/non-operative rehabilitation and prevention of complications.
5. Concomitant management of complications and sequalae of paraplegia.
6. Rehabilitation, mobilization and occupational therapy.
7. Care must start at scene of injury to reduce injury, preserve function

8. Rapid assessment of ABC (airway, breathing, circulation)
9. Immobilize and stabilize head and neck
10. Use cervical collar before moving patient.
11. Secure head and maintain patient in supine position.
12. IV fluids
13. Catheterization of patient if urinary retention is suspected and also to monitor urine output.
14. Screening for concomitant injury to other organ systems and prompt management of any serious injury.

Treatment

Aims of treatment
  i. Avoid any deterioration of neurological status.
  ii. Achieve stability of spine.
  iii. Rehabilitate the paralysed patient.

Treatment of spinal shock
1. Maintain adequate intravascular volume
2. Maintain blood pressure (spinal cord arterial pressure).
3. Keep bladder well decompressed; attend to bowel routine.
4. Surgical stabilization if indicated or surgical decompression.
   Phase 1: Emergency care at the scene of accident or in emergency department.
   Avoid any movement of injured spine during transportation, support the neck with cervical collar.
   Log rolling of the patient should be done for change of lateral position.
   Phase 2: Definitive care depending upon stability of injury and presence of neurological deficit.

Treatment of Cervical Injuries
  i. **Ligamentous instability**
     a. *Conservative:* Skull traction by Crutch field tong (Fig. 10.9a), head-halter

(Fig. 10.9b), Minerva jacket to immobilize the cervical spine (Fig. 10.9c).

   b. *Operative:* Treatment of mainly osseous injuries is bracing while mainly ligamentous injuries are treated with posterior fusion.

   For unstable spine and persistence of subluxation, it is treated by anterior/posterior spinal fusion.

  ii. **Wedge compression:** Immobilization of spine in skull traction, Minerva jacket, 4 poster collar.

  iii. **Burst fracture:** Conservative/operative depending on neurological status and stability.

  iv. **Care of quadriplegia:** Care of back, bowel and bladder.

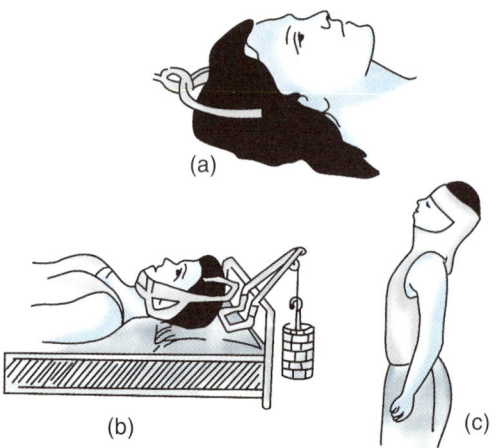

(a)

(b)   (c)

Figs 10.9a to c: (a) Crutch field tong, (b) Head halter, (c) Minerva jacket

Treatment of Thoracic and Lumbar Spine Injuries

Conservative (for stable injuries without neurological deficit)

- Bedrest, regular turning of patient, care of bladder, bowel, back (use of water-air mattress), prevent complications e.g. bed sores,

- Physiotherapy of joints,
- Use of braces (External orthosis for 8–12 weeks Serial radiographs every 2–3 weeks for the first 3 months, then 4–6 week intervals until 6 months and at 3 month intervals for 1 year)
- Orthoses: Orthoses are used to relieve pain, to support weakened or paralysed muscles and unstable joints, to immobilize the vertebral column in the best functional position, to prevent the occurrence of deformity, and to correct an existing deformity. They can be divided into two groups:

- **Supportive**
  Fabric: It is the most commonly prescribed orthosis. These orthoses encircle the sacral region and extend a variable distance upwards, the term applied to them depending on their depth posteriorly.
  – Sacroiliac
  – Lumbosacral
  – Thoracolumbar (Figs 10.10a to c).

RIGID

1. *Taylor's brace:* It limits forward flexion, extension, and lateral flexion of the thoracolumbar region of the thoracolumbar spine. It increases movement at the lumbo-sacral junction.
2. Fisher spinal brace
3. Thomas–Jones brace
4. Ash brace
5. Moulded spinal jackets.

Corrective

- Rehabilitation
  Operative (for unstable injuries/neurological deficit)
  Indications for surgery: Commonly sited indications for surgery are either
    i. Angular deformity >15–40 degrees
    ii. Canal compromise >40–70%

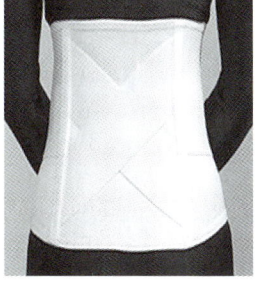

Fabric LS belt

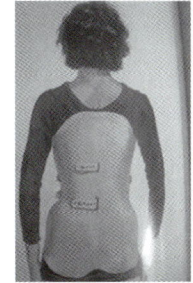

TLSO jacket

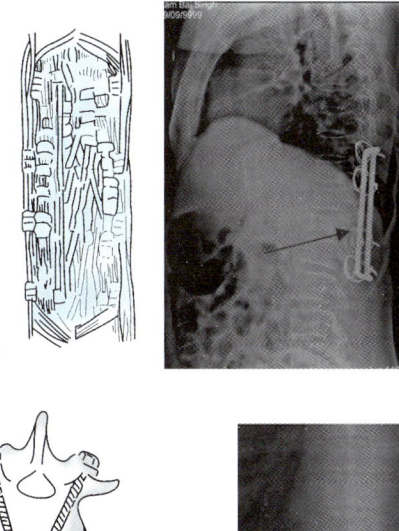

(a)

(b)

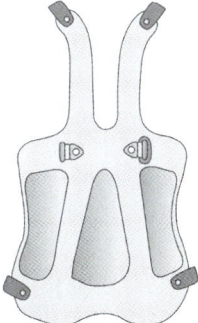

Taylor's brace

Figs 10.10a to c

iii. Worsening of neurological deficit.
iv. Partial neurological deficit with CT proven loose body in canal.
v. For better nursing care.

Principle

Decompression of cord and internal fixation by either posterior or anterior approach with fusion.

Different techniques to restore integrity of the vertebral column
1. Vertebroplasty
2. Balloon kyphoplasty
3. Specific instrumentation
   Harrington rod and sublaminar wire (Fig.10.11a).
   Hartshill rectangle fixation (Fig. 10.11b).
   Pedicle screw instrumentation (Fig. 10.11c).

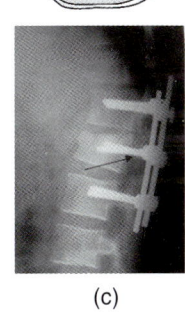

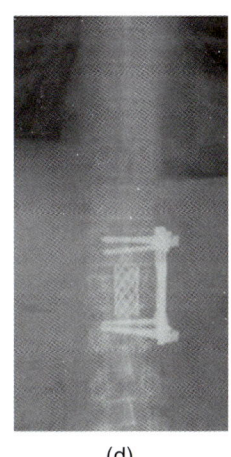

(c)   (d)

Figs 10.11a to d: (a) Harrington rod with sublaminar wire (b) X-ray showing Hartshill rectangle fixation (arrow) (c) X-ray showing pedical screw fixation (Moss miami) (d) Titanium cage and bone graft

Anterior spinal instrumentation:
Kaneda instrumentation
Anterior plate fixation
4. Anterior vertebral body excision with titanium cage and bone grafts (Fig. 10.11d).
Rehabilitate the patient keeping his physical, mental, social and occupational needs in mind.

Complications

1. *Skin breakdown:* Skin breakdown (also termed "decubitus ulcers" or "pressure

sores") are a major complication associated with spinal cord injury.

- They occur as a result of excessive pressure, primarily over the bones of buttock.
- Following a spinal cord injury, there are not only changes in muscle tone and sensation, but shift in the supply of blood to the skin and subcutaneous tissue.
- Additionally there is a loss of the normal elastic nature of the tissues underlying the skin.
- Increased stiffness, vascular alteration and alteration in muscle tone combine to significantly reduce the skin's ability to withstand pressure.

2. Osteoporosis and fractures
3. Pneumonia, atelectasis, aspiration
4. Heterotopic ossification
5. Spasticity
6. Autonomic dysreflexia
7. Deep vein thrombosis
8. Cardiovascular disease
9. Syringomyelia
10. Neuropathic pain
11. Respiratory dysfunction.

Never loose hope, patients of spinal injury have tremendous will power and can out shine normal individuals in many fields despite the handicaps (Figs 10.12a and b).

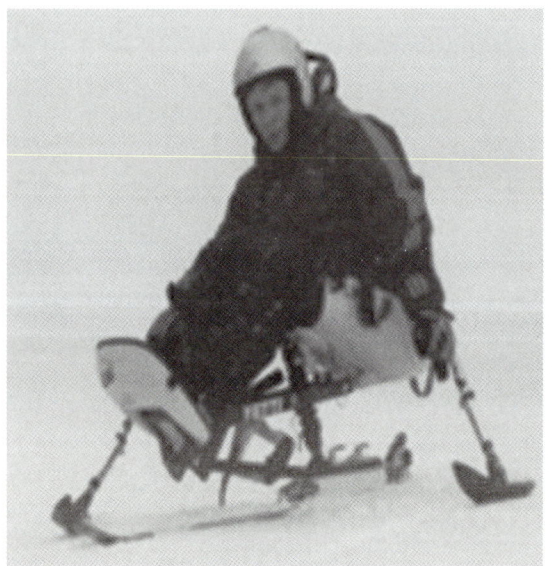

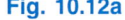
Fig. 10.12a

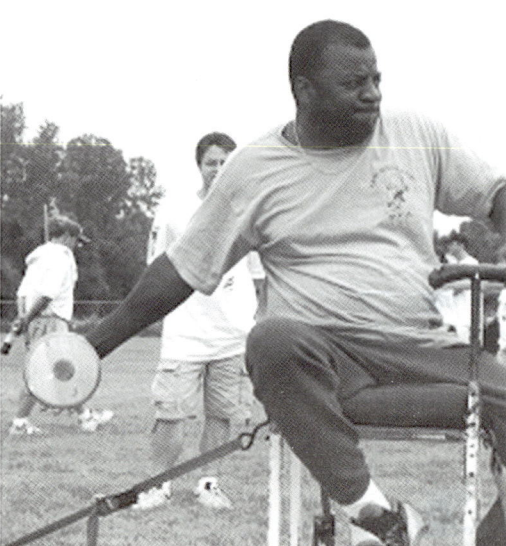
Fig. 10.12b

BRACHIAL PLEXUS INJURY (Fig. 10.13)

The brachial plexus lies in the lower part of the posterior triangle of neck, behind the clavicle, and in upper part of axilla. It is formed by anterior rami of C_5 to T_1 nerves; the first thoracic ganglion connects with T_1 ramus which carries sympathetic fibres. The plexus consists of roots, trunks, division, cords and branches (Fig. 10.13).

Roots

These are constituted by the anterior primary rami of spinal nerves C_{5-8} and T_1, with contribution from the anterior primary rami of C_4 and T_2.

Trunks

- **Upper trunk** is formed by C_5 and C_6 roots
- **Middle trunk** is formed by C_7 root
- **Lower trunk** is formed by C_8 and T_1 roots
  Each trunk divides into ventral and dorsal divisions.

Cords

- *Lateral cord:* It is formed by the union of the ventral division of the upper and middle trunks.
- *Medial cord:* It is formed by the ventral division of the lower trunk.
- *Posterior cord:* It is formed by the union of the dorsal division of all the three trunks.

Branches of the cords:

- **Lateral cords** *gives off lateral pectoral, musculocutaneous and lateral root of median nerve.*
- **Medial cord** *gives off medial pectoral, median cutaneous nerve of arm and forearm, ulnar nerve and medial root of median nerve.*
- **Posterior cords** *gives off upper subscapular, nerve to latissimus dorsi, lower subscapular, axillary and radial nerve.*

Mechanism of injury:

- *Traction:* Head fall and lateral stretching of neck, birth trauma, breech delivery

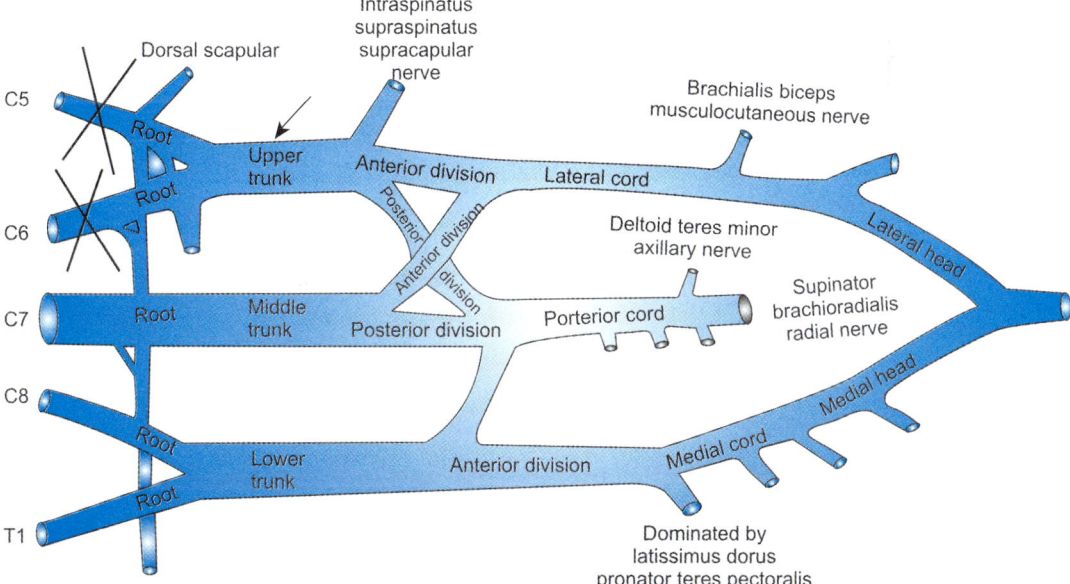

Fig. 10.13: Brachial plexus; note: arrow pointing the Erb's point

- *Compression:* Fracture clavicle, infection in the neck.
- *Penetrating injury:* Gun shot/stab injury in the neck.

Upper Cord Type
(Erb–Duchenne Paralysis C₅₋₆)

Due to obstetrical injury, traction injury, fall on shoulder joint; upper cord injury may occur (Fig. 10.14).

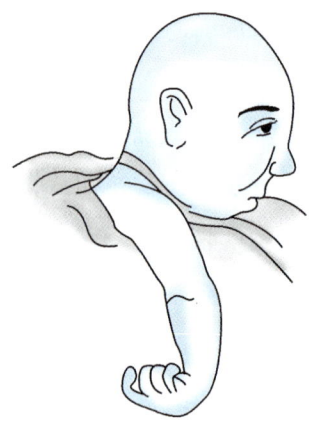

Fig. 10.14: Erb's palsy

Clinical Features

It involves injury to C_{5-6} nerve roots

- **Muscles affected are** deltoid, the biceps, brachialis, brachioradialis and supinator
- **Deformity:** The affected limb becomes internally rotated, extended at the elbow and pronated in the well-known position of '*Policeman taking a tip*'.
- There may be sensory loss over the outer side of the arm and upper part of the lateral aspect of the forearm.

Treatment

Wait and watch, recovery takes 2–3 years.
  i. **Early:** Splintage, hand to occiput position.
  ii. **Late:** If recovery is not complete, explore and repair the roots of brachial plexus.

Tendon and nerve transfers with shoulder arthrodesis should be done if hand functions are spared.

Lower Cord Type
(Klumpke's Paralysis C₈–T₁)

Such injury occurs due to forceful abduction of the shoulder, which may occur during breech presentation with arms above the head. In adult this injury may occur when a falling person clutches at an object or a person failing to obtain a foothold on a passing bus may forcefully hyper abduct his arm.

The C8 and T1, nerve roots may be affected though T1 is more often involved.

Clinical Features

Deformity

Claw hand (paralysis of the intrinsic muscles of the hand and features of combined median and ulnar nerve palsy) with anaesthesia of the innerside of the forearm, head and inner 1½ finger

Horner's syndrome: Preganglionic lesion due to avulsion of roots from the cord (Sympathetic fibres through T1 ganglion are damaged).
  i. Ptosis
  ii. Miosis
  iii. Enophthalmos
  iv. Anhidrosis
  v. Loss of spinocilliary reflex.

Prognosis
Poor

Treatment
Same as that of Erb's paralysis.

PERIPHERAL NERVE INJURY

A peripheral nerve has motor, sensory and sympathetic components. A nerve can be myelinated/unmyelinated. An axon has myelin sheath, Schwann cells and node of Ranvier. Axon collection is called funiculus, which is covered by endoneurium, some bundles are covered by perineurium and some collections are covered by epineurium.

Classification

According to Seddon
  i. *Neuropraxia:* Damage to myelin sheath—complete recovery.
  ii. *Axonotmesis:* Axon and endoneurium—variable recovery.
  iii. *Neurotmesis:* Axon, endoneurium, perineurium and epineurium are damaged, hence prognosis is poor.

Pathology

After injury, degeneration starts after 24 hours. Swelling occurs, axons break up and myelin sheath is filled with granules. After 7–8 days, macrophages creep in and engulf debris, sheath shrinks in size. Schwann cell starts multiplying and sprouting of axons from proximal nerve occurs and recovery starts.

Degeneration occurring proximally is retrograde or primary, up to first proximal node of Ranvier. Degeneration occurring distal to injury is wallerian degeneration.

The rate of recovery is 1 inch /month.

Investigations

Strength duration curve: To know the excitability of a muscle in relation to the current strength and its duration, the muscle is stimulated by decreasing the duration of the current from 300 ms to 1 ms and a consequent increase in the strength of the current required is detected and plotted on a graph as the *strength duration curve*.

Electromyography: In electromyography, the study of the electrical activity of contracting muscle gives information regarding the structure and function of the motor units.

Nerve conduction study: It is a measure of the conduction velocity of impulse in a nerve.

Stimulation of a peripheral nerve by an electrode placed on the skin overlying the nerve will readily evoke a response from the muscle innervated by that nerve. The velocity of the conduction of the impulse between any two points of the nerve can be calculated.

Faradic and Galvanic stimulation test.

Muscle power estimation done by MRC grading. This is done to assess the status of injury and measure the progress of recovery.

MRC Grading

Grade **V**   : Contraction against powerful resistance (normal and 100%).
Grade **IV** : Contraction against gravity, some resistance (75%).
Grade **III** : Contraction against gravity only (50%).
Grade **II** : Movements possible (entire range of movements) with gravity eliminated (25%).
Grade **I**   : Flicker of muscle (10%).
Grade **0**   : Complete paralysis.

Treatment
  i. **Closed injury**
     • If associated with fracture with neurological deficit, treat conservatively and reduce fracture and wait for recovery.
     • If associated with fracture and injury after manipulation, explore immediately.
  ii. **Open injuries**
     • If clean cut incised wound then primary repair is done.
     • If clean cut wound but delayed presentation then delayed primary repair is done after 5–7 days.
  iii. **If crush/contaminated wound**
     Debridement of wound and secondary repair during the intervening period, treat by splintage, passive movements of all joints.

To close nerve gaps

- Mobilization of nerve from soft tissues proximally and distally.
- Transportation of nerve subcutaneously.
- Flexing the joints, positioning of extremity.
- Bone resection.
- Nerve grafting (the most commonly used donor is sural nerve).

Guidelines for Management of Peripheral Nerve Injuries

1 **If nerve cut and exposed** ----------
   - Repair the nerve (a) **Primary** if wound clean and fresh (b) **Secondary** or delayed if wound potentially contaminated
2. **If wound closed** ----------*wait and watch* for 3–6 weeks
3. **If no recovery** by the end of 3 –6 weeks do *EMG and nerve conduction velocity*
   a. If there is no motor or sensory response and EMG shows No voluntary motor Potential, positive Positive sharp waves and fibrillation potentials ---------*Explore and repair the nerve*
   b. EMG shows Positive sharp waves, fibrillations potentials and a few voluntary muscle potentials --------- the *nerve is on its way to recovery*
   See Chapter 8 for details of EMG and NCV

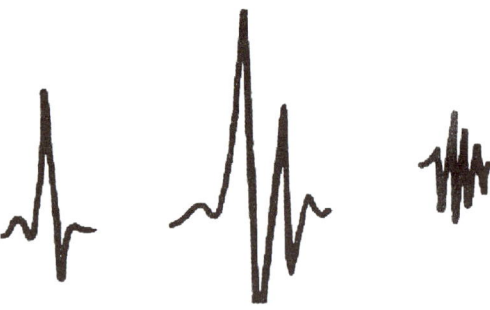

(a) Normal waves
(b) Positive waves pattern
(c) Fibrillation potentials

Prognosis

Purely motor or purely sensory nerves recover better that mixed nerve because there is less likelihood axonal confusion. Radial has best prognosis while ulnar has worst.

Axillary Nerve Injury

This nerve arises from posterior cord of the brachial plexus.

Clinical Features

i. *Weakness of deltoid:* Abduction of shoulder impaired.
ii. Sensory loss in *regimental badge area* (deltoid insertion).

Cause

Fracture and fracture dislocations around shoulder or due to injection injury.

Treatment

Conservative

RADIAL NERVE INJURY

This nerve receives twig from the C5, C6, C7, C8, and T1. This nerve is a branch of the posterior cord of the brachial plexus.

Causes

i. Fracture of humerus shaft.
ii. Gun shot and injection injury to the arm.
iii. Compression of posterior interosseous nerve.
iv. Saturday night palsy due to prolonged local pressure.

Site of injury: According to the side of the injury the various muscles will be paralyzed. As for example when the radial nerve is injured in the axilla all the muscles supplied by the radial nerve will be paralyzed and the cutaneous sensation of the regions supplied by the cutaneous branches of the radial nerve will be abolished.

When injury affects the radial nerve at the radial groove the triceps muscle escapes, similarly the posterior cutaneous nerve of arm when the posterior interosseous nerve is injured, all the muscle supplied by the radial nerve itself and the cutaneous branches escapes as also the supinator and the extensor carpi radialis brevis which are supplied before the site of injury.

Clinical Features

i. Wrist drop as shown in Fig. 10.15.
ii. Weakness of extensor of elbow, wrist, forearm, IP joints, all the fingers and thumb.
iii. Weakness of supination.
iv. Sensory loss in first dorsal web space (autonomous zone). In high radial nerve palsy triceps is also involved.

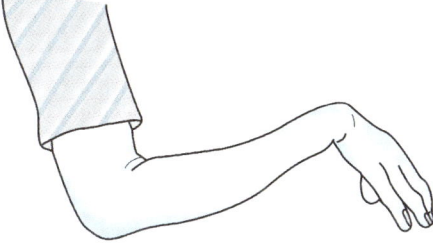

Fig. 10.15: Wrist drop

Treatment

i. **Conservative**
   Cockup splint, electrical stimulation and physiotherapy.
ii. **Surgery**
   a. **Early**
   • If incised wound with nerve injury then do repair.
   • If caught between fracture ends then exploration and internal fixation of fracture is done. Expose the nerve and repair it, if damaged.

b. **Late**
   • Bunnell's tendon transfers (flexor to extensor) at the wrist or arthrodesis of the wrist.

ULNAR NERVE INJURY

This nerve arises from the medial cord of brachial plexus comprising of C8 and T1.

Causes

i. Supracondylar fracture (malunited with cubitus valgus)
ii. Dislocation of elbow
iii. Osteoarthritis overgrowths
iv. Lacerations
v. Leprosy (leads to palsy).

TARDY ULNAR NERVE PALSY

Ulnar neuritis may occur, due to continuous stretching.

Causes

i. Cubitus valgus deformity.
ii. Rheumatoid arthritis.
iii. Chronic repetitive blunt injury.

Clinical Features

i. Claw hand: Extension at metatarsophalangeal joint and flexion at PIP joint (Fig. 10.16a).
ii. Card test positive due to paralysis of interossei.
iii. Froment's sign positive (Fig. 10.16b).

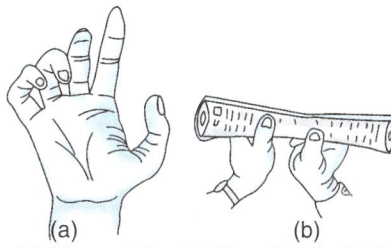

Figs 10.16a and b: (a) Claw hand; (b) Froment's sign

Flexor pollices longus (FPL) acts to overcome paralysis of adductor pollicis (AP).

iv. Sensory loss in ulnar nerve distribution (little finger and medial half of ring finger).

v. Weakness in the power of pinch.

Prognosis

Poor and recovery is usually incomplete.

Treatment

i. Splintage.

ii. Decompression of nerve and anterior transposition.

iii. If clean cut then primary repair is done.

iv. In claw hand: Tendon transfers to restore thumb adduction, pinch and grasp.

MEDIAN NERVE INJURY

This nerve arises by two roots, one from the lateral cord (C5–7) and the other from the medial cord (C8 and T1) of the brachial plexus

Causes

i. Fracture of humerus.

ii. Supracondylar fracture.

iii. Posterior dislocation of elbow.

iv. Compression neuropathy at the wrist due to carpal tunnel syndrome.

v. Volkmann's ischaemia.

Clinical Features

- **Pointing index finger:** Flexor digitorum superficialis and profundus (lateral half) are paralyzed when the median nerve is injured at the elbow or above. When the patient is asked to clasp the hands, the index finger of the affected side fails to flex. Other fingers are flexed by the medial half of the profundus muscle, which is supplied by the ulnar nerve. This test is called *Ochsner's clasping test* and the index finger, which fails to flex, is called the *'pointing index'* (Fig. 10.17).

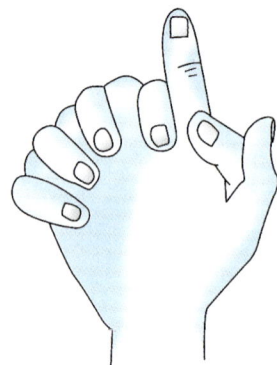

Fig. 10.17: Ochsner's clasping test *(Pointing index)*

- Weakness of flexion of wrist and opponens of thumb, thenar wasting **(Simian or Ape-like hand)**.
- **Pen test:** To test Abductor pollicis brevis. The patient is asked to lay his hand flat on the table, a pen is held above the palm and the patient is asked to touch the pen with his thumb—"the pen test". In median nerve injury the muscles will be paralyzed cell and this test will be negative.
- **Sensory loss** in autonomous zone-dorsal and volar surfaces of distal phalanges of index, middle finger (Fig. 10.17).

Treatment

- Fresh incised cut: Primary repair.
- For opponens weakness: Opponens-plasty, tendon transfers.

INTRINSIC MINUS HAND

The proximal phalanges remain fully extended. The middle and distal phalanges are partially flexed. Abduction and adduction of finger is lost, the thumb cannot be adducted or opposed across the palm. There is flattening of carpal and metacarpal arches. This is a typical claw hand (Fig. 10.16a) and is due to the involvement of ulnar and sometimes ulnar and medial nerve.

INTRINSIC PLUS HAND

This is due to contracture of intrinsic muscle (interossei or lumbricals or both). There is flexion at the metacarpophalangeal joint and extension at proximal interphalangeal joint. The thumb is similarly involved and is adducted into the palm. This is due to contracture of intrinsic muscles, collagen diseases, lumbrical over activity following severance of long flexor tendons distal to the origin of lumbrical muscle, ischaemic hand injuries (Fig. 10.18).

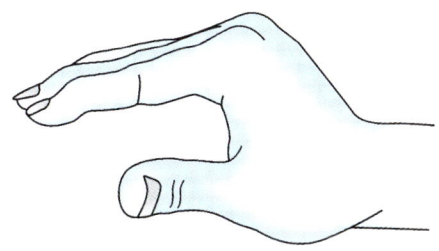

Fig. 10.18: Intrinsic plus hand

SCIATICA 'N' INJURY

The common peroneal part of the sciatic nerve is more often affected than the medial tibial part in injury to the sciatic nerve.

Causes

i. Post dislocation of hip.
ii. Lacerations around hip.
iii. Penetrating injuries.
iv. Operative procedures around the hip.

Clinical Features

i. *Foot drop:* Weakness of extensor and evertor.
ii. High steppage gait.
iii. Sensory loss along the sciatic distribution.

Treatment

i. **Conservative:** Foot drop splint.

ii. **Surgery**
   a. *Early*
   • If incised: Primary repair.
   • If gap: Nerve grafting.
   b. *Late:* Tibialis posterior tendon transfer for foot drop. Arthrodesis of ankle.

LATERAL POPLITEAL 'N' INJURY

Causes

i. Fracture of head and neck of fibula.
ii. Cut or penetrating injuries.
iii. Iatrogenic (traction, surgery).
iv. Hansen's neuropathy.

Clinical Features

i. Foot drop.
ii. Unable to stand on heels.
iii. Unable to dorsiflex ankle.
iv. Sensory loss along the distribution of the nerve.

Treatment

i. Foot drop splint.
ii. Treat the cause by decompression, neurolysis, tendon transfers, and stabilization of foot.

CEREBRAL PALSY (Little's Disease)

Cerebral palsy is due to cerebral hypoxia during pregnancy, labour or immediately after birth, causing a variety of neuromuscular incoordination with or without mental retardation.

In cerebral palsy with mental retardation (MR), the child is grossly handicapped; recovery and prognosis is very poor. Cerebral palsy can be divided into six physiological types: spastic, athetoid, ataxic, hypotonic, rigid, and mixed. Spastic cerebral palsy is the most common type, occurring in about 70% to 80% of patients with cerebral palsy. Athetoid cerebral palsy is the next most common type, accounting for about 10 to 15%

of cases. Athetoid cerebral palsy is further subdivided into five groups, each characterized by a type of abnormal posture movement: tension athetosis, dystonia, choreiform, ballismus, and rigidity.

The lesions in the brain that cause abnormality in movement or posture occur primarily in the following four areas: the cerebral cortex (spasticity), the midbrain or base of the brain (athetosis), the cerebellum (ataxia), and widespread brain involvement (mixed).

Types of Cerebral Palsy

i. Spastic 75% (due to damage to cerebral cortex).
ii. Athetotic (damaged basal ganglia) with writhling movements
iii. Ataxic (due to damage to cerebellum) with incoordination
iv. Hypotonia
v. Rigid
vi. Mixed
  The involvement may be:
i. Whole body
ii. Quadriplegia
iii. Paraplegia, hemiplegia
iv. Monoplegia

Clinical Features

i. The child has abnormal looks and gestures with clumsy movements.
ii. Delayed milestones with scissoring of legs.
iii. All the jerks are exaggerated with ankle clonus and extensor plantar reflex.
v. Mentally retarded child has abnormal facial expression, dribbling saliva, unable to sit up, stand or walk incontinence of urine, faeces, and aphonia.

The most common clinical type of cerebral palsy is spasticity resulting from an injury to the pyramidal tracts in the immature brain. An exaggerated stretch reflex is pathognomonic of spasticity. In an exaggerated stretch reflex, resistance is felt as a sudden passive movement of the muscle, followed by relaxation of the muscle. This tightening and relaxation may become cyclical, with a fast passive stretch of the muscle resulting in clonus.

The second most common clinical type of cerebral palsy is athetosis. Athetosis is a type of dyskinesia (abnormal movement caused by an extrapyramidal brain lesion). The movement disorder is one of continuous motion, and hypotonia may or may not be present. Joint contractures are not common in this type of cerebral palsy... . Athetotic cerebral palsy can be subdivided into the following five patterns.

Tension athetosis: This condition results from deposition of bilirubin in the infant's basal ganglia. In the past this was more commonly the result of erythroblastosis fetalis, which was almost completely eradicated in developed countries over the past several generations; however, this condition is being seen again. Patients with tension athetosis are hypertonic but not hyperreflexive. There are no signs of clonus or other signs of spasticity; the tension in these muscles can literally be "shaken out." Associated problems in patients with tension athetosis include deafness and absence of an upward gaze.

Dystonic athetosis: These patients are in a continuous, tortuous, slow, twisting type of motion. All extremities, as well as the neck and trunk, tend to be involved.

Choreiform athetosis: More common than dystonic athetosis, this pattern is characterized by continual movement of the patient's wrist, fingers, ankles, toes, and tongue.

Dramatic ballismus athetosis: This type is characterized by trunk flailing that persists throughout the wakened state. These patients can injure themselves or their caregivers by

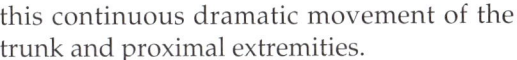

this continuous dramatic movement of the trunk and proximal extremities.

Rigid athetosis: Patients with this type are the most hypertonic of all patients with cerebral palsy, yet there are no signs of spasticity and no evidence of clonus or hyperreflexia. These patients have extreme muscle stiffness, which may be of the "lead pipe" or "cogwheel" variety. When these patients undergo tendon release or neurectomy, the orthopaedic surgeon must use extreme caution so as not to create a fixed reversal of the deformity by overweakening an agonist and allowing the muscles' antagonists to drive the patient's rigidity in the opposite direction.

Aims of treatment

Rehabilitate the child depending on his IQ level so as to make him, self sufficient for daily activities and bread earning.

Modes

i. Physiotherapy, speech therapy, occupational therapy.
ii. Surgery tendon lengthening in children with athetosis often is unpredictable, and can result create an opposite deformity that is more difficult to treat
   a. Release of contracture, especially T. Achilles, adductors of hip.
   b. Tendon transfer to restore muscle imbalance.
   c. Arthrodesis to stabilize flail joints.

POLIOMYELITIS

It is an endemic disease caused by echovirus of three types (Leon, Lancing and Burnhilde) and within 2–4 weeks of the infection, clinical manifestation occurs.

Stages

Incubation, prodromal, paralytic and residual phase. The poliovirus causes damage to brain-

stem and anterior horn cells of spinal cord. So there is LMN type of paralysis (flaccid type) with normal sensation.

It involves mainly the antigravity group of muscles.

Acute

- Stages of fever, arthralgia, malaise.
- Injection or exercise may precipitate the stage of paralysis.
- In bulbar paralysis, respiratory failure occurs.

Treatment

Rest, analgesics, respiratory assistance, warm moist packs, proper positioning and gentle physiotherapy treatment should be given.

Chronic

Causes of deformities are muscle imbalance, faulty positioning during recovery, gravity, contracture of fascia/capsule, growth disturbance due to uneven growth of epiphyseal plate.

a. *Principles of treatment*
   i. Prevention of deformities.
   ii. Re-establishment of muscle power by tendon transfer, muscle transplant.
   iii. Stabilization of loose/flail joints by arthrodesis/braces/calipers.
   iv. Release of contractures—fascia, ligaments, capsule, etc.
   v. Correction of deformity by tendon lengthening and osteotomy.
   vi. Limb length discrepancy by shoe raise, Illizarov lengthening.

b. *Surgical Management*
   i. *Upper limb*
     - *Deltoid paralysis:* Shoulder arthrodesis in 60° abduction and 30° of flexion.
     - *Wrist drop:* Arthrodesis of the wrist to improve hand functions.
   ii. *Lower limb*
     - **Hip**

– Flexion, abduction contracture corrected by Soutter's release.

– Associated pelvic/knee deformity-Yount's release of fascia lata.

- **Knee**
  – Strong quadriceps and poor hamstrings results in **genu recurvatum** which is corrected by supracondylar posterior wedge osteotomy of the femur.

  – Strong hamstrings and poor quadriceps results in flexion contracture which is corrected by hamstring release hamstring to quadriceps transfer or supracondylar anterior wedge osteotomy.

  – Biceps dominance causes **triple deformity** (flexion, external rotation, posterior subluxation) treated by soft tissue release.

- **Ankle**
  – Poor dorsiflexion and strong T. achillis results in **equinus** which is treated by T.A. release calipers (below knee with toe raising device). Tibialis post-transfer anteriorly and arthrodesis for flail ankle.

  – Poor gastrocnemius results in **Calcaneo cavus** deformity treated by transfer of tibialis anterior to T. Achilles.

- **Subtalar**
  – Varus/valgus treated by Subtalar Grice extra-articular arthrodesis and Dunn's triple arthrodesis.

- **Flail foot**
  – This is treated by plantar arthrodesis.

iii. *Spine*

Kyphoscoliosis treated by anterior/posterior spinal fusion, spinal braces.

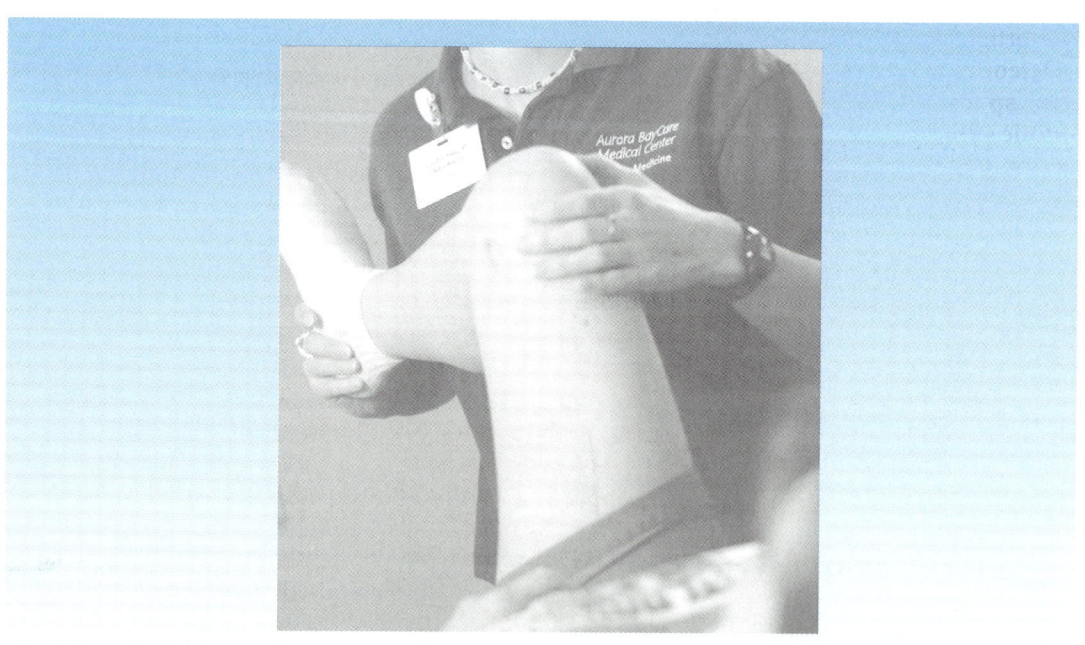

Regional Orthopaedic

SPINE

CERVICAL SPONDYLOSIS

It is a type of osteoarthritis involving the spine of the body due to degeneration of inter-vertebral disc and the posterior facet joints leading to local pain, spasm, radiculopathy and vertigo.

Osteophyte formation and reduction of canal space is seen with loss of normal lordotic spinal curvature (Fig. 11.1). *Rule out diabetes, if the changes are too advanced for the age*

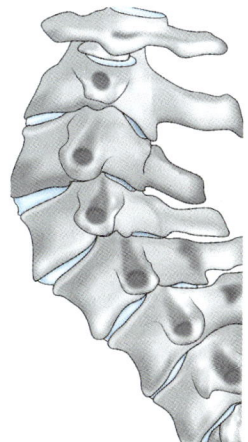

Fig. 11.1: Cervical spondylosis

of the patient. Patient may present with (a) severe radicular pain along the neck, shoulder, arm and forearm extending to the hand requiring traction (b) muscle spasm requiring muscle relaxants (c) vascular in the form of vertigo requiring stabilization by collar and drug like cinnarazine

Management

i. **Conservative:** Cervical collar, traction, anti-inflammatory drugs muscle rela-xants, injection B1, B6, B12 and cervical exercises.
ii. **Surgical:** For root or cord compression, surgery in the form of discectomy and fusion by anterior approach.

TORTICOLLIS

This is also known as **wry neck**. This is a rotational deformity of the cervical spine with secondary turning, tilting of the head, neck and face.

The common causes are congenital, acquired (post-traumatic, spasmodic, inflam-matory, neurotic, paralytic and at times ocular).

Types

Congenital torticollis: This is observed at birth, often unilateral tightness of sterno-cleidomastoid muscle with a tumorous swelling involving the muscle, which is usually a birth trauma. It may be as a result of congenital anomalies of the cervical spine like Klippel–Feil syndrome. The child usually suffers trauma of the neck during assisted delivery, soon a swelling at the junction of upper two-thirds and lower one-third of sternomastoid muscle appears. The haema-toma in due course of time shrinks and causes fibrosis of the muscles leading to the deformity. As the child grows, the deformity increases which can be seen as a tight prominent band in the neck. If this goes on unattended, secondary changes in the face starts appearing with hemiatrophy of the involved side (Fig. 11.2).

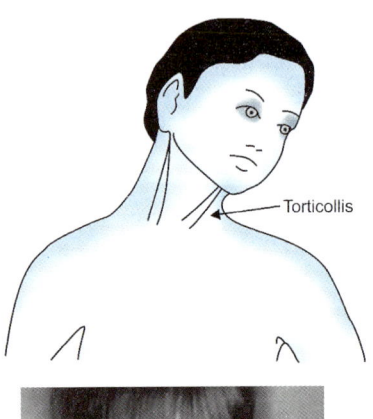

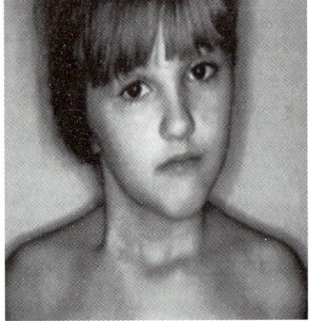

Fig. 11.2: Congenital torticollis

Treatment

In the neonates, manipulations and correction of head position by 4 post cervical collar can improve the deformity. In established late cases, bipolar release of sternocleidomastoid muscle is done.

Sometimes, following correction of the deformity, ocular problems like compensatory squint develops.

Traumatic torticollis: This is usually seen after the sprain, dislocation or fracture of the cervical spine. The patient has history of injury of the neck; spontaneous subluxation occurs in children between 6 and 12 years of age following upper respiratory infection and is the most common cause of torticollis in young children.

Miscellaneous: This is because of spasm, infection, paralysis of cervical muscle or ocular defects.

CERVICAL RIB (THORACIC INLET SYNDROME)

This causes symptoms of compression involving the lower trunk of brachial plexus and the subclavian vessels leading to pain and numbness in the shoulder and neck region which radiates into the arm with subsequent weakness and wasting. It may be due to a congenital cervical rib (Fig. 11.3) vigorous exercise or can be post-traumatic.

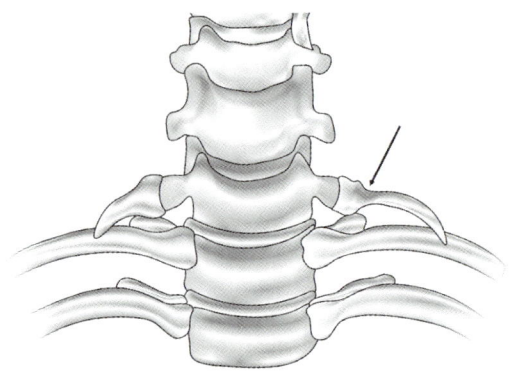

Fig. 11.3: Cervical rib (arrow)

Adson's sign (the symptoms are exaggerated by turning the chin to the affected side, hyper extending the neck and taking a deep breath, which causes obliteration of the radial pulse) is usually positive, the rib may be seen on X-ray and for neurological involvement, nerve conduction study may be done.

Treatment

i. Conservative treatment by developing the shoulder elevators.
ii. Surgical treatment by excision of cervical rib.

KYPHOSIS

This is an exaggeration of the normal spinal primary curves (dorsolumbar).

Causes

- *Congenital*
- *Developmental:* Scheuermann's disease
- *Metabolic:* Ricket, osteoporosis
- *Degenerative:* Osteoarthritis
- *Traumatic:* Wedge compression
- *Neoplastic:* Primary (osteoclastoma, eosinophilic granuloma), secondary (from gut, breast).

Types

i. *Angular:* This is due to
  a. Fracture; collapse of the vertebral body
  b. Tuberculosis of spine
  c. Secondaries.
ii. *Gentle curve:* This is due to developmental or degenerative causes
  a. Postural
  b. Scheuermann's disease (Fig. 11.4)
  c. Senile osteoporosis.

LORDOSIS

This is an exaggerated lumbar curve.

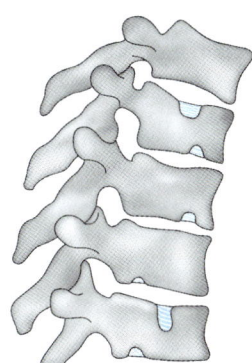
Fig. 11.4: Scheuermann's disease

Types

i. **Primary**
  This is due to:
  a. Advanced pregnancy
  b. Potbelly seen in rickets/cretinism
  c. Spondylolisthesis : Osteochondrosis of the vertebral epiphysis in children.
ii. **Secondary**
  This is compensatory type; due to:
  a. Kyphosis
  b. Flexion contracture of hip
  c. CDH, coxa vara
  d. Bilateral short tendo Achilles.

SCOLIOSIS

This is defined as lateral deviation of the spine, causing deformity, disfigurement and displacement of viscera.

The causes may be non-structural (postural, compensatory) or structural (idiopathic, congenital, neuromuscular, post-traumatic, mesenchymal disorders, etc.) (Fig. 11.5).

Types

i. **Mobile Scoliosis**
  a. *Postural:* This is usually seen in young girls with a mild curve usually convex to the left side. The important

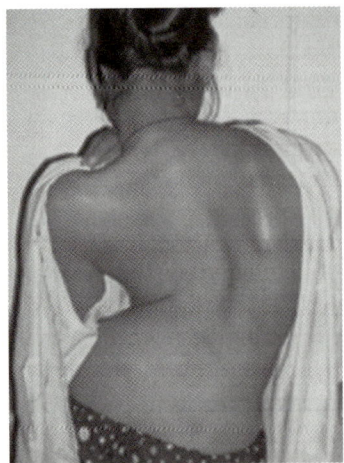

Fig. 11.5: Dorso lumbar scoliosis

diagnostic feature is that on forward bending the spine straightens completely. Recovery is spontaneous.

b. *Compensatory:* This is usually because of obvious deforming reasons like limb length discrepancy, short sternomastoid, ocular disorders and empyema.

c. *Sciatic:* This is a lateral tilt of the spine associated with lumbar disc prolapse and paraspinal spasm.

ii. **Idiopathic scoliosis**

This accounts for 75% of the cases, generally females undergoing rapid precocious growth. It may appear in the following types

a. **Infantile type:** It occurs during the first 3 years of life with male predominance having a left thoracic curve invariably resolving spontaneously.

b. **Juvenile type:** It occurs between 3 to 10 years of age with right thoracic curve equally involving both sexes (Fig. 11.6a).

c. **Adolescent type:** It occurs between 10 and 15 years of age with right thoracic and thoracolumbar curves. First occurs during growth spurt and usually progressive. The younger the child, the worse the outlook (Fig. 11.6b).

• *Simple curve:* When a single spinal deviation occurs.

• *Compound curve:* When displacement occurs in both left and right direction.

• *Primary curve:* The one which develops first.

• *Secondary curve:* The one which develops in response to balance the primary curve. When the curve is flexible and corrects by bending towards the convex side it is non-structural curve, when it fails to correct by side bending it is a structural curve, implying changes in the vertebrae in soft tissues, which have already occurred.

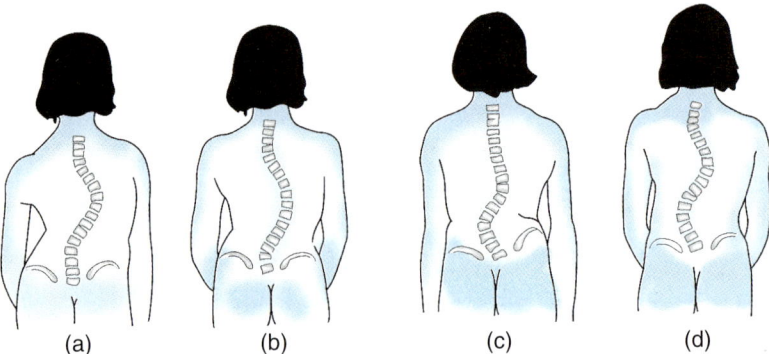

(a)   (b)   (c)   (d)

Figs 11.6a to d: Patient with kyphoscoliosis

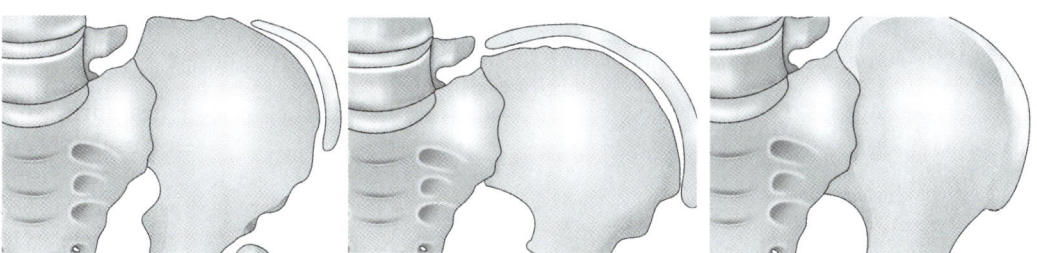

Fig. 11.7: Iliac apophysis in progressive ossification (Risser's sign)

- *A major curve* is the one with significant structural change and is the main curve of greatest degree.
- *The compensatory curves* occur in opposite direction to the major curve in an effort to balance it (Figs 11.6c and d).

When the stage of maturity is reached, the rate of spinal growth is minimum and thereby reducing the progress of deformity. The maturation is assessed by:

- Risser's sign, i.e. completion of ossification of iliac apophysis anterior to posterior (Fig. 11.7).
- X-rays of the wrist.
- Completion and fusion of vertebral apophyseal ring (Fig. 11.7).

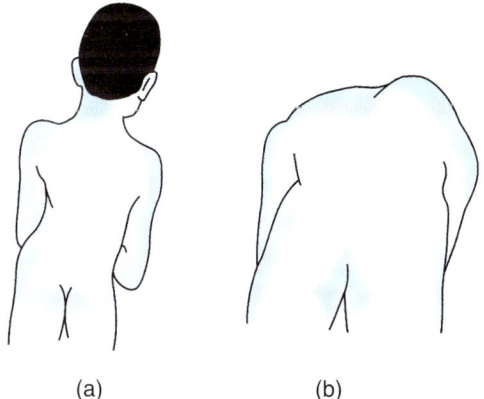

(a)   (b)

Figs 11.8a and b: **Razorback** (deformity increases on forward bending)

Clinical Features

The patient is usually a young girl with obvious deformity of the spine and ribs called the **razorback** involving the thoracic region with secondary curve in the lumbar region. This deformity increases on forward bending, as shown (Figs 11.8a and b).

One should always look for associated skin pigmentation, muscle weakness, neurological disorder, limb length discrepancy and cardiothoracic diseases.

An assessment of pulmonary function is always beneficial.

X-rays are done to see congenital anomalies, type of scoliosis and measurement of angles to decide the progress of the disease and treatment modalities.

Measurement of curve is done by following methods:

Cobb method (Fig. 11.9a): The vertebrae, with wedges on the concave side are considered, horizontal line is drawn at the superior border of the top vertebrae, and another line along the inferior border of lower vertebrae is drawn, perpendicular lines are then drawn erected from these horizontal lines and the intersecting angle is measured.

Risser–Fergusson method (Fig. 11.9b): A small dot is placed at the centre of upper and lower vertebrae and the centre of apical vertebrae. Straight lines are then drawn to join these dots and the intersecting angle is measured.

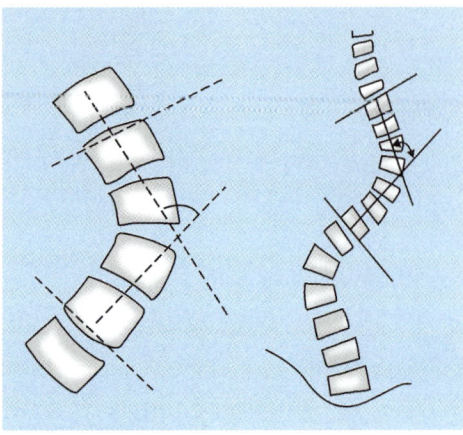

(a)   (b)

Figs 11.9a and b: (a) Cobb method (b) Risser-Fergusson method

Treatment

Protocol based on the degree of the curve and Cobb angle (Fig. 11.9c). Principles of treatment are basically aimed to prevent progress of the deformity and to correct the existing ones. Prognosis is poor in cases of neurofibromatosis and a high curve in a young child with paralytic or idiopathic curves.

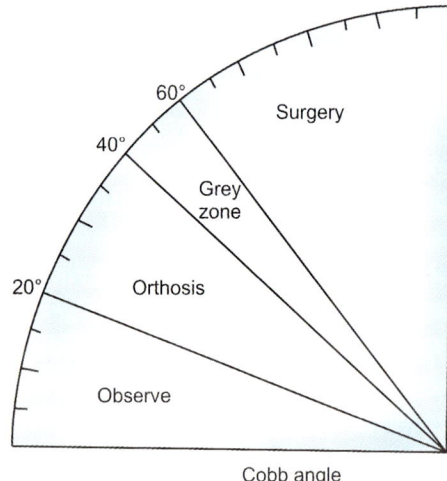

Fig. 11.9c

i. **Conservative**

Indications are as follows

a. Patient should be kept under observation.

- If the curve is less than 20° in a young child.
- Less than 40° in a skeletally matured patient.
- Non-progressive curve.

b. Halo pelvic traction (Fig. 11.10a), Risser's cast and Cotrel cast corrections.

c. Braces : It is indicated in patients who are skeletally immature, who have a progressive curve, provided it is flexible and the patient is cooperative.

Milwaukee brace: This utilizes the forces of distraction and lateral compression combined with these active corrective forces provided by exercises done in the brace. Numerous modifications have been made in the brace to increase its effectiveness and minimize the complications (Fig. 11.10b).

Newer jackets like TLSO (Fig. 11.10c), which gives an excellent fit and are cosmetically accepted. Boston's brace is also used.

It is contraindicated in curves more than 40° and thoracic lordosis. Complications of orthosis are pressure sore, skin allergy and neuralgias.

ii. **Surgery**

Indications are

a. Curves more than 50° in skeletally mature patients.

b. Curves more than 40° in skeletally immature patients.

c. Thoracic lordosis.

d. Pain, failure of brace, and cosmesis. MRI is useful to rule out bony and soft tissue anomalies prior to surgery. A complete blood and pulmonary function analysis is mandatory.

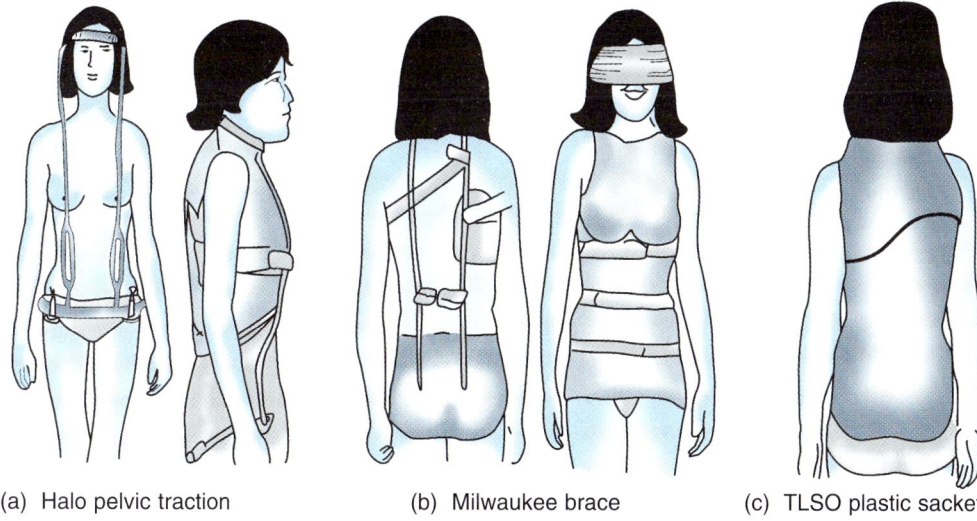

(a) Halo pelvic traction   (b) Milwaukee brace   (c) TLSO plastic sacket

Figs 11.10a to c

Preoperative Cotrel's traction correction by head halter, halo pelvic traction is useful.

- **Posterior surgical correction** by Harrington rods with intermediate wire loops and posterior spinal fusion (Fig. 11.11a).
- **Anterior Dwyer technique** is useful for lumbar and thoraco-lumbar curves, especially in paralytic ones.

In this procedure a series of wedges are excised including intervertebral discs and adjoining vertebral plates. Staples and screws are fixed to the body through which cables are tightened to correct the curve (Fig. 11.11b).

- **Other procedures:** Growth control by excision of growth plates on the convex side, electrical stimulation of muscles and excision of rib hump for cosmetic improvement.

Complications

In spite of the best surgical procedures there is always a fear of spinal cord damage at any time during or after surgery. At times acute high

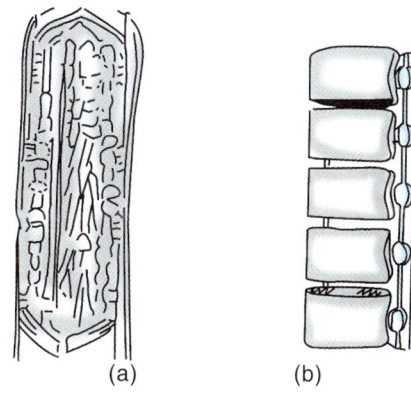

(a)   (b)

Figs 11.11a and b

intestinal obstruction, failure of implant, infection and pseudoarthrosis can occur.

SCIATICA

Pain along the sciatic nerve is often due to lumbar spondylitis, sacralization of L5, lumbar disc prolapse or peripheral neuropathy in diabetics.

Clinical Features

a. Pain may start in the lumbar zone, gluteal area, back of the thighs, calf and lateral side of the foot.
   Paresthesia along the distribution of L5 dermatome
   Straight leg rising is positive and painful.
b. Decreased power of EHL and diminished sensation in the first web indicates disc prolapse.
c. Lumbar tilt or body list (Figs 11.12a and b).

Nerve Root Compression (Table 11.1)

Investigations

i. **X-ray**
   a. *LS spine:*

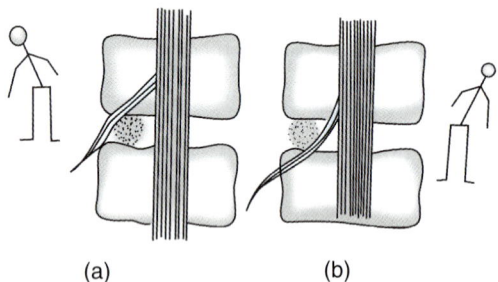

(a)   (b)

Figs 11.12a and b: (a) Paracaudal prolapse causes tilt to the same side. (b) Pararadicular prolapse causes tilt to opposite side.

- AP/Lateral view: To see degenerative spondylitis changes (Fig. 11.13a). Occasional findings are spina bifida, sacralization L5.
- Oblique view: For spondylolisthesis (Fig. 11.13b).

b. *Pelvis:* To see sacroiliac joint, secondaries, osteoporosis and systemic disease.

ii. **Myelography:** To see for disc prolapse (Fig. 11.13c).

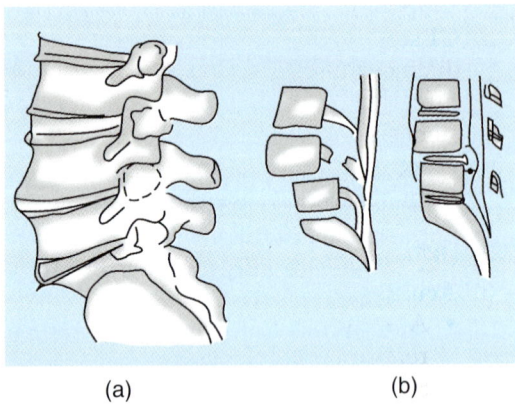

(a)   (b)

Figs 11.13a and b: (a) Degenerative spondylitis change (b) Spondylolisthesis

Table 11.1						
Disc prolapse between	Pain	Radiation	Motor loss	Sensory loss	Reflexes loss	SLRT
L3 and L4 (L4 root is involved)	Lumber region	Along the Antero-medial aspect of thigh	Quadriceps	Medial shin	Knee jerk	Normal
L4 and L5 (L5 root is involved) commonest	Lumber, sacroiliac region	Lateral thigh, leg, dorsum of the foot and hallux	Extensor hallucis muscle	Hallux area	Medial hamstrings	Reduced
L5 and S1 (S1 root is involved)	Same as above	Buttocks, posterior thigh, leg and lateral foot	Gastroc-nemius	Lateral foot	Ankle jerk	Reduced

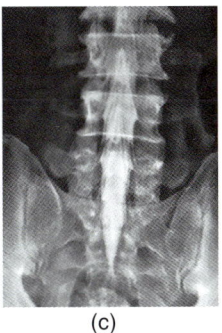 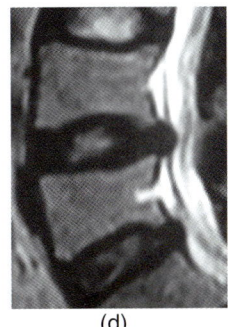

(c)   (d)

Figs 11.13c and d: (c) Myelography showing disc prolapse (d) MRI showing disc prolapse

iii. **CT scan and MRI:** For early non-invasive diagnosis of disc degeneration, prolapse, infection, tumour, and lumbar canal stenosis.

iv. **Electrodiagnostic studies:** For assessment of nerve damage.

Management

i. **Acute**
   - Absolute bedrest, analgesics, muscle relaxants, sedative, hot fomentation. Shortwave diathermy in the lumbar region, injection B1, B6, B12, pelvic traction may ensure bedrest.
   - After the pain is relieved maintain lumbar corset and spinal exercises. Working habits and lifestyle should be changed.

ii. **Chronic:** If associated with root compression.
   - *Lumbar discectomy:* Lumbar decompression by laminectomy (Fig. 11.14a), hemilaminectomy, fenestration surgery, microdiscectomy/endoscopic discectomy.
   - Stabilization for severe lumbar degeneration/spondylolisthesis by fusion which can be anterior interbody or posterior with Steffi plate and bone grafting (Figs 11.14b and c).

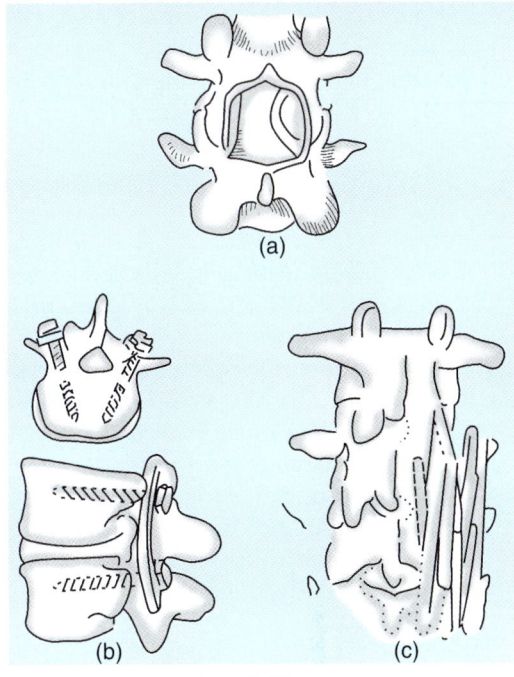

Figs 11.14a to c

In spite of best of treatment a certain amount of backache often prevails due to inadequate surgery, adhesions, and relapse.

Spondylolisthesis

This is forward slipping of the proximal part of the vertebral column on the subjacent lower vertebrae, commonly associated with a defect in the pars interarticularis, invariably appearing between L4 and L5 and at times between L5 and S1. Normally the laminae and facet form a locking mechanism, which prevents vertebral slipping.

The common causes are

i. **Dysplastic (20%):** The superior sacral facets are congenitally defective, slow but inexorable forward slip leads to severe displacements.

ii. **Degenerative (25%):** Degenerative changes in the facet joints and the discs permit forward slip (nearly always at L4-L5) despite an intact lamina.

iii. **Isthmic (50%):** Usually the lamina is in two pieces (spondylolysis) with a gap in the pars interarticularis. It is difficult to exclude a genetic factor because spondylolithesis often runs in families and is common in certain races, notably Eskimos; but the incidence increase with age, so an acquired factor probably coexists. The acquired factor is almost certainly stress; the repeated falls of the toddler or continual stress imposed in later life by the upright posture might well be the damaging forces.

iv. **The remaining 5%** of the cases comprise of traumatic spondylolisthesis following a single major injury and pathological spondylolisthesis due to bone disease or neoplasm.

SPINAL CANAL STENOSIS

Clinical Features

The patient presents with insidious onset of deformity, pain and paresthesia involving the L5 root invariable and at times L4/S1. There is usually numbness and tingling over the great toe with weakness of extensor hallucis longus (EHL).

The patient has a stiff back with limited lumbar movement and a positive step sign at L4–L5 junction with symptoms of sciatica.

A large number of industrial patients are malingerers due to occupational problems, they will have changing site and pattern of pain and its character.

For malingerers see for Aird's/Magnuson's test, which is usually positive.

X-ray

i. **Spondylolysis:** A defect in the pars interarticularis but no slipping (collar around the dog's neck picture) (Fig. 11.15a).

ii. **Spondylolisthesis (forward slip)**
   a. *First degree:* Less than 25% of forward slip (Fig. 11.15b).
   b. *Second degree:* 25%–50% of slipping.
   c. *Third degree:* More than 50% of slip with anterior subluxation.
   d. *Fourth degree:* More than 75% slip with eburnation of the anterior third of lower vertebrae (Fig. 11.15c).

Treatment

i. **Conservative:** Spinal exercise and braces.
ii. **Surgical:** Spinal decompression, reposition of displaced vertebrae, posterior spinal fixation by pedicle screws and fusion by bone grafts (Figs 11.16a and b).

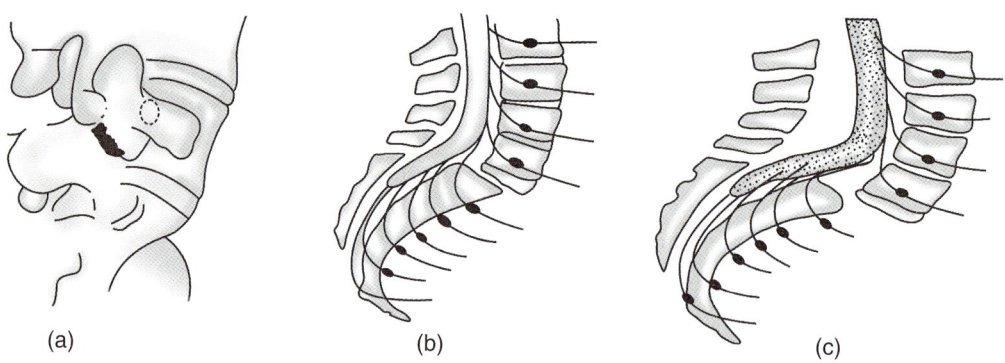

(a) (b) (c)

Figs 11.15a to c: (a) Spondylolysis, (b) first degree, (c) fourth degree

LOW BACK PAIN

A continuous pain in the lower back or lumber region. This is perhaps the price we pay for being erect and a large number of causes are responsible for it. They may be broadly grouped as under:

 i. Vertebral (10 %)
   a. *Congenital:* Spina bifida.
   b. *Developmental:* Spondylolisthesis.
   c. *Inflammatory:* Tubercular, pyogenic spondylitis.
   d. *Degenerative:* Osteoarthritis of the lumbar vertebrae.
   e. *Tumorous:* Primary, secondary deposits.
   f. *Trauma:* Causing fracture and ligament injuries.
 ii. Lumbar disc degeneration and subsequent prolapse (85 %).
iii. *Sacroiliac joint:* Strain, degeneration, infections.
iv. Myofascial inflammation and strain.
 v. *Metabolic:* Osteomalacia, senile osteoporosis.
vi. Diabetes mellitus, Paget's disease, rheumatoid, ankylosing spondylitis.
vii. Peripheral neuropathy, compression radiculopathy (disc prolapse).
viii. *Psychosocial and occupational:* In labourers and industrial workers.
ix. Spinal canal stenosis.
 x. *Referred:* Renal, colon, tubo-ovarian, paraspinal abscess.
   It is important to take a detailed history, thorough clinical examination and relevant investigations like X-ray, CT scan, myelography, MRI, etc. to reach the appropriate diagnosis.

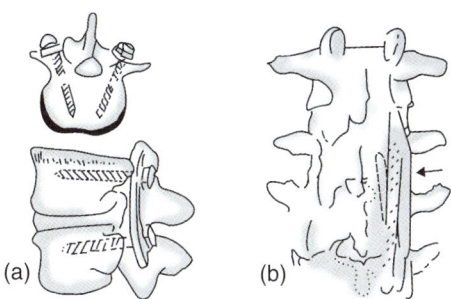

Figs 11.16a and b: (a) Spinal fixation (by pedicle screws) (b) Spinal fusion (by bone grafts)

Treatment is directed at **rest** and **relief of pain** by:
   a. Managing the basic cause.
   b. Spinal strengthening exercises, spinal braces, physical therapy.
   c. Analgesics, muscle relaxants, local steroid and analgesic injections.
   d. *Surgery:* (Decompression and stabilization) for the following conditions:
     • Infection: Tubercular, pyogenic.
     • Instability: Due to trauma, spondylolisthesis, degenerative.
     • Compression: Disc prolapse, tumours.

NEW IN THE TREATMENT OF LOW BACKACHE

• MISS (Minimally invasive spinal surgery): It consists of endoscopic spine surgery discectomy.
• Laser discectomy
• Percutaneous discectomy
• Total disc replacement: using a prosthetic disc nucleus. It has a hydrogel core and is encased in a polyethylene jacket. It restores disc height and ensures normal range of mobility.

UPPER LIMB

PERIARTHRITIS/FROZEN SHOULDER

This is due to post-traumatic immobilization or as a part of cervical spondylitis, there is terminal limitation of shoulder movement. Overhead abduction and rotation is limited and painful.

Phases

Initially there is excruciating pain and limitation of movements. Over a period of time, the pain gradually subsides and the patient develops a frozen shoulder in which the patient is unable to lift up the arm or brush his back. The pain at times disturbs the patient's sleep (Fig. 11.17).

Treatment

i. **Early:** Analgesics, hot fomentation, short-wave diathermy and physiotherapy.
ii. **Late:** Treated with intraarticular steroid injections and mobilization of shoulder.

PAINFUL ARC SYNDROME

This is painful abduction of shoulder between 45° and 160°.

The causes are
i. Supraspinatus tendinitis, partial tear of supraspinatus tendon, calcific tendinitis.
ii. Subacromial bursitis.
iii. Osteoarthritis of acromioclavicular joint.

Treatment is local fomentation, steroid injections and physiotherapy.

TENNIS ELBOW

This is due to tear and subsequent inflammation of the common extensor origin at the lateral epicondyle, usually following strain of the extensors. There is tenderness at the lateral condyle which radiates down the forearm and incapacitates the person even to lift small objects. Positive Cozen's sign and Mill's manoeuvre.

Treatment is in the form of hot fomentation, ultrasonic therapy, local steroid injection and in recalcitrant cases surgical excision of the origin of extensor carpi radialis brevis.

MADELUNG'S DEFORMITY

This deformity develops during puberty, consists of volar curving of distal end of radius carrying with it the carpus forward leaving the ulna behind (Fig. 11.18). The cause is retarded

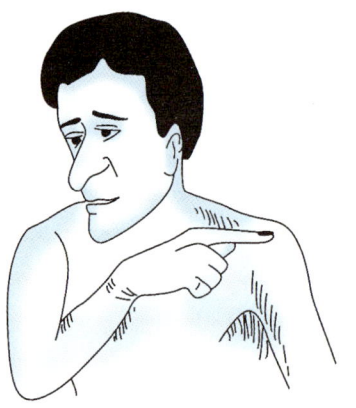

Fig. 11.17

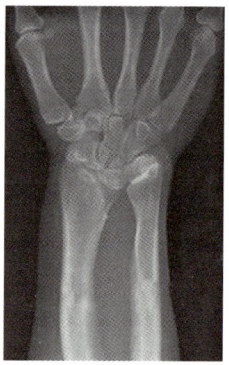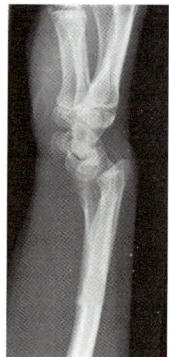

Fig. 11.18: Madelung's deformity

asymmetric growth of the distal radial epiphysis leading to presentation of deformity between 10 and 15 years in females, often bilateral. Usually presents as progressive deformity, pain, muscle cramps and feeling of weakness. At times audible clicks during wrist movement.

Treatment

Surgical excision of lower end of ulna and wedge-corrective osteotomy of radius.

CARPAL TUNNEL SYNDROME

Definition

Syndrome characterized by the compression of median nerve as it passes beneath the flexor retinaculum at wrist leading to excruciating pain in the palm, especially in the thumb and index finger as well as atrophy of the thenar muscles.

Causes

i.	**Idiopathic**	: Most common.
ii.	**Inflammatory**	: Rheumatoid arthritis, osteoarthritis.
i.	**Post-traumatic**	: Bone thickening after Colles' fracture.
i.	**Systemic**	: Myxoedema, diabetic neuropathy, acromegaly.

Clinical Features

Middle-aged women, complaining of tingling, numbness or discomfort in the thumb and radial two and a half fingers. The symptoms are excruciating at night and after kitchen work.

Phalen's test: Flexing the wrist causes median nerve compression and precipitates the symptoms.

Investigations

Nerve conduction study shows delayed or absence of conduction of median nerve at the level of wrist.

Treatment

Rest, splintage and injection of steroid in the carpal tunnel. Surgical decompression of median nerve is done by dividing the flexor retinaculum.

de QUERVAIN'S TENOSYNOVITIS

Characterized by pain and swelling over the radial styloid process due to inflammation of the common sheath of abductor pollicis longus and extensor pollicis brevis tendons.

Clinical Features

Tenderness over the radial styloid process with small tender bony hard lump.

Finkelstein's test: If wrist is passively adducted or thumb is ulnar deviated, pain increases.

Treatment

i. Early stage of treatment: Rest, analgesics, ultrasonic radiation, injection of hydrocortisone.

ii. In chronic cases, slitting and excision of common tendon sheath of abductor pollices longus and extensor pollices brevis. *Take precautions to avoid damage to the superficial branch of radial nerve.*

GANGLION

Herniation of the synovial lining of a joint or tendon as a cystic lesion arising from the dorsum of the wrist or palmar crease, sometimes from the dorsum of the foot or along any tendon generally following trauma.

It appears as a small peanut size swelling which is tense and gradually increases in size, fixed to the deeper structures, smooth surface with free overlying skin. Pain is continuous and aggravates with joint movements and strain (Fig. 11.19).

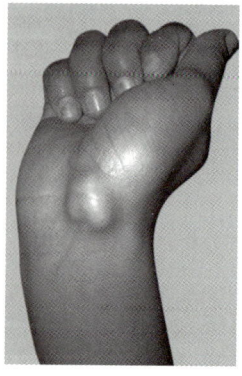

Fig. 11.19: Ganglion at the wrist joint

Treatment

The cyst may be aspirated and then infiltrated with hydrocortisone. Threading can also be done with the help of non-absorbable suture. The main aim is to re-epithelize the track. The best treatment is excision followed by repair of the capsule and a plaster support for about two weeks.

DUPUYTREN'S CONTRACTURE

This is hypertrophy and nodular contracture of palmar aponeurosis with consequent flexion deformity of the distal palm and fingers (Fig. 11.20). This disease starts, in the second decade, invariably following trauma and has a familial tendency. It is usually bilateral, starts as a small nodule in the palm and gradually progressive involvement of the palmar fascia and the overlying skin, which becomes adherent. The medial three fingers

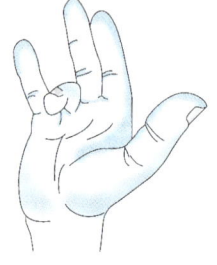

Fig. 11.20: Flexion deformity of the distal palm and fingers (Dupuytren's Contracture)

are more severely involved. The patient usually comes with pain, deformity and loss of hand function. ***Rule out diabetes.***

Treatment

Surgery is the only answer requiring excision of the thick fibrous facial bands and nodules, partial or complete in the form of fasciectomy with Z-plasty of the involved skin.

MALLET FINGER

This is due to avulsion of the extensor tendon at the base of the distal phalanx causing inability to extend the distal phalanx which in due course ends up with a flexion deformity of the terminal phalanx (Figs 11.21a and b).

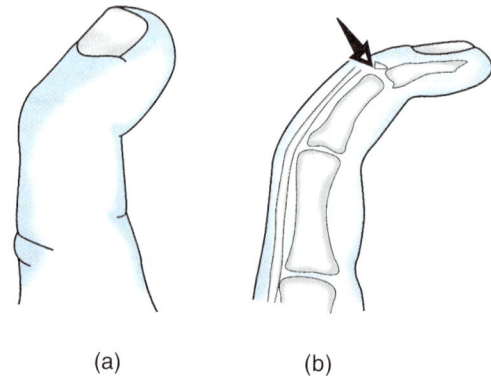

(a)   (b)

Figs 11.21a and b: (a) Flexion deformity of the terminal phalanx (b) Avulsion of the extensor tendon at the base of the distal phalanx

It is best treated in a frog splint which keeps the proximal interphalangeal joints in flexion and the distal joint in hyperextension so as to repose the avulsed tendon along with its bony insertion in the distal phalanx. This is kept for 3 weeks.

PERTHES'S DISEASE/COXA PLANA

This is avascular necrosis of the ossification centre of the capital femoral epiphysis occurring in children. This is a progressive but self-limiting disease in which the head of femur undergoes necrosis, resorption and replacement, resulting in a deformed head with restricted movement.

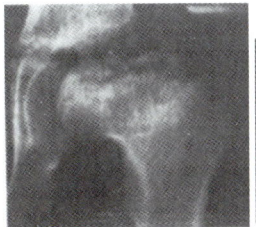 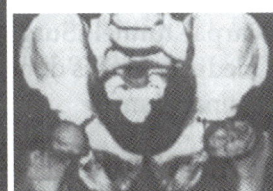

(a) X-ray   (b) 3D CT scan

Clinical Features

Usually starts around 5 years of age in a male child bilateral in about 15% (following trauma). The child presents with limp, pain and stiffness of the hip, which gradually progresses.

Examination reveals a tender hip with severe muscle spasm with restriction of all movements. For early diagnosis MRI is very helpful.

X-ray shows a wide range of changes depending on the stage of the disease (Fig. 11.22a).

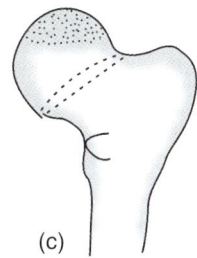

(c)

Figs 11.22a to c: (a) Increased joint space with slight lateral subluxation (Gage's sign); Segmental fracture of the superolateral aspect of the head, (b) 3D CT scan feature as discussed in X-rays (c) Avascular necrosis and anterolateral segmental collapse of the femoral head (schematic diagram)

i. **Early**
  a. Increased joint space with slight lateral subluxation.
  b. Failure of the ossification centre to increase.
  c. A convex, rounded enlargement of superior margin of the femoral neck (Gage's sign), segmental fracture of the superolateral aspect of the head.

ii. **Late**
  a. Avascular necrosis and anterolateral segmental collapse of the femoral head.
  b. Entire ossific centre becomes necrotic, fragmented, deformed, flattened, mushroomed, broadened, etc.
  c. The neck becomes short and wide with rarefaction of the metaphysis below the growth plate.

  d. Early osteoarthritic changes of the hip and symmetrical adaptive changes in the acetabulum occur depending on the deformity of the head.
  e. **Cattell** has classified the changes in the head of the femur as seen radiologically into 4 groups :
  1. Epiphysis damaged on the anterior part but no collapse.
  2. Sequestration and collapse of the above.
  3. The entire epiphysis is damaged except the small posterior segment (head within the head picture).
  4. Collapse of the entire head seen as a linear opacity completely replacing the head with severe metaphyseal changes.

Treatment

i. **Early:** This is basically aimed at an effort to preserve the containment of the head, eliminate load bearing initially and mobilize the hip and ambulation in abduction.

ii. **Late:** Patients usually come with deformity of the neck and osteoarthritic changes due to the damaged head and acetabulum.

Femoral varus-rotation osteotomy is advised in early cases, in late cases THR is done.

SLIPPED CAPITAL FEMORAL EPIPHYSIS (Muller's Disease)

This is seen in young chubby boys during the growth spurt around 15 years, usually following trauma with bilateral involvement in 25% cases. The femoral epiphysis along with the head of femur gradually slips backwards and ultimately separates.

The child usually presents with pain, limp which becomes gradually progressive.

On examination, the child has abduction, external rotation deformity and real shortening with a positive Trendelenburg sign and in bilateral involvement a typical **waddling gait**.

X-ray: AP view of the hip will show that the **Klein's line** (along the upper border of the neck of femur) passing above the head of femur, due to the slip **(Trethowan's sign)** (Fig. 11.23b). Normally it cuts through the upper third of the head of femur (Fig. 11.23a). Skiagram taken in frog leg position shows slipping of the epiphysis.

Treatment

i. **Early stage:** Fixation by Knowle's pins.
ii. **Late cases:** Wedge correction osteotomy of the neck of femur.

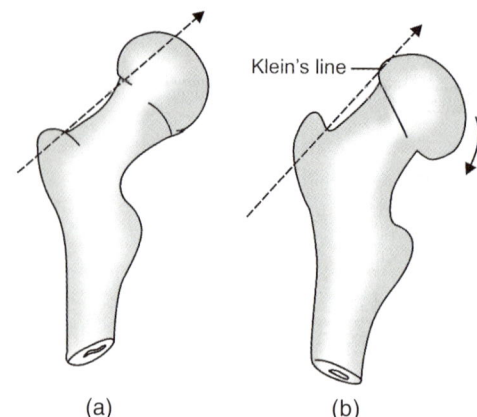

Klein's line

(a)   (b)

Figs 11.23a and b: (a) Normal (b) Slipped

PAINFUL KNEE

Chondromalacia Patellae

This is commonest cause of anterior knee pain in young women usually following prolonged sitting. On clinical examination, there is medial retropatellar tenderness, obvious patellar lesion and loose body can be seen on X-ray and arthroscopy. It is treated by arthroscopic shaving of the damaged patellar cartilage and if necessary removal of the loose body.

Recurrent Subluxation of Patella

This is due to the tight lateral retinaculum causing the patella to subluxate laterally in flexion, causing severe pain and discomfort in young girls with mild knee valgus, a high riding patella or hypotrophic lateral femoral condyle.

Treatment

a. Campbell's procedure (lateral retinacular release with medial double breasting).
b. Shifting of the insertion of ligamentum patellae proximally.

Fat-Pad Syndrome

This is due to inflammation and impingementation of the fat pad around the ligamentum patellae.

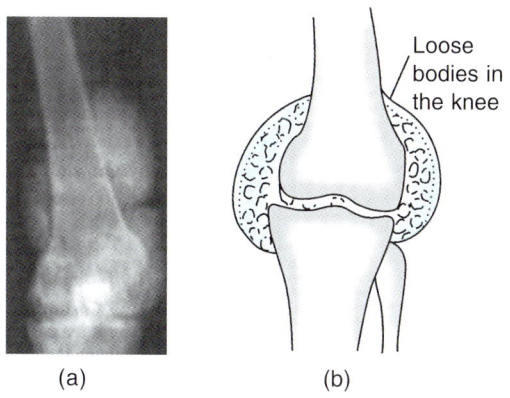

(a)   (b)

Fig. 11.24: Multiple loose bodies as in case of synovial osteochondromatosis

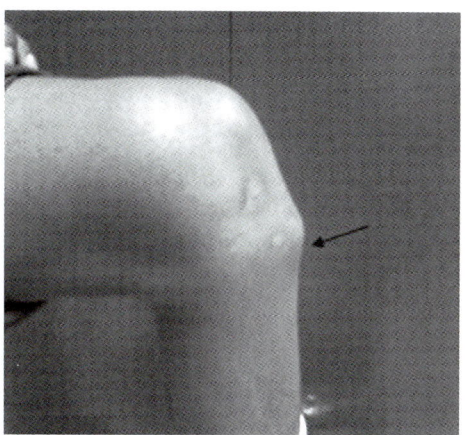

Fig. 11.25: Clinical photo of Osgood–Schlatter disease

Loose Bodies in the Knee (Fig. 11.24)

Patient presents with features of acute pain, effusion and recurrent locking. The loose bodies may be (a) **few** as in cases of intra-articular chip fracture, chondromalacia patellae, osteoarthritis or may be (b) **multiple** as in case of synovial osteochondromatosis/villonodular synovitis and neuropathic joint.

Investigation

X-ray shows multiple loose bodies like a bunch of grapes or solitary one. Keep in mind "fabella". This is an ossification in the lateral head of gastrocnemius.

Treatment

Arthroscopic removal of loose bodies.

Osgood–Schlatter Disease

This is apophysitis involving the tibial tuberosity, common in young boys of adolescent age, preventing with pain and progressive

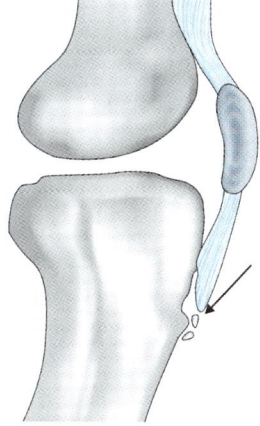

Fig. 11.26: Schematic diagram to show avulsion

swelling in the area of insertion of the ligamentum patellae (as shown below), X-ray shows avulsion and fragmentation of the tuberosity in different stages, the condition is self limiting and need assurance, rest and limitation of outdoor sports. A knee immobilizer and analgesics often helps.

In advanced cases surgical excision of the fragments and fixation of the tuberosity may be required (Figs 11.25 and 11.26).

PAINFUL FOOT

i. **Forefoot pain:** This is usually due to hallux valgus, hallux rigidus, hammer toes, splayed foot, ingrowing toenail, paronychia and plantar corns.

ii. **Metatarsal pain:** After a stress fracture of 2/3 metatarsal, Morton's metatarsalgia (neuritis involving digital nerves between 3/4 toes), Freiberg's disease (crushing osteochondritis of 2nd/3rd metatarsal head).

iii. **Midfoot:** Pes cavus, flat foot, plantar fascitis, varicose veins.

iv. **Hindfoot:** Calcaneal spur (heel pad), tendo Achilles bursitis, is usually due to gout, diabetic tendonitis.

- *Painful heel/Plantar fasciitis:* Pain at the heel is due to inflammation of the plantar fascia due to overweight, faulty footwear, long hours of standing or diabetes mellitus. Skiagram may show calcaneal spur. Management is alternate hot/cold dip, ultrasonography and padded heel in the footwear or local hydrocortisone injection.

- *Hallux valgus:* This is a valgus deformity of the metatarsophalangeal joint. The first metatarsal is in varus position while the proximal phalanx deviates laterally. The head of the first metatarsal becoming prominent with overlying skin and soft tissue developing recurrent bursitis (Bunion) and callosity (Fig. 11.28a).

This may be congenital or acquired as a result of gout or faulty footwear.

Treatment

Conservative: by splints (Fig. 11.27)

Surgical

i. **In young patients**
   a. Simmonds' procedure, which requires osteotomy of first metatarsal and wedge resection of the medial side of the first metatarsal head (Fig. 11.28 b).
   b. Wilson's operation: Oblique osteotomy through the distal third of the metatarsal (Fig. 11.28c).

ii. **In Adults**
   a. Bevelling of the medial prominence of the metatarsal head (Fig. 11.28d).
   b. *Keller's operation:* Excision of proximal third of the phalanx and prominent portion of the metatarsal head, combined with proximal metatarsal osteotomy (Fig. 11.28e).
   c. *Mayo's operation:* Excision of metatarsal head and prominent part of proximal phalanx (Fig. 11.28f).

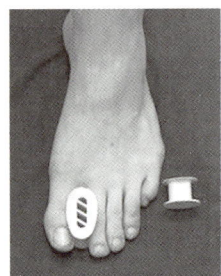 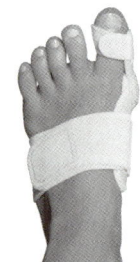

Toe spreader   Hallux valgus splint

Fig. 11.27: Splints used in hallux valgus

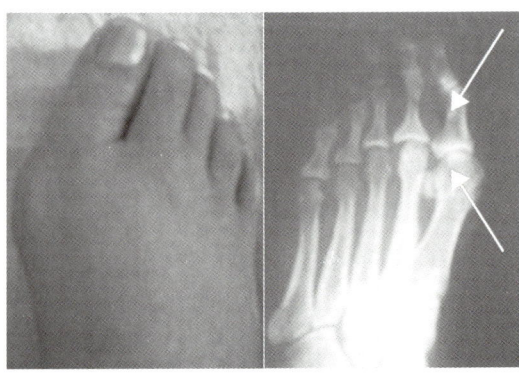

Fig. 11.28a: Hallux valgus

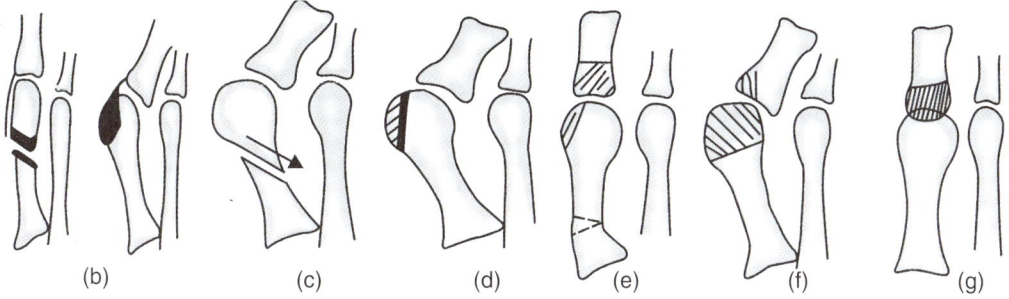

Figs 11.28b to g: (b) Simmonds' procedure, (c) Wilson's operation, (d) Bevelling of the medial prominence, (e) Keller's operation, (f) Mayo's operation, (g) Arthrodesis

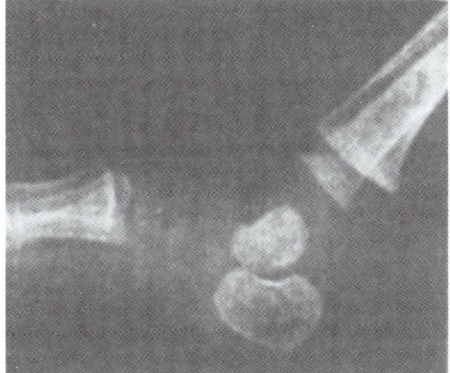

Fig. 11.29: Congenital vertical talus

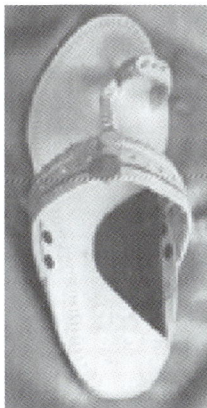

Fig. 11.30: Arch support footwears

d. *Arthrodesis:* Surgical refashioning of the deformed joint and fusion (Fig. 11.28g).

In spite of all treatments, the most important thing is attention to proper footwear.

Pes Cavus

This is exaggerated medial arch of the foot, with clawing of the toes in the severe form. The causes may be myopathy, neuropathy or muscle imbalance.

Treatment in young children is by suitable footwear, exercises. In adults, Steindler's release of plantar fascia and if necessary Japa's 'V' dorsolateral wedge tarsectomy.

Pes Planus

This is flat foot due to collapse of the medial arch seen in, congenital vertical talus (Fig. 11.29), physiological in toddlers, paralytic in polio, compensatory to genu valgum, spasmodic as a result of muscle spasm, or acquired following trauma or diseases.

Detailed history, clinical examination and relevant investigations are necessary to understand the pathology involved and plan correction. Treatment is aimed at arch support (Fig. 11.30) in the footwear, inversion exercises and if necessary surgical correction.

12

Congenital Anomalies

CONGENITAL ANOMALIES

The anomalies may be broadly grouped as under.

Absence

i. *Amelia:* The congenital absence of a limb or limbs.
ii. *Phocomelia:* A congenital malformation in which limb represented as short stubs – only hand, fingers.
iii. *Hemimelia:* Absence of part of limb-transverse, axial-medial, lateral or ectromelia.

Extra

i. *Polydactyly:* A developmental anomaly characterized by extra fingers, toes, thumb.
ii. *Syndactyly:* Common congenital anomaly of fused fingers and toes.

Upper Limb

i. *Cleidocranial dysostosis:* There is defective ossification of the membranous bones involving vault of skull, maxilla, clavicle, etc.
ii. *Sprengel's deformity:* Undescended scapula or congenital elevation of scapula.

iii. *Syndactyly or polydactyly*
iv. *Radioulnar synostosis:* Fusion of radio-ulnar joint completely/incompletely
v. *Radial club hand:* Absence of radius and radial ray, i.e. thumb
vi. *Lobster claw hand:* Cleft hand.

Lower Limb

1. *CDH:* Dysplastic hip joint.
ii. *Coxa vara:* Reduced neck shaft angle.
iii. *Pseudoarthrosis of tibia:* Kyphos-coliotic tibia with non-union of fractured tibia.
iv. Congenital absence of tibia.
v. CTEV.
vi. *Flat foot:* A condition in which the medial arch of the foot is flat developmentally or due to congenital vertical talus.
vii. Syndactyly, lobster foot and polydactyly.

Spine

i. *Torticollis:* Damaged sternomastoid muscle leading to bent, rotated neck.
ii. *Klippel–Feil syndrome:* Fused lamina of cervical spine with short webbed neck.
iii. *Spina bifida:* Developmental anomaly in the spinal column, involving the posterior arch of vertebra.

Joints

- *Stiff:* Arthrogryposis multiplex congenita (multiple deformities, stiff joints, and CTEV).
- *Lax:* Marfan's syndrome.
- *Rigid:* Cerebral palsy.

CLUB FOOT

Club foot is a complex congenital anomaly still incompletely understood and hence a wide-ranging etiopathology and equally large number of surgical variations are seen.

Relevant Anatomy

To understand the aetiology and/or management of clubfoot, it is essential to know relevant anatomy, which can be divided into related joints, ligaments, and tendons.

Joints

Joints related to clubfoot are

Ankle joint: Synovial joint of hinge variety.

- The upper articular surface is formed by (i) the lower end of tibia including the medial malleolus; (ii) the lateral malleolus of the fibula; and (iii) the inferior transverse tibiofibular ligament.
- The inferior articular surface is formed by articular areas on the upper, medial and lateral aspects of talus.

Subtalar or talocalcanean joint is a plane synovial joint between the concave facet on the inferior surface of the body of the talus and the convex facet on the middle one-third of the superior surface of the calcaneum

Talonavicular joint between the talus and navicular

Caleoneocuboid joint: This is a saddle joint. The opposed articular surfaces of the calcaneum and cuboid are concavoconvex.

Ligaments: The related ligaments are:

- **Spring ligament** (or plantar caleaneonavicular) is a powerful ligament. It is attached posteriorly to the anterior margin of the sustentaculum tali, and anteriorly to the plantar surface of the navicular bone between its tuberosity and articular margin. This is the most important ligament for maintaining the medial longitudinal arch of the foot.
- **Deltoid ligament (medial):** This is a very strong triangular ligament present on the medial side of the ankle. The ligament is divided into superficial and deep part.
- **Capsular ligaments:** Play important role in pathology of clubfoot.
- **Plantar ligament (long and short):** Strong ligament whose importance in maintaining the arches of foot is surpassed only by the spring ligament. It is attached posteriorly to the plantar surface of the calcaneum, and anteriorly to the lips of the groove on the cuboid bone, and to the bases of the middle three metatarsals.

Tendons: Mainly on medial side of foot

Tibialis posterior: Most important muscle in causing deformity. The tibialis posterior is inserted chiefly into the tuberosity of the navicular bone; the tendon also gives off slips to all tarsal bones except talus and to 2nd, 3rd, and 4th metatarsal bone, is an invertor and powerful flexor.

Other being: Flexor hallucis longus, flexor digitorum longus.

On the posterior side tendon Achilles (is the thickest and strongest tendon of the body).

Deformities

Before proceeding it is essential to know the exact definition of various deformities.

- *Equinus:* The foot is fixed in plantar flexion (walk on toes with the heel raised)
- *Calcaneus:* The foot is fixed in dorsiflexion.
- *Varus:* The foot is inverted and adducted at the mid-tarsal joint
- *Valgus:* The foot is everted and abducted at the midtarsal joint

- *Planus:* Absence or collapse of the arches leads to flat foot
- *Cavus:* The longitudinal arch of the foot is exaggerated.

Talipes equinovarus and talipes calcaneovalgus are the two common combinations and among the mixture of two different deformities stated above talipes equinovarus is the commoner of the two (Fig. 12.1).

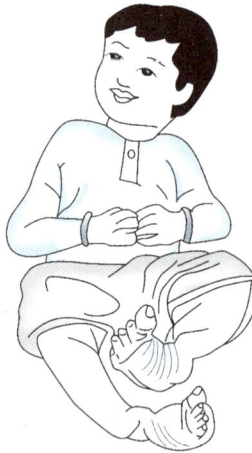

Fig. 12.1: Child with bilateral CTEV

Clubfoot may be:
i. *Congenital Talipes Equinovarus (CTEV)*
   a. *Isolated or primary:* Unilateral, at times it is bilateral in 30% cases.
   b. *Part of a complex:* Spina bifida, diastometamyelia, arthrogryposis multiplex congenital, Friedreich's ataxia, tibial amelia.
ii. *Acquired*
   Cerebral palsy, polio, myopathy, peripheral nerve injury, amyotrophic lateral sclerosis, infantile spastic haemiplegia. The foot may be clinically categorized as mild, moderate or severe, depending on the soft tissue pliability on passive correction.

Pathology

The deformities are as follows (Figs 12.2a and b)

Deformity	Joint	Structures responsible
Equinus	Ankle joint	Tendo Achilles and posterior capsule of ankle, subtalar joint
Cavus	Mid tarsal joints	Plantar fascia and small muscles of the foot
Inversion	Subtalar joint	Tibialis posterior
Heel varus	Subtalar joint	Deltoid ligament
Forefoot adduction	T/M joint	Abductor hallucis

Clinical Features

In a patient of CTEV always do general examination to rule out other deformities / anomalies.
   i. *Incidence:* 1 per 1000 live births.
   ii. *Age:* The child is born with the deformity, which develops *in utero.*
  iii. *Sex:* M:F : 2:1.
   iv. *Side:* Bilateral in 30% of the cases.
   v. *Deformity:* The foot is small with updrawn heel, a thin calf and tight tendo Achilles, the sole faces inwards with deep furrows along the medial border, the toes are adducted and as the child starts walking on the dorsolateral aspect of the foot, callosities develop on the skin (Fig. 12.2).

INVESTIGATIONS

   i. *Cardiac:* To rule out anomalies and fitness for surgery.
   ii. *CNS:* For secondary causes of CTEV, e.g. meningocele, Friedreich's ataxia.
  iii. *X-ray*
   Foot: This is done before and after the correction. Both, AP and stress dorsiflexion lateral view for talocalcaneal axis, known as KITE'S angle (25°–55°) (Figs 12.3a and b).
   Spine: For spina bifida, etc.

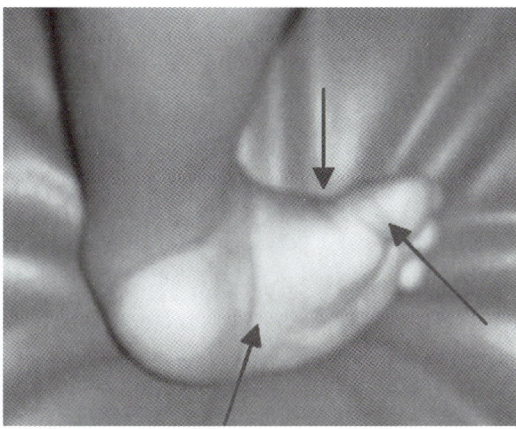

Fig. 12.2a: Typical deformities of CTEV

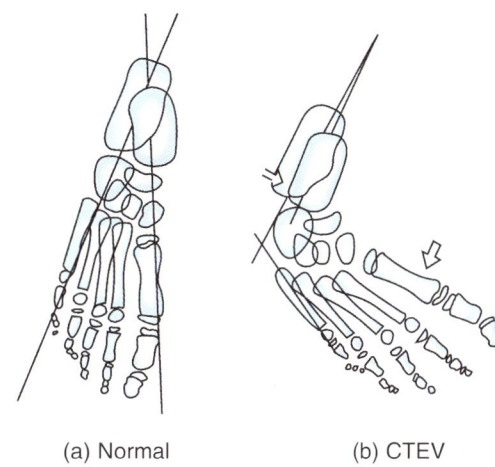

(a) Normal   (b) CTEV

Figs 12.3a and b: KITE'S angle

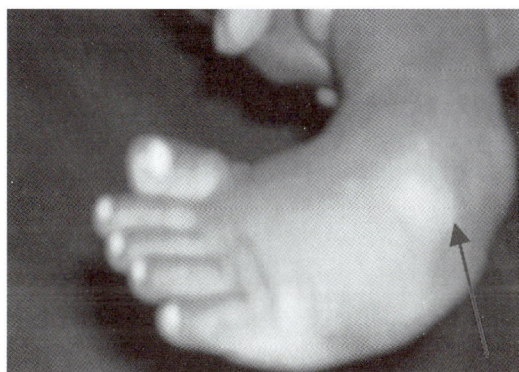

Fig. 12.2b: (1) Equinus of the heel, (2) Varus of the calcaneum, (3) Cavus of the foot, (4) Inversion: The sole faces inwards with deep furrows along the medial border, (5) Clawing of toes and forefoot in adduction with callosities on the skin (arrow) as seen in the figure

Management

The principles of management are correction of the deformity and subsequent maintenance of the correction achieved by appropriate footwear, till the child starts walking and regains the muscle balance.

   i. **Conservative:** Manipulations and serial corrective POP casts.

   ii. **Surgery**
      a. Soft tissue release.
      b. Tendon transfer.
      c. Bony operations.
   iii. JESS distractor, correction by differential distraction.

Conservative

   i. *Manipulative correction:* By mother.
   ii. *Corrective cast:* Start correcting fore-foot adduction and heel varus first and subsequently cavus and equinus last of all. The cast is well-padded with cotton and applied above knee, knee flexed at 90° to avoid slipping out, extending up to the toe tips. The cast is changed every three weeks till maximum correction is achieved.

   Caution: Don't forcefully dorsiflex the foot initially otherwise complication of ROCKER BOTTOM may occur due to break in the mid foot.

Ponseti Technique: A New Technique of Corrective Cast

This method is particularly suited for developing countries where there are few orthopaedic surgeons. The treatment is economical and easy on the babies. If well implemented, it will greatly decrease the number of clubfoot cripples.

First Four or Five Casts (more if necessary)

Start as soon after birth as possible. Make the infant and family comfortable.

First cast: The first element of management is correction of the cavus deformity by positioning the forefoot in proper alignment with the hind foot.

Second, third, and fourth casts: During this phase of treatment, the adductus and varus are fully corrected.

Manipulation

The manipulation consists of abduction of the foot beneath the stabilized talar head. Locate the head of the talus (which is the fulcrum for correction). All components of clubfoot deformity, except for the ankle equinus, are corrected simultaneously (Fig. 12.4).

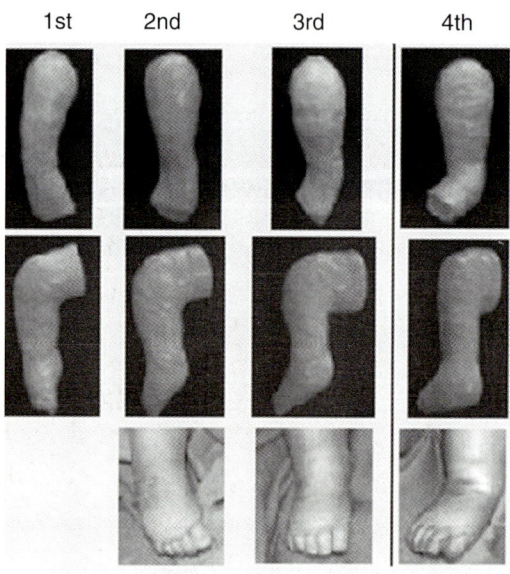

Figs 12.4: Appearance of casts and foot

Equinus correction and fifth cast: Perform the tenotomy approximately 1.5 cm above the calcaneus with the foot held in maximal dorsiflexion by the assistant (Fig. 12.5).

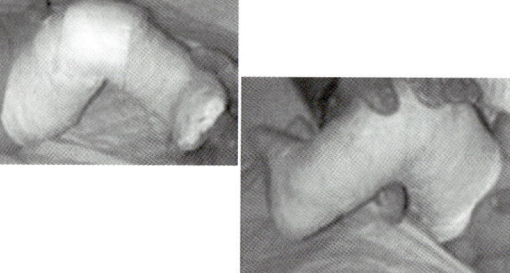

Fig. 12.5: Appearance of cast after tenotomy (foot held in maximum dorsiflexion)

Surgery

A fair trial of corrective POP cast must always be done before embarking on any surgical intervention, nevertheless, I agree with suggestion of Lovell [1970] who suggested that if correction is not achieved within 3 months of conservative management, then surgery should be done.

The ideal time for soft tissue release is 3 months to 1 year.

Aims of surgical management is to provide a painless plantigrade and flexible foot with near normal gait and lasting correction of the deformity.

The surgical options available are depending on the deformity and age of the child.

- Posteromedial soft tissue release (3 months to 1 year).
- Tendon transfer (5 to 8 years).
- Soft tissue differential distraction by JESS/Illizarov apparatus (3 months to adulthood).
- Bony procedures
  - *Immature foot:* Evans/Dwyer's osteotomy (5 to 10 years).
  - *Mature foot:* Triple arthrodesis/talectomy (>15 years).

Posteromedial Soft Tissue Release

The structures released are as follows
 i. *Posterior:* Z-plasty lengthening of tendo achillis, capsule/ligaments of ankle and subtalar joint.
 ii. *Medial:* Tibialis posterior tendon insertions, abductor hallucis deltoid ligament (superficial layer).
 iii. *Plantar:* Plantar fascia, spring ligament.
  Shortcomings of posteromedial release are:
 i. Mild forefoot adduction (because of unattended T/M and calcaneocuboid joints).
 ii. Heel varus (due to subtotal release of subtalar joint).

Tendon Transfer

The principle is to transfer the deforming force of tibialis posterior as an inverter to the dorsum of the foot so that it works as a dorsiflexor.

Tibialis posterior is transferred anteriorly and attached to the dorsum of 3rd cuneiform, this transfer is done after the child is 5 years old and mature enough to understand tendon retraining.

Bony Operations

Required to correct residual deformity
 i. **Forefoot adduction**
  a. Cuboid decancellation < 3 years.
  b. Evan's procedure (dorsolateral wedge resection of calcaneocuboid joint) > 5 years.
  c. Tarsometatarsal capsulotomy < 5 years.
  d. Metatarsal osteotomy > 5 years.
 ii. **Heel varus:** Dwyer's osteotomy of the calcaneum – 3 to 10 years.

Neglected CTEV

 i. **Early:** JESS/Illizarov distractors to stretch out the contracted soft tissues.
 ii. **Late:** Triple arthrodesis/talectomy with dorsolateral calcaneocuboid wedge resection.

Criteria For Correction

Clinical Features

 i. The child walks with a full plantigrade foot
 ii. No limp/in-toeing
 iii. Painless cosmetic scar
 iv. The child can wear a normal footwear.

Radiological Features

 i. Restoration of normal talocalcaneal angle in both AP and LAT view
 ii. Talocalcaneal index > 40.

Maintenance of Correction Achieved

 i. *Non-ambulatory child:* NOVA shoes, Dennis Browne night splint (Fig. 12.6).
 ii. *Ambulatory child:* Surgical shoes with broad toe box.
  • Straight medial border of sole.

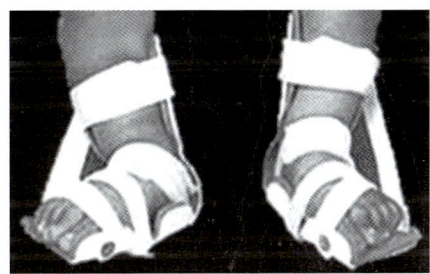
(a)

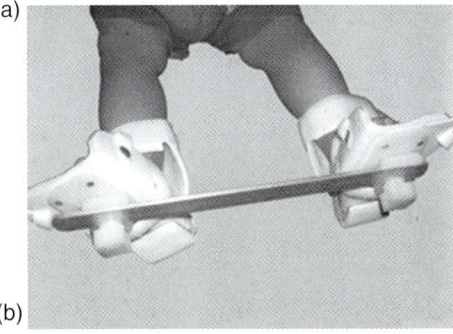
(b)

Figs 12.6a and b: (a) Nova shoes (b) Denis Browne night splint

- Thomas heel (lateral wedge extension).
- Inside iron and outside T-strap.

There is no fixed procedure for all feet. Each foot has to be examined on its own merit and surgery best suited for it, decided depending on the age of presentation and the dominating factor responsible for the deformity.

CONGENITAL DISLOCATION OF HIP

It is a disabling disorder present at birth which is invariably missed, if diagnosed early and treated adequately can provide good long-term result. It is uncommon in Asian and African countries where it is habit of the mother to carry the child cross-legged which is in itself a good corrective mode of treatment. It is common in girls and often unilateral.

Clinical Features

i. An observant mother notices the limb length discrepancy, an extra groin crease (Fig. 12.7a) or a click during hip massage.
ii. On examination there is a shortening of the thigh as seen by Allis test (Fig. 12.7b) and extra groin crease, a positive Ortolani's sign (Fig. 12.7c), audible click during abduction of flexed hip. Barlow's test (the head can be pushed out and

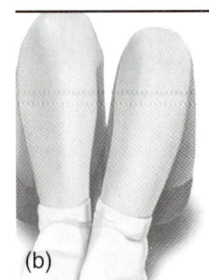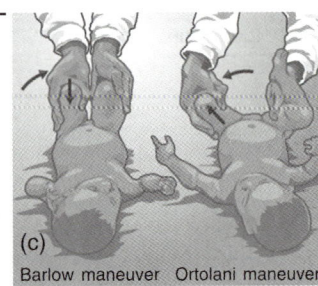

(b)

(c) Barlow maneuver Ortolani maneuver

Figs 12.7b and c: (b) Allies or Galeazzi test: difference of limb length as showing by line (c) Barlow and Ortolani test

relocated during adduction and abduction by giving trochanteric pressure).
iii. A positive telescoping test and Trendelenburg sign, if the patient is able to stand and walk. The gait becomes waddling, if it is bilateral.

X-ray

Since the head of the femur is visible only after a year, it is better to do an ultrasonography to see the position of the head in neonates.

An X-ray of the pelvis would show the head area in the upper and outer quadrant of the Perkins square with breach in Shenton's line and dysplasia of the acetabular roof (Figs 12.8a and b).

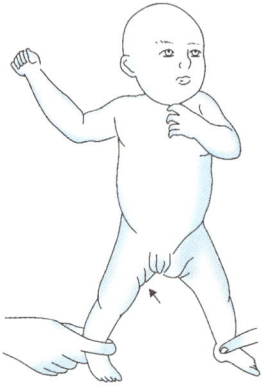

Fig. 12.7a: An extra groin crease (arrow)

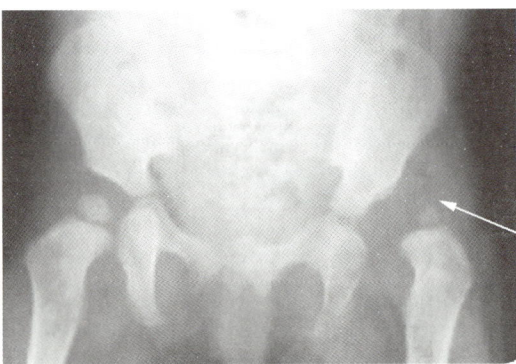

Fig. 12.8a: X-ray features of dislocated hip (marker)

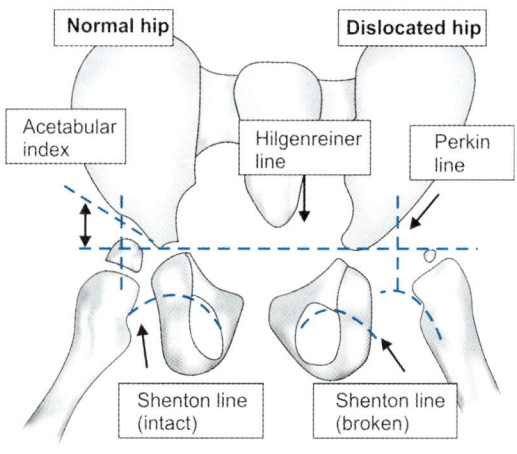

Figs 12.8b: Normal and dislocated hip

Treatment

i. *Neonates:* Double diapers/von Rosen's splint Pauvlics harness (Fig. 12.8c) keep the hip in abduction.
ii. *6 months:* Abduction hip spica/splint. (Fig. 12.9)
iii. *12 months:* Traction, adductor tenotomy followed by hip spica.

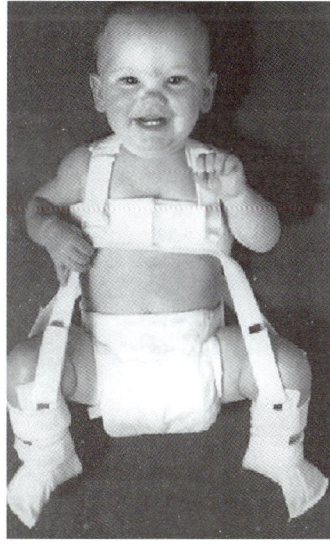

Fig. 12.8c: Pauvlic harness

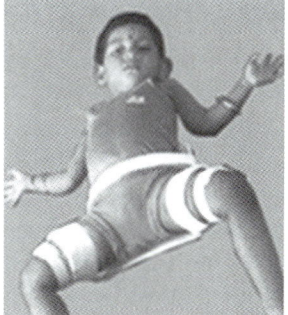

Fig. 12.9: Abduction splint

iv. *3 years:* With neck in valgus and anteversion requires a femoral varus derotation osteotomy (Fig. 12.10a).
v. *5 years:* Femoral osteotomy or Salter's innominate (Fig. 12.10b), to provide an acetabular roof by Pemberton pericapsular (Shelf) osteotomy (Fig. 12.10c) or by Chiari's pelvic osteotomy (Fig. 12.10d).

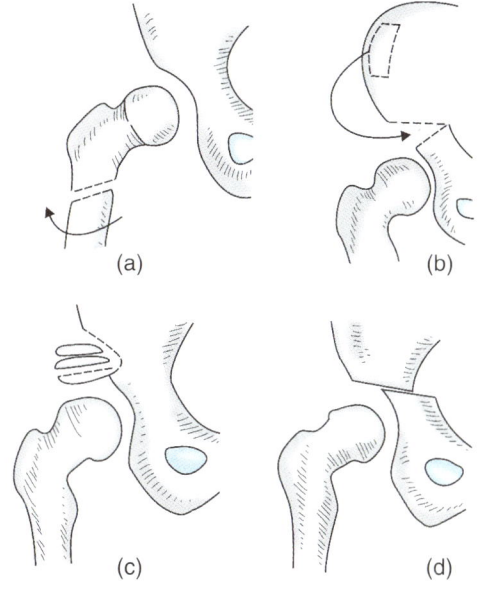

Figs 12.10a to d: (a) Femoral osteotomy (b) Salter's innominate (c) Shelf (d) Chiari's pelvic osteotomy

Complications

Chronic dislocations, avascular necrosis of femoral head and osteoarthritis

SPRENGEL'S SHOULDER

This is a failure of the descent of the scapula from the neck downward during the development, it may be associated with Klippel-Feil syndrome (the fusion of cervical vertebrae with a short neck and low hair line). Treatment is surgical reposition and tenodesis of the scapula.

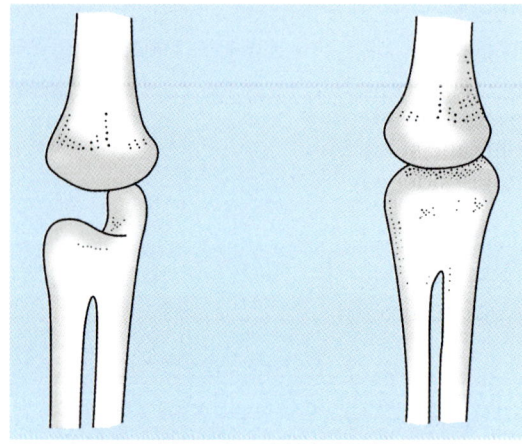

(a) Partial   (b) Complete

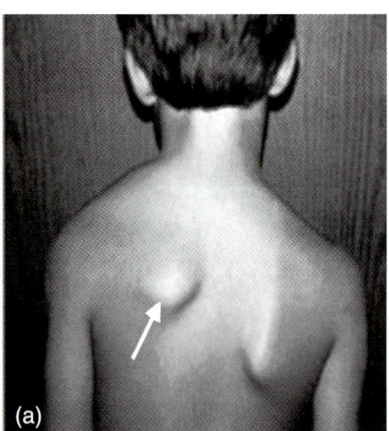

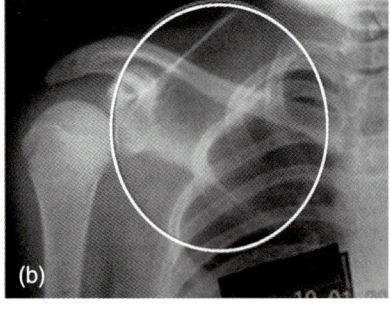

Figs 12.11a and b: (a) High riding scapula on the left side (b) X-ray showing Sprengel's shoulder

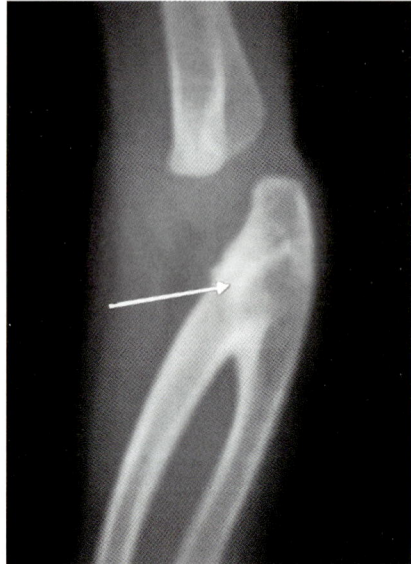

(c) X-ray showing congenital fusion of radioulnar joint (arrow)

Fig. 12.12a to c: Congenital radioulnar synostosis

CONGENITAL RADIOULNAR SYNOSTOSIS

This is a bilateral congenital fusion of the superior radioulnar joint (Figs 12.12a to c). The child being unable to supinate the forearm. It is a difficult situation to treat because of malformation and undeveloped supinator muscle. A derotation osteotomy of the radius can be tried.

RADIAL CLUB HAND

This is congenital absence of part or whole of the radius and thumb leading to deviation of the wrist outwards with curved overgrown ulna and subluxated wrist. The muscles on the radial side may be absent (Fig. 12.13).

Treatment

JESS distractor on the radial side followed by centralization of ulna.

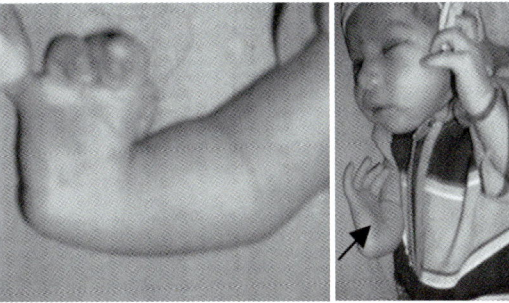

Fig. 12.13: Radial club hand

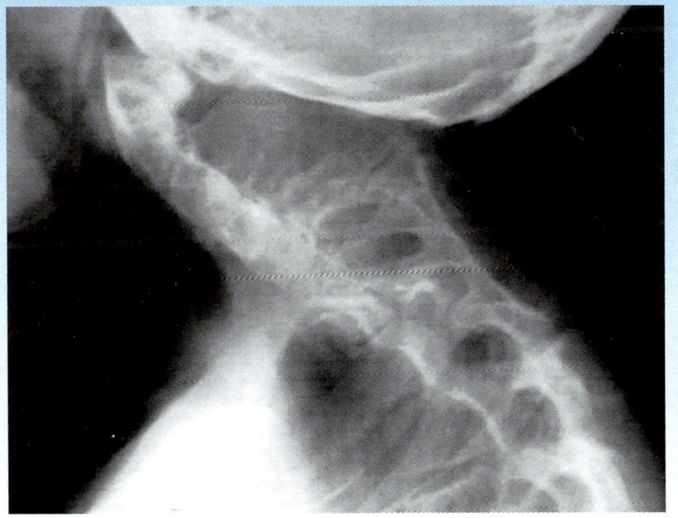

13

Bone Tumours

CLASSIFICATION BASED ON CELL OF ORIGIN

1. Primary

	Benign	Malignant
A. Osseous		
a. Cartilage	Osteochon-droma	Chondro-sarcoma
	Chondroma	
	Chondro-blastoma	
	Chondro-myxoid Fibroma	
b. Osteoid	Osteoma	Osteogenic
	Osteoid osteoma	sarcoma
	Periosteal fibroma	
c. Resorptive	Fibrous dysplasia	
Bone cysts	Giant cell tumour	Giant cell tumour
B. Non-osseous		
a. Marrow	Solitary plasma cytoma	Leukemia, M. myeloma
	Reticulo-endotheliosis	Reticulum cell sarcoma
	Xanthoma	Ewing's sarcoma
b. Muscle	Myoma	Myosarcoma
c. Inclusion	Chordoma	
	Fibroma	Fibrosarcoma
	Angioma	Angiosarcoma
	Synovioma	Synovial cell sarcoma
	Adamantinoma	Squamous cell carcinoma

2. Secondary
   i. *Osteoblastic:* Brain, bronchus, breast, bowel, bladder, prostrate.
  ii. *Osteolytic:* Colon, thyroid, kidney, etc.

WHO CLASSIFICATION OF PRIMARY BONE TUMOURS AND TUMOUR LIKE LESIONS

  I. **Bone forming tumours**
      A. *Benign*
          1. Osteoma
          2. Osteoid osteoma
          3. **Osteoblastoma**
      B. *Malignant*
          1. Osteosarcoma (osteogenic sarcoma)
          2. **Juxtacortical osteosarcoma (periosteal osteosarcoma).**
 II. **Cartilage forming tumours**
      A. *Benign*
          1. Chondroma
          2. Osteochondroma (osteocartilaginous exostosis)
          3. Chondroblastoma
          4. Chondromyxoid fibroma
      B. *Malignant*
          1. Chondrosarcoma
          2. Juxtacortical chondrosarcoma
          3. Mesenchymal chondrosarcoma

III. Giant cell tumour (osteoclastoma)
IV. Marrow tumours
    1. **Ewing's sarcoma**
    2. Reticulosarcoma of bone
    3. Lymphosarcoma of bone
    4. Myeloma.
V. Vascular tumours
    A. Benign
        1. **Haemangioma**
        2. Lymphangioma
        3. Glomus tumour (Glomangioma)
    B. Intermediate or indeterminate.
        1. **Haemangioendothelioma**
        2. Haemangiopericytoma
    C. Malignant
        1. **Angiosarcoma**
VI. Other connective tissue tumours
    A. Benign
        1. Desmoplastic fibroma
        2. Lipoma.
    B. Malignant
        1. **Fibrosarcoma**
        2. Liposarcoma
        3. Malignant mesenchymoma
        4. Undifferentiated sarcoma.
VII. Other tumours
    1. Chordoma
    2. Admantinoma
    3. Neurilemoma
    4. Neurofibroma.
VIII. Unclassified tumours
IX. Tumour like lesions
    1. **Solitary bone cyst**
    2. Aneurysmal bone cyst
    3. Juxta-articular bone cyst
    4. Metaphyseal fibrous defect
    5. **Eosinophilic granuloma**
    6. Fibrous dysplasia
    7. Myositis ossificans
    8. 'Brown tumour' of hyperparathyroidism.

Primary bone tumours account for only 2% of total body tumours, 98% of all tumours metastasize in the bone. Of the large number

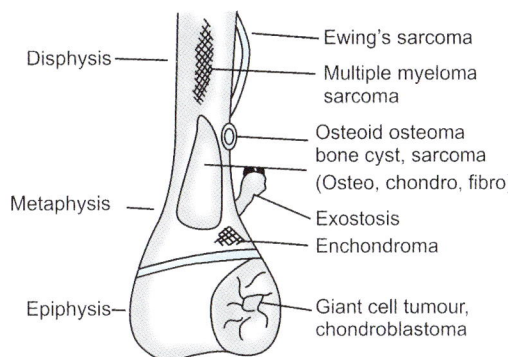

Fig. 13.1: Anatomical location of some common bone tumours

of bone tumours, only the common ones have been described.

GENERAL APPROACH TO MUSCULOSKELETAL NEOPLASMS

History

An adequate history and physical examination are the first and most important steps in evaluating a patient with a musculoskeletal tumour. Patients may present to the orthopaedic oncologist with

a. **Pain**, patients with bone tumours most frequently present with pain. The pain initially may be activity related, but the patient with a malignancy of bone often complains of progressive pain at rest and at night. Other benign lesions, most notably osteoid osteoma, may initially cause night pain.
b. **Swelling**
c. **Abnormal radiographic** finding detected during the evaluation of an unrelated problem.

INVESTIGATIONS

Plain Roentgenograms

Compared with any other test, conventional roentgenography provides more useful diagnostic information for evaluation of bone lesions. Often, the patient's age and plain roentgenographic findings are sufficient to arrive at a specific diagnosis.

- An epiphyseal lesion in a skeletally mature patient is likely to be a giant cell tumour, whereas an epiphyseal lesion in a skeletally immature patient is likely to be a chondroblastoma.
- Diaphyseal lesions include Ewing's sarcoma, histiocytosis, lymphoma, fibrous dysplasia, and adamantinoma (especially in the tibia).
- Most vertebral lesions in adult patients are metastases, myelomas, or hemangiomas.
- In the sacrum, chordoma is at the top of the list of differential diagnoses.
- In younger patients with a vertebral body lesion, the most likely diagnosis is histiocytosis; if the lesion is in the posterior elements, the differential diagnoses include aneurysmal bone cyst, osteoblastoma, and osteoid osteoma.
- Inactive lesions usually are well marginated, often with a surrounding rim of reactive bone formation.
- Aggressive lesions usually have a less well-defined zone of transition between the lesion and the host bone. Cortical expansion can be seen with aggressive benign lesions, but frank cortical destruction usually is a sign of malignancy.
- Periosteal reactive new bone formation results when the tumour destroys cortex and may take the form of a *Codman's triangle*, "*onion-skinning*," or a "*sunburst*" pattern. It usually is a sign of malignancy but may be present with infection or histiocytosis.

Computed tomography (CT) is most helpful in assessing ossification and calcification and in evaluating the integrity of the cortex. It also is the best imaging study to localize the nidus of an osteoid osteoma, to detect a thin rim of reactive bone around an aneurysmal bone cyst, to evaluate calcification in a suspected cartilaginous lesion, and to evaluate endosteal cortical erosion in a suspected chondrosarcoma.

CT of the lungs also is the most effective study to detect pulmonary metastases.

Technetium Bone Scans

These are indicated to detect skeletal metastases and to determine the presence of multiple lesions in such entities as osteochondroma, enchondroma, fibrous dysplasia, and histiocytosis. Bone scans frequently are falsely negative in multiple myeloma. With the exception of myeloma, however, virtually all malignant neoplasms of bone demonstrate increased uptake on technetium bone scans. A normal bone scan is therefore very reassuring; however, the converse statement is not true because most benign lesions of bone also demonstrate increased uptake.

Magnetic Resonance Imaging (MRI)

It has replaced CT as the study of choice to determine the size, extent, and anatomical relationships of both bone and soft tissue tumours. It is the most accurate technique for determining the limits of disease both within and outside bone. MRI may yield a specific diagnosis with tumours such as lipoma, hemangioma, hematomas, or pigmented villonodular synovitis, all of which have very characteristic appearances.

Ultrasonography

It is useful for distinguishing cystic from solid soft tissue lesions.

Angiography

Angiography previously was used to determine the relationship of a neoplasm to the vessels, has been supplanted by MRI. However, angiography still is useful to rule out non-neoplastic conditions, such as pseudoaneurysms or arteriovenous malformations, and for preoperative embolization of highly vascular lesions, such as renal cell carcinoma and aneurysmal bone cysts.

Gallium scans are the most sensitive tests for locating nonpulmonary metastases.

Blood and Urine Tests

A basic metabolic panel may be indicated to evaluate the overall health of a patient. Risk of wound-healing problems and infection have been shown to be significantly greater in patients whose serum *albumin is less than 3.5 g/dl or whose total lymphocyte count is less than 1500/ml.*

A complete blood count may be helpful to rule out infection and leukemia. The erythrocyte sedimentation rate usually is elevated in infection, metastatic carcinoma, and small "blue cell" tumours such as Ewing's sarcoma, lymphoma, leukemia, and histiocytosis.

A serum protein electrophoresis should be ordered if multiple myeloma is part of the differential diagnosis. Likewise, a prostate-specific antigen should be ordered if prostate carcinoma is a possibility.

Hypercalcemia may be present with metastatic disease, multiple myeloma, and hyperparathyroidism.

Alkaline phosphatase may be elevated in metabolic bone disease, metastatic disease, osteosarcoma, Ewing's sarcoma, or lymphoma. Blood urea nitrogen and creatinine may be elevated with renal tumours, and a urinalysis may reveal hematuria in this setting. Brown tumours of hyperparathyroidism can sometimes look like giant cell tumours and can be evaluated with serum calcium and parathyroid hormone levels. Finally, Paget's disease may be in the differential diagnosis and can be evaluated by serum alkaline phosphatase and urinary pyridinium cross-links.

STAGING

Both benign and malignant tumours of bone and soft tissue can be staged according to the Enneking staging system

Benign tumours are staged as follows: Stage 1 latent; stage 2 active; and stage 3 aggressive.

Stage 1: are intracapsular, usually asymptomatic, and frequently incidental findings. Roentgenographic features include a well-defined margin with a thick rim of reactive bone. There is no cortical destruction or expansion.

Stage 2: also are intracapsular but are actively growing and therefore can cause symptoms or lead to pathological fracture. They have well-defined margins on roentgenograms but may expand and thin the cortex. Usually they have only a very thin rim of reactive bone.

Stage 3: lesions are extracapsular. Their aggressive nature is apparent both clinically and roentgenographically. They usually have broken through the reactive bone and possibly the cortex. MRI may demonstrate a soft tissue mass, and metastases may be present in up to 5% of patients with these lesions.

BIOPSY

A biopsy should be planned as carefully as the definitive procedure. Biopsy should be done only after clinical, laboratory, and roentgenographic examinations are complete.

A biopsy can be done by fine needle aspiration, core needle biopsy, or an open incisional procedure. Complications are greater with incisional biopsy; however, this procedure is least likely to be associated with a sampling error, and it provides the most tissue for additional diagnostic studies such as cytogenetics and flow cytometry. In experienced hands, a core needle biopsy can provide an accurate diagnosis in up to 90% of cases. However, the limited amount of tissue obtained may not be adequate for accurate grading or for any additional studies that may dictate subsequent treatment. Fine needle aspiration may be up to 90% accurate at determining malignancy; however, its accuracy at determining specific tumour type is much lower. In addition, the absence of malignant cells on fine needle aspiration is less reassuring than a negative incisional biopsy.

Primary Resection

A small (<5 cm) subcutaneous mass that is unlikely to be malignant may be marginally resected primarily. In the rare circumstance that the lesion turns out to be malignant, the tumour bed may be re-excised with wide margins without adversely affecting the outcome.

Some benign bone lesions, such as osteoid osteoma and osteochondroma, have a characteristic roentgenographic appearance and can be primarily resected if indicated without biopsy.

Management

The goal of treatment in a patient with a primary malignancy of the musculoskeletal system is to make the patient *free of disease*.

The goal of treatment of a patient with metastatic carcinoma to bone is to *minimize pain and to preserve function*.

In either circumstance, the optimal treatment of the tumour often requires a combination of radiation therapy, chemotherapy, and surgery.

RADIATION THERAPY

Radiation causes cell death by inducing the formation of intracellular free radicals that subsequently cause DNA damage. The goal of radiation treatment is to deliver the highest possible dose of radiation to the tumour cells while trying to minimize toxicity to normal tissues.

Most primary bone malignancies are relatively radioresistant. Exceptions are the marrow cell tumours including multiple myeloma, lymphoma, and Ewing's sarcoma, which are each exquisitely sensitive. Carcinoma metastatic to bone also is frequently sensitive to radiation treatment radiotherapy for tumours that were once surgically inaccessible.

In addition to conventional external beam radiation, radiation also can be delivered by **brachytherapy**. By this method, hollow catheters are implanted in the tumour bed at the time of resection. These catheters exit through the skin. Postoperative roentgenographic evaluation and computer calculations determine the optimal loading of the catheters with radioisotopes. This technique allows for high doses to be delivered to the target tissues. The radiation levels fall off rapidly at the edges of the field, thus sparing normal tissues.

CHEMOTHERAPY

With the use of modern chemotherapy protocols, the current 5-year survival rate for osteosarcoma is approximately 70%. Similar numbers are available regarding the treatment of Ewing's sarcoma.

"Adjuvant" chemotherapy refers to chemotherapy administered postoperatively to treat presumed micrometastases.

"Neoadjuvant" chemotherapy refers to chemotherapy administered before surgical resection of the primary tumour.

AMPUTATION VERSUS LIMB SALVAGE

Advances in diagnostic imaging, chemotherapy, radiation therapy, and surgical technique for resection and reconstruction now allow limb salvage to be a reasonable option for most patients with bone or soft tissue sarcomas.

Most patients with osteosarcoma around the knee are treated with one of three surgical procedures—wide resection with prosthetic knee replacement (or allograft-prosthesis composite), wide resection with allograft arthrodesis, or transfemoral amputation

RESECTION AND RECONSTRUCTION

Currently most musculoskeletal malignancies are treated with local resection and reconstruction. Aggressive benign neoplasms also can be treated in this manner. The goal of resection of a malignancy is to achieve wide surgical margins if possible.

Osteoarticular allografts offer several attractive advantages including the ability to replace ligaments, tendons, and intra-articular structures Allograft-prosthetic composites may provide a long-term solution for some patients. They avoid the complications of degenerative joint disease and articular collapse while still preserving the ability to directly attach soft tissue structures such as the patella tendon or the hip abductors. However, they are associated with fatigue fracture, infection, and nonunion at the graft-host junction. Although many surgeons use this as their primary method of reconstruction, our main indication for an allograft-prosthesis composite is an inadequate length of host bone to cement an endoprosthesis securely.

Endoprosthetic reconstruction also may provide long-term function for some patients and is associated with its own complications. Endoprosthetic reconstruction provides the advantage of predictable immediate stability that allows for quicker rehabilitation with immediate full weight-bearing. Most endoprostheses are modular, thus allowing for incremental limb lengthening as an immature patient grows. Improvements in implant materials have greatly increased the durability of modern endoprostheses.

COMMON BONE TUMOURS

Osteochondroma (Exostosis)

It is a mushroom-like protrusion in the metaphyseal zone growing away from the growth plate, the growth of this tumour stops, once the patient attains skeletal maturity.

It could be
- *Solitary*, as an isolated growth, or
- *Multiple*, as a triad of multiple osteochondroma, wide deformed trumpet-shaped metaphysis and stunted growth, this condition is called **diaphyseal achalasia**.

Clinical Features

Tumour of growing children, hard, smooth and lobulated surface progressively growing away from the joint attached to the metaphysis, with the overlying skin freely mobile.

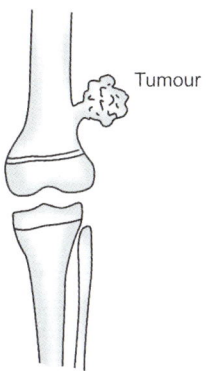

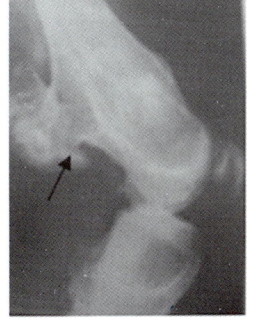 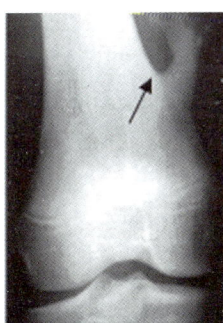

Fig. 13.2: Osteochondroma of distal femur

Rate of malignant transformation to chondrosarcoma and osteosarcoma is less than 1%. Features suggesting malignant transformation include:

If the cartilaginous cap is thicker than 1 cm.

If there is fracture of the stalk

If the cartilaginous cap shows snowstorm appearance

If there is rapid growth.

Treatment

Surgical excision along with periosteal cover is the only option.

Indications for surgery: Pain, fracture of the stem, pressure symptoms, interference with joint function, cosmetic excision especially in females only after completion of longitudinal growth.

Osteoid Osteoma

This is a benign tumour involving the enchondral bones usually the long, short bones and spine. In young adults, between 10 and 25 years, it is a solitary lesion presenting with pain, worse at night, palpable bony swelling and spasm.

X-ray shows small rarified lesion less than 2 cm involving the cortex or subperiosteal area with surrounding reactive new bone formation (Figs 13.3a and b), occasionally a small dense centre of ossification may be seen in the nidus. CT scan (Fig. 13.3b), ^{99m}Tc uptake (Fig. 13.3c) for better visualization.

It should be differentiated from Brodie's abscess, osteomyelitis and syphilitic periostitis.

Treatment

1. Excision of the nidus
2. Radiofrequency ablation of osteoid osteoma under imaging.

Enchondroma

This is a benign cartilaginous growth involving short bone of the hand, the generalized variety is called **Ollier's disease** (Fig. 13.4). The patient presents with multiple growths and deformity of hand.

Maffucci's syndrome: Multiple enchondromata with soft tissues haemangiomata and skin pigmentation

Treatment (Surgical Indication)

i. Pathological fracture requiring curettage and bone grafting
ii. A malignant change in a long-standing case, requiring amputation.

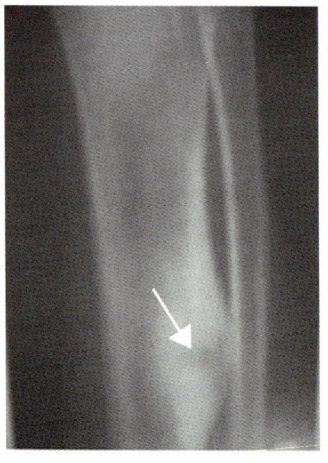

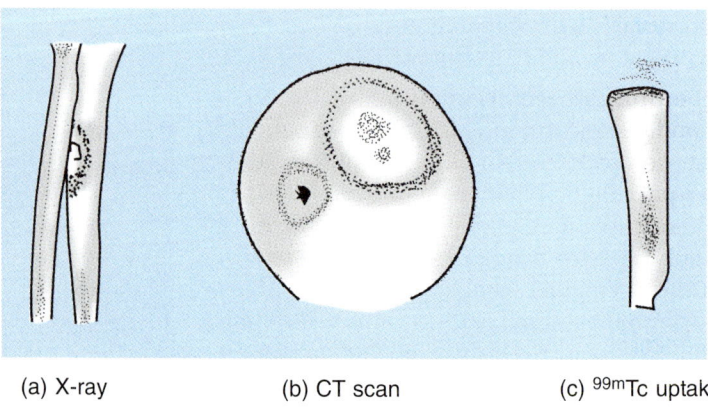

(a) X-ray   (b) CT scan   (c) ^{99m}Tc uptake

Figs 13.3a to c

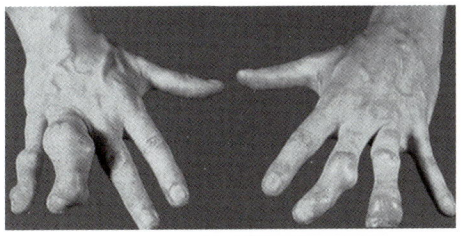

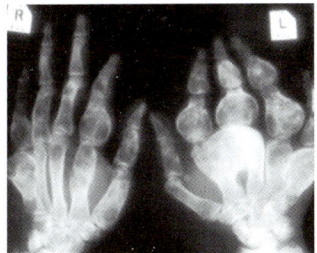

Fig. 13.4: Ollier's disease

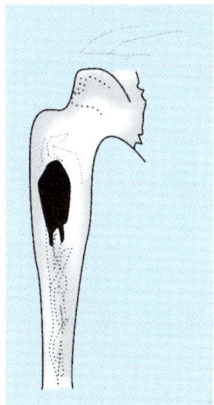

Fig. 13.5: Unicameral bone cyst

Unicameral Bone Cyst (Fig. 13.5)

This is also known as a **solitary bone cyst**. It is seen as an oval, cystic, expanding lesion in the long axis of the long bones. It is metaphyseal in location occurring in the humerus or femur of a young child usually presenting after a pathological fracture and healing occurs spontaneously. Surgical treatment in the form of curettage and bone grafting may be done. Small lesions can be aspirated and cured by repeated injections of Methyl prednisolone.

Aneurysmal Bone Cyst

This is a solitary rapidly progressive lesion of the epiphyseometaphyseal area after the second decade involving the long bones and posterior vertebral area. The patient presents with pathological fracture.

X-ray shows metaphyseodiaphyseal, osteolytic, expansile, eccentric lesion in the bone.

Treatment

i. Surgical excision, cauterization and bone grafting.
ii. Radiotherapy for vertebral areas.

Osteoclastoma or Giant Cell Tumour

It is an osteolytic tumour of young adults arising from the epiphysis seen after closure of the growth plate.

Clinical Features

i. **Age:** 15–35 years, **Sex:** females are more affected, **Site:** lower femur, upper tibia, lower radius, **Skin:** tense and shiny with dilated veins (Fig. 13.6a).
ii. **Palpation:** Tender swelling with variable consistency, *eggshell crackling* due to thin expanded cortex.

Sequence of events: Trauma ® pain ® swelling (tumour) ® pathological fracture.

Investigations

i. **X-ray:** Osteolytic lesion at epiphysis (Fig. 13.6b) of a mature skeleton. Cortex thin expanded eccentrically and eroded, medulla is destroyed with few remnants of trabeculae seen as *soap bubble* appearance. Pathological fracture may occur at the junctional zone, with the diaphysis. The tumour rarely crosses the articular cartilage.

No periosteal/endosteal new bone formation is seen in the tumour area.

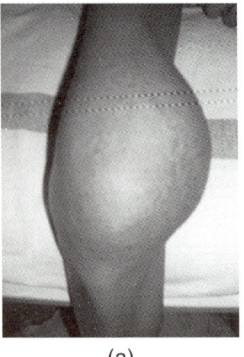 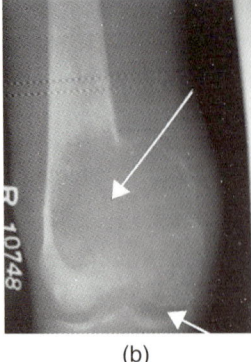

(a)　　　　　　　　　(b)

Figs 13.6a and b: Osteoclastoma lower end femur

Callus may be seen after pathological fracture occurring at the junctional zone.

ii. **Histopathologically:** Two types of cells are seen:

　a. Spindle-shaped cells, pleomorphic with loose network and mitotic figures (Fig. 13.6c).

　b. Giant cells containing 10–100 centrally placed nuclei. *These cells contain only acid phosphate.* More the number of giant cells better prognosis, this statement is not always true since even grade-I tumour which contains 75% of giant cells can present with metastasis while grade-III with 25% giant cells may remain benign. Hence, it is treacherous and unpredictable.

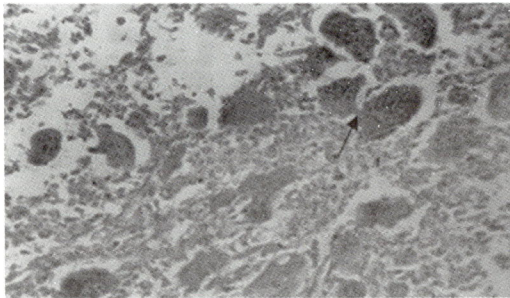

Fig. 13.6c: Slide: Giant cell tumour showing giant cells and stromal cells

Treatment

i. **Surgical**
　a. Complete excision of tumour with adjoining healthy bone with or without replacement by bone transplant/ prosthesis. Lower end of radius may be excised and replaced by proximal fibula which closely resembles it.
　b. Curettage of cavity, cauterization of wall with carbolic acid and bone grafting.

ii. **Radiotherapy:** The tumour is radioresistant and may convert to secondary osteosarcoma/malignant fibroma histiocytoma with radiation of 3000 gy or above. For inaccessible lesions of the vertebrae or sacrum tumour embolization may be done.

Ewing's Sarcoma

This is a highly malignant diaphyseal tumour of childhood.

Clinically, pathologically and radiologically closely resembling subacute osteomyelitis. Extremely radiosensitive and invariably a fatal course.

Clinical Features

i. **Age:** 5–15 years.
ii. **Site:** Diaphysis of long bones, tumour presents as a painful and tender swelling, diffuse, fixed to bone, indurated zone all around. Features of high vascularity (as dilated veins) (Fig. 13.7a).
iii. **Course:** Phases of remission and relapses in the size and pain related to tumour. Spreads by blood and lymphatics.

Investigations

i. **X-ray:** Shows corticomedullary destruction of diaphysis, periosteal reaction (onion peel appearance) (Fig. 13.7b).
ii. **MRI and CT scan:** Excellent soft tissue extension of the tumour (Figs 13.7c and d).

iii. **Histopathology:** Sheets of polyhedral cells, high vascularity and mitotic figures (Fig. 13.7e).

Treatment

Tumour is invariably fatal. When diagnosed, tumour is well spread all over the body:

i. *Radiotherapy:* Tumour is highly sensitive (*melts like an ice*) only to reappear again.
ii. *Radical surgery:* Amputation of the full length of bone.
iii. Multi-drug chemotherapy with Vincristine, Adriamycin and cyclophosphamide are the major drugs.

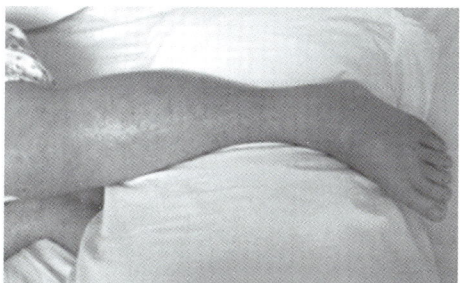

Fig. 13.7a: Ewing's sarcoma of the tibia [swelling, indurated zone all around. Features of high vascularity (as dilated veins)]

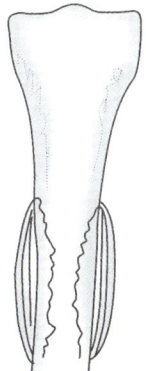 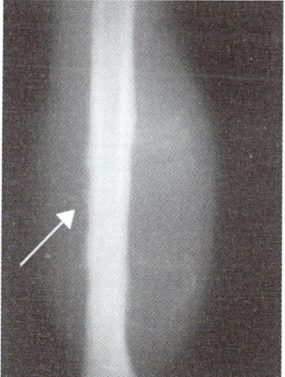

Fig. 13.7b: X-ray showing corticomedullary destruction with periosteal reaction (onion peel appearance).

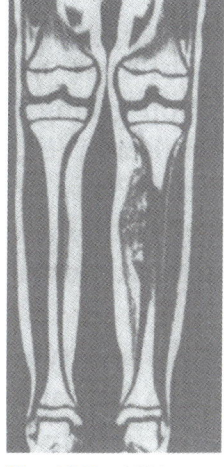 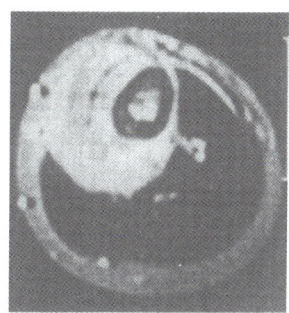

Fig. 13.7c: MRI   **Fig. 13.7d:** CT scan

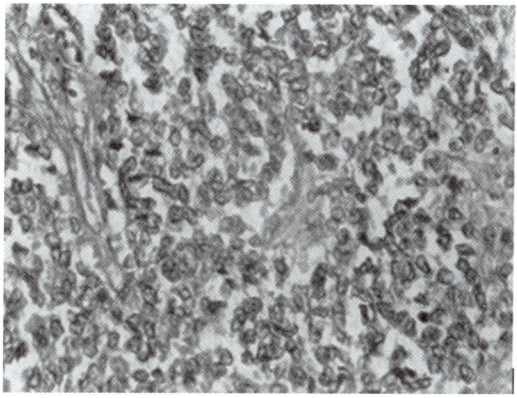

Fig. 13.7e: Microphotograph of Ewing's tumour showing small monotonous round cells separated by fibrous septa

Multiple Myeloma

This is a tumour arising from the **plasma cell of the bone marrow**, and is found in all the areas where red marrow exists. As a solitary lesion, or multiple involvement closely mimicking multiple secondaries. The plasma cell under the microscope has a large eccentric nucleus with spoke like arrangement of chromatin.

Clinical Features

The patient is usually between 40 and 60 years and comes with severe bone pain, backache, weakness and pathological fracture. In long-standing cases anaemia, cachexia and chronic renal failure.

Investigations

i. **X-ray**
   a. In solitary type, it may show a solitary punched out lesion in one bone with multilocular expansion.
   b. In the generalized variety **multiple punched** out defects in the skull, pelvis, long bones and vertebral involvement is seen as biconcave vertebrae and collapse with extensive rarefaction giving it **a disappearing vertebrae** picture, without any marginal new bone formation. One should think about multiple secondaries as differential diagnosis.

ii. **Sternal puncture:** Will show typical cartwheel myeloma cells in the marrow.

iii. **Blood:** Will show raised ESR, **hypercalcemia with low alkaline phosphatase** in spite of extensive bone destruction and a typical pattern on serum electrophoresis showing abnormally elevated gamma globulin.

iv. **Urine:** Will show positive **Bence Jones** protein in 50% of the patients (on boiling, a white precipitate appears at about 50°C which disappears on further boiling and reappears on cooling).

v. **M band** on electrophoresis of serum.

Treatment

i. **For local lesions:** Radiotherapy, internal fixation of fractures and spinal decompression.

ii. **For generalized:** Chemotherapy and spinal braces.

This myelomatosis is invariably fatal within 3 to 5 years.

Osteogenic Sarcoma

Highly malignant tumour arising from the metaphysis of adolescent child is characterized by tumour new bone formation.

This may be (1) primary or (2) secondary to pre-existing tumours, Paget's disease or following radiation of benign tumours.

Clinical Features

i. **Age:** 10–20 years, **Sex:** males are more affected, **Site:** lower femur, upper tibia, upper end humerus and mandible.

ii. **Local:** Skin is tense, shiny with dilated veins. Tumour present as a warm swelling, painful, variegated, diffuse margins with soft tissue involvement (Fig. 13.8a).

Investigations

i. **X-ray:** Shows corticomedullary destruction of metaphysis, diffuse involvement of bone and soft tissues (Fig. 13.8b).
   New bone formation within the tumour tissue and Codman's triangle, sunray appearance of tumour new bone formation (the cells grow along the periosteal vessels which travel horizontally from the periosteum to the bone).
   X-ray chest: May show features of secondaries. Canon ball appearance, pleural effusion or lobar collapse.

ii. **CT scan, ^{99m}Tc uptake and MRI:** For early diagnosis and to know exact extent of the primary and secondaries in the body.

iii. **Blood:** Hb decreased, ESR increased, alkaline phosphatase–very high (indicates the course and prognosis).

iv. **Histopathology:** Features are pleomorphic, multipotent, spindle cells with

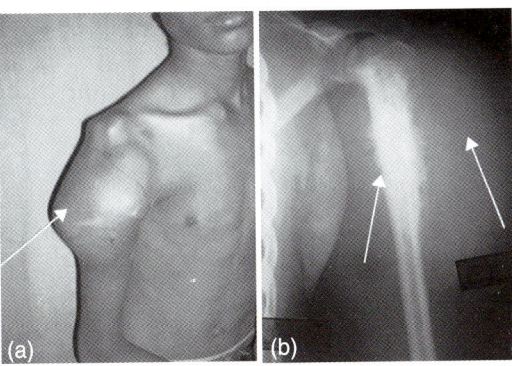

Figs 13.8a and b: (a) Osteosarcoma upper end of humerus; (b) X-ray showing corticomedullary destruction of metaphysis, diffuse involvement of bone and soft tissue involvement (arrow). New bone formation within the tumour tissue, sunray appearance of tumour new bone formation (arrow)

mitotic figures and evidence of tumour new bone formation with remnants of a few trabeculae (Fig. 13.8c).

Treatment

For extracompartmental tumours radical amputation and for unicompartmental radical excision is the treatment combined with neoadjuvent and adjuvant chemotherapy. For tumour with metastasis only chemotherapy or radiotherapy may be done.

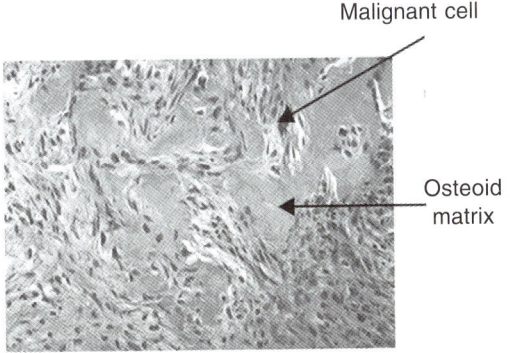

Fig. 13.8c: Histopathological features of osteosarcoma

i. **Surgery**
 a. Primary tumour amputation with full-length excision of involved bone.
 b. Lobectomy for secondaries in lungs.
ii. **Radiotherapy:** 6000–8000 rads over a period of 6–8 weeks (mega voltage irradiation).
iii. **Chemotherapy:** Multidrug, multi-cyclic regimen. HDMT (High dose methotrexate therapy).

Chondrosarcoma

This is a malignant tumour of cartilagineous origin arising (i) primarily (ii) secondary from pre-existing cartilage tumour like exostosis or enchondroma. The patients present with a hard lobulated swelling arising from the femur or ilium around the fourth decade of life.

i. **X-ray:** Shows expanded corticomedullary destruction with a cauliflower type of picture with patchy calcification.
ii. **Histologically:** Malignant cartilage cells are seen all over.
iii. **Treatment:** Surgical excision is the only choice, since this tumour does not respond to chemotherapy or radiotherapy.

Synovial Cell Sarcoma

This is a malignant tumour arising from the synovial lining of joints, tendons and bursa, around the second decade of life.

Treatment is wide surgical excision and amputation, if necessary.

Secondary Bone Tumours

Twenty-five percent of patients of cancer who die have bone metastasis.

The common metastasis are from:
i. breast 60%,
ii. lungs 20%, (iii) kidney 12%, (iv) others 8%.

Metastasis are most commonly located in (i) vertebrae 50%, (ii) pelvis 30%, (iii) femur 15%, (iv) others 5%.

- *Osteoblastic:* Prostrate, bladder, breast, carcinoid.
- *Osteolytic:* Thyroid, bronchus, colon, etc.

Clinical Features

i. Pain, pathological fracture, hyper-calcemic.

Investigations

i. **X-ray, MRI, Body scan with ^{99m}Tc,** to know the extent of secondaries.
ii. **Biopsy** to know the tumour histology.
iii. **Blood:** Increased calcium and alkaline phosphatase.

Treatment

i. Care of the primary tumour.
ii. Radio/chemotherapy for management of secondaries.
iii. Fixation of pathological fractures.
iv. Surgical excision with prosthetic replacement.
v. Hormonal treatment to relive pain in secondaries for testis/ovary/breast.

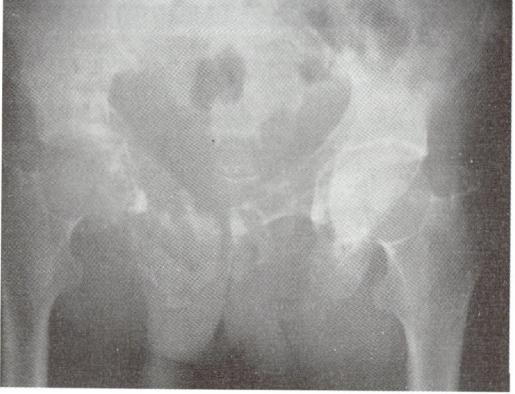

Fig. 13.9: X-ray showing multiple secondaries

Bone Grafts

This is utilization of bone tissue live or preserved for a variety of indications:

i. To provide osteogenic tissue in delayed union and non-union.
ii. To fill up gap in areas of bone loss following trauma.
iii. To fill up cavities following curettage of tumours, defects in the bone.
iv. To provide stability and osteogenic potential in pseudoarthrosis.

The grafts may be cortical, cancellous, or both.

Types

i. **Autograft:** These are grafts taken from the patient himself and the usual sites of harvesting are:
   a. *Cortico cancellous:* Iliac crest.
   b. *Cortical:* Fibula and ribs.
   c. *Unicortical:* Upper tibia.
ii. **Allografts (homografts):** These are taken from other person's like relatives or fresh corpse. The bone is deep frozen, stored in antiseptic solution, boiled and autoclaved. The disadvantage of using this is slow incorporation and the possibility of rejection.
iii. **Xenografts** (heterografts): These are animal bones which are denatured.

AMPUTATIONS

DEFINITION

Surgical removal of part or the whole limb and refashioning the mobile stump with intact sensation, fit for a prosthetic device and subsequent function.

This may be done as **Guillotine** amputation which is done in emergency for grossly crushed and infected limbs, all the tissues are cut at the same level and the stump left open

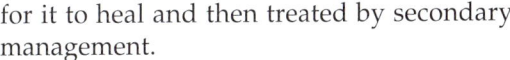

for it to heal and then treated by secondary management.

In planned closed amputation, proper flaps are designed and then skin, muscle and fascia followed by bone are cut stepwise and then closed over a drain.

Indications

Dead limb – Severely crushed and devitalized.

Dying limb – Diabetic, gangrene, Buerger's disease.

Infections – Gas gangrene, Madura foot, leprosy.

Tumours – Osteogenic sarcoma, Ewing's sarcoma.

Congenital – Deformed and useless limb.

Always give a chance of survival, take a second surgical opinion before amputation

While doing any amputation keep in mind the following :

- The level should be above the safe margin in tumours and vascular lesions, all the same good enough for prosthetic fitting. The suture line should be anterior or posterior.

- Cut the bone and cover it with periosteal sleeve, pull the nerve before cutting it with a knife.

- Double ligate the artery and vein separately to avoid A-V fistula.

- In potentially contaminated and crushed limbs, it is preferable to debride and leave the wound open for secondary closure.

- Remove the tourniquet before closure and keep a closed suction drain, apply compression dressing.

- Mobilize the stump as early as possible and fit the prosthesis for early ambulation and rehabilitation.

SOME COMMON SITES OF AMPUTATION

Upper Limb

a. *Fingers and thumb:* All possible lengths should be preserved.

b. *Wrist:* Disarticulation is an excellent functional unit and does not require above elbow cuff. If done through the transcarpal zone, it provides flexion and extension of the stump.

c. *Forearm* amputation should always be done at the junction of upper two-thirds and lower one-third, since rotation is preserved and cine plastic procedures can be done.

d. *Mid arm:* An ideal stump is 2 inches proximal to the elbow, to allow the elbow lock mechanism and permit rotation with a prosthesis.

Cineplastic procedure: This consists of creating a surgical canal through the muscle belly for insertion of a rod which is connected to a cable. Contraction of the muscle belly provides the motor function for the cable attached to the distal part of the prosthesis.

Lower Limb

a. Amputation through the toes/metatarsal gives satisfactory results.

b. **Lisfranc's** (tarsometatarsal) is unacceptable because of the resulting inversion-equinus deformity.

c. **Chopart's** (tarsal amputation proximal to insertion of tibialis anterior) results in equinovalgus deformity corrected by TA lengthening.

d. **Syme's:** This is done through the ankle and the heel flap is brought over the lower end of tibia forming an excellent end bearing stump, but prosthetic fitting requires a bulk tissue which is cosmetically not accepted.

e. **Through leg:** This requires about 6 inches or more of the tibia for an adequate prosthetic fit, preferably if the fibula is excised 3 cm proximal to the level of tibial resection. This is an excellent weight bearing stump.

f. **Disarticulation of knee:** This is an excellent end-bearing stump in children as it preserves the growth plate in the distal femur and prosthetic fitting can be made easy by resecting the condylar flare.

g. **Through thigh:** This is done 3 inches proximal to the knee joint and the closure is done either by **tendoplasty** (the patella is excised and the tendinous part of the quadriceps is sutured across the femoral stump) or **myodesis** (muscles are attached to the end of the bone providing a dynamic stump). This cylindrical stump is ideal for modern total contact prosthesis.

h. **Hip disarticulation:** This is done in cases of malignant tumours of the bone and is best fitted with Canadian hip disarticulation prosthesis or an ischial weight bearing prosthesis.

In general the level of amputation: The standard amputations are designed to be non-end bearing. The traditional site for ideal stumps is as follows:

- **Above knee:** 11 inches from the top of greater trochanter
- **Below knee:** 51/2 inches below the tibial plateau
- **Above elbow:** 8 inches from the tip of acromian process
- **Below elbow:** 7 inches below the tip of olecranon process.

Complications

a. Infections leading to secondary haemorrhage, wound dehiscence and osteomyelitis of the bony stump.

b. Stump neuroma, phantom limb, contractures, bony overgrowth in children.

c. Skin blisters ulceration and dermatitis.

Tourniquets

A pneumatic tourniquet with a hand pump and an accurate pressure gauge is probably the safest, but a constantly regulated pressure tourniquet is quite satisfactory if it is properly maintained and checked. A tourniquet should be applied by an experienced person.

Several sizes of pneumatic tourniquets are available for the upper and lower extremities. The upper arm or the thigh is wrapped with several thicknesses of smoothly applied cotton cast padding. An assistant manually grasps the flesh of the extremity just distal to the level of tourniquet application and firmly pulls this loose tissue distally before the cast padding is placed. Traction on the soft tissue is maintained while the padding and tourniquet are applied and the latter is secured. The assistant's grasp is then released, resulting in a greater proportion of the subcutaneous tissue remaining distal to the tourniquet. This bulky tissue tends to support the tourniquet and push it into an even more proximal position. All air is expressed from the sphygmomanometer or pneumatic tourniquet before application. When a sphygmomanometer cuff is used, it should be wrapped with a gauze bandage to prevent its slipping during inflation. Every effort is made to decrease tourniquet time; the extremity often is prepared and ready before the tourniquet is inflated. The extremity is then elevated for 2 minutes, or the blood is expressed by a sterile sheet rubber bandage or a cotton elastic bandage. Beginning at the fingertips or toes, the extremity is wrapped proximally to within 2.5 to 5.0 cm of the tourniquet. If a Martin sheet rubber bandage or an elastic bandage is applied up to the level of the tourniquet, the latter will tend to slip distally at the time of inflation. The tourniquet should be inflated quickly to prevent filling of the superficial veins before the arterial blood flow has been occluded.

The correct pressure depends somewhat on the age of the patient, the blood pressure, and the size of the extremity pneumatic tourniquet pressures determined by the pressure required to obliterate the peripheral pulsations then add, 50 to 75 mm Hg above the systolic blood pressure for surgery in the upper extremity and 100 to 150 mm Hg for surgery in the lower extremity, wide tourniquet cuffs are more effective at lower inflation pressures than are narrow ones.

In an average healthy adult under 50 years of age, we prefer to leave the tourniquet inflated for no more than 2 hours. If an operation on the lower extremity takes longer than 2 hours, it is better to finish it as rapidly as possible than to deflate the tourniquet for 10 minutes and then reinflate it. It has been found that up to 40 minutes is required for the tissues to return to normal after prolonged use of a tourniquet. Consequently, the previous practice of deflating the tourniquet for 10 minutes appears to be inadequate

Any solution applied to the skin must not be allowed to run beneath the tourniquet, or a chemical burn may result. Sterile pneumatic tourniquets are available for operations about the elbow, and the limb may be prepared and draped before the tourniquet is applied. Rarely, a superficial slough of the skin may occur at the upper margin of the tourniquet in the region of the gluteal fold. This usually occurs in obese individuals and is probably related to the use of a straight instead of a curved tourniquet.

Pneumatic tourniquets should be kept in good repair, and all valves and gauges must be routinely checked. The inner tube should be completely enclosed in a casing to prevent the tube from ballooning through an opening, allowing the pressure to fall or causing a "blowout." The cuff also should be carefully inspected. On older tourniquets, the firm plastic band that keeps the tourniquet from rolling must lie superficial to the inflatable cuff to prevent damage to the underlying structures. Damage has been reported when the plastic band had been inserted between the skin and the inflatable cuff.

One of the greatest dangers in the use of a tourniquet is an improperly registering gauge in a number of tourniquet injuries.

Complications

1. *Tourniquet paralysis* can result from (1) excessive pressure, (2) insufficient pressure, resulting in passive congestion of the part, with hemorrhagic infiltration of the nerve, (3) keeping the tourniquet on too long, or (4) application without consideration of the local anatomy. This complication is thought to be related to the duration of ischaemia and not to the mechanical effect of the tourniquet.

2. *Post-tourniquet syndrome,* is a common reaction to prolonged ischaemia and is characterized by oedema, pallor, joint stiffness, motor weakness, and subjective numbness. Spontaneous resolution usually occurs within 1 week.

3. *Compartment syndrome*, rhabdomyolysis, and pulmonary emboli are rare complications of tourniquet use.

4. *Vascular complications* can occur in patients with severe arteriosclerosis or prosthetic grafts. **A tourniquet should not be applied over a vascular graft**.

The Esmarch tourniquet is still in use in some areas and is the safest and most practical of the elastic tourniquets. It is only in the middle and upper thirds of the thigh. This tourniquet has a definite although limited use in that it can be applied higher on the thigh than can the pneumatic tourniquet. The Esmarch tourniquet is applied in layers, one on the top of the other; a narrow band produces less tissue damage than a wide one.

The Esmarch tourniquet should not be applied until the patient is well anesthetized; otherwise, persistent adductor muscle spasm may cause the tourniquet to be too loose after the muscles have relaxed. A hand towel, folded lengthwise in four layers, is wrapped snugly as high as possible around the upper thigh. The tourniquet is then applied over the towel as follows. The chain end is held over the lateral surface of the thigh with one hand; the other hand is passed under the thigh and grasps the rubber strap near the chain and pulls it taut. The strap is allowed to slip between the thumb and fingers as the hand is brought under and around the thigh; properly performed, this slipping produces a singing sound from friction. When it completely encircles the thigh, the tourniquet is overlapped layer on layer, with no skin or towel caught between the layers. This is repeated, keeping constant tension on the strap, until its application is complete. The hook on the end of the strap is then caught in one of the links of the chain. Care must be taken that excessive tension is not built up gradually as the tourniquet is applied.

Rubber bands and strips of Glove ends can be used for short procedures in the fingers.

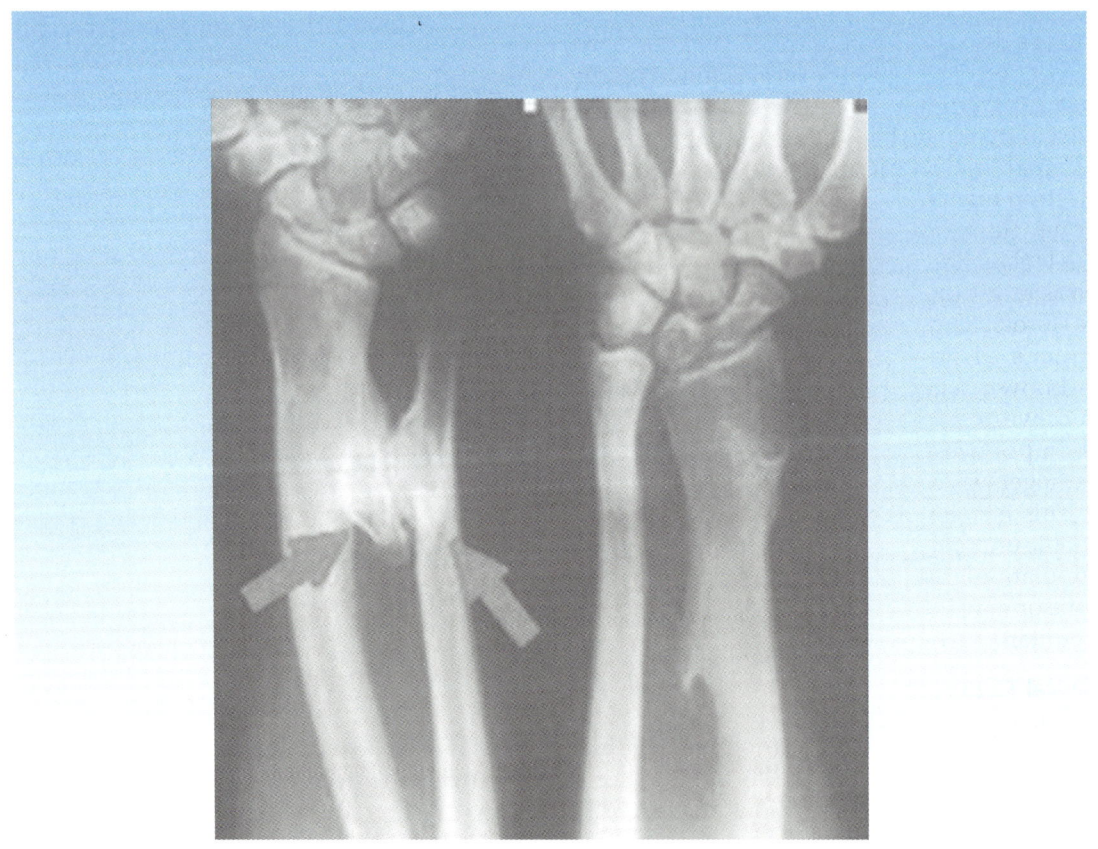

Miscellaneous Diseases

PAGET'S DISEASE (Osteitis Deformans)

Paget's disease is characterized by excessive resorption of bone by osteoclasts, followed by the replacement of normal marrow by vascular, fibrous connective tissue. Intra-nuclear inclusions have been found by electron microscopy in osteoclasts in pagetic bone. Some of the inclusions resemble nucleocapsids of viruses belonging to the measles group. Different *paramyxovirus* may have role in the initiation or propagation of Paget's disease. The exact cause is still unknown whether it is inflammatory or infective or there are genetic factors that might be important in the predisposition to and pathogenesis of Paget's disease.

This is a generalized skeletal; disease of people under the age of 50 involving 3% of the population; it remains localized to a part of bone or may involve a large number of bones simultaneously.

Clinical Features

Local: The bone is painful (more severe at night), bent, thickened, and deformed. The pelvic bones are most commonly involved, followed by femur, skull, tibia, lumbosacral spine, dorsal spine, clavicles, and ribs. Males are most often affected.

General: This usually presents with headache, deafness, deformity, stiffness, pain in the limbs with fracture and heart failure. The skull progressively enlarges. Otosclerosis causes deafness and optic nerve pressure causes blindness. The patient develops progressive kyphotic deformity and appears shorter, ape-like. There may be obvious coxa vara and anterolateral bowing of tibia (Fig. 14.1).

X-ray may show symmetric involvement of bones of the skull and lower limb, the bone is thickened, bent, and sclerotic. The trabeculae are coarse and widely separated (honey combed) and fine subperiosteal cracks may be seen (Fig. 14.2). Some important radiological features are:

- Soldier helmet (cranium is so heavy that it become difficult for the patient to hold the head erect)
- Ivory vertebrae
- Cotton-wool appearance
- Picture window frame vertebra
- Blade of grass appearance (in long bones).

Special investigation: Very high alkaline phosphate (the other condition with such high alkaline phosphatase is hereditary hyper-phosphatasia) and hydroxyproline in the plasma are noted features. Hydroxyproline is

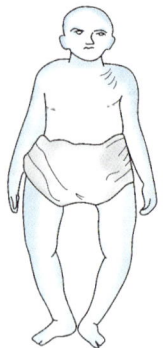

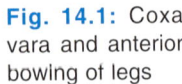

Fig. 14.1: Coxa vara and anterior bowing of legs

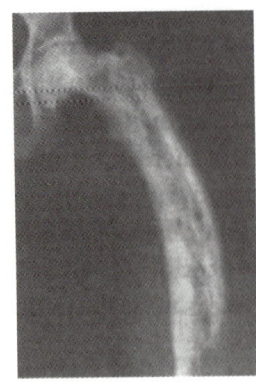

Fig. 14.2: Honeycombs appearance and subperiosteal cracks

also excreted in the urine in high quantity. But the serum calcium and phosphorus level remain within normal limits.

Complications

High output cardiac failure, deafness, blindness, pathological fracture (common in femur, of which subtrochanteric is the commonest), hyperuricemia and gout are common in men with Paget's disease, and calcific periarthritis may occur. Osteosarcoma is the dread complication (1–10%). Pagetic osteosarcoma is lytic in appearance on radiographs, in contrast to the sclerotic appearance of radiation-induced osteosarcoma.

Treatment

i. **Medical:** Medicines, which suppress bone turnover, e.g. calcitonin, diphosphonates, glucagon, mithramycin.
ii. **Surgical:** Treatment in the form of correction of deformities by osteotomy and internal fixation in patients developing fractures.

In spite of all complications patients of Paget's disease often live up to a ripe old age.

INFANTILE CORTICAL HYPEROSTOSIS (Caffey's Disease)

This is an idiopathic condition characterized by swellings, which may be tender on the mandible, clavicle, and long bones and sometime scapula due to subperiosteal ossification and signs of fever, elevated ESR and leukocyte count. The cause of disease is unknown but a virus infection has been suggested.

It should be differentiated from
i. Hypervitaminosis which shows involvement usually after 1 year of age and the mandible is never involved
ii. Scurvy, in which a characteristic ground glass osteoporotic picture with dense lines around (Wimberger's line) is seen
iii. Osteomyelitis
iv. Syphilitic hyperostosis.

STORAGE DISEASES

A generic term that includes any accumulation of a specific substance within tissues, generally because of congenital deficiency of an enzyme necessary for further metabolism of the substance.

EOSINOPHILIC GRANULOMA

This is solitary benign bone destroying lesion characterized by the presence of eosinophils. It is clinically characterized by acute onset of bone pain, swelling, fever, leukocytosis with sudden pathological fractures involving the bones of the limbs and vertebral collapse. Radiologically well localized radio translucent areas of corticomedullary destruction, expansion and periosteal reaction may be seen. Histopathologically, tissues from the lesion will show a highly cellular granuloma in which eosinophils and macrophages dominate, a few lymphocytes, plasma cells and foam cells are also seen. The macrophages are large mononuclear, containing blood pigments. As the lesion heals, the eosinophils disappear and the foam cells dominate.

Treatment

The lesion is radiosensitive. In accessible sites, it is preferable to do curettage of the lesion and packing the cavity with bone grafts is done. Radiation is given for inaccessible areas.

CALVÉ DISEASE (VERTEBRA PLANA)

This is an involvement of single vertebra due to eosinophilic granuloma. The patient usually presents with backache and knuckle deformity. X-ray shows destruction of vertebral body with subsequent collapse. This is best treated by rest, spinal brace and local irradiation.

LETTERER–SIWE DISEASE (XANTHOMATOSES)

This is an acute generalized reticuloendothelial disease of infants, invariably fatal. It involves the red marrow of flat bones, vertebrae and skull, due to rapid proliferation of reticulum cells, mononuclear cells and vacuolated cells. These histiocytes display malignant appearing nuclei. The patient usually presents with bone pain, fever, respiratory infection, generalized lymphadenopathy, hepatosplenomegaly, haemorrhages, progressive anaemia and death. No known treatment works.

HAND–SCHÜLLER–CHRISTIAN DISEASE

This is a congenital condition characterized by destruction of skull due to proliferation of reticuloendothelial tissue.

Radiologically, large well demarcated defects are seen in the skull, flat and long bones with resulting multiple defects, cortical thinning, but no periosteal reactions. The neoplastic tissue destroys and replaces the bone and protrudes into the soft tissue. There may be exophthalmos. Histologically the tissue consists of highly cellular reticuloendothelial tissue, macrophages, eosinophils, plasma cells and lymphocytes. The macrophages are characteristically xanthoma foreign body giant cells loaded with cholesterol and blood pigments.

Treatment

The lesions are radiosensitive following which the lesions may completely reossify.

GAUCHER'S DISEASE

This is a common familial metabolic disease characterized by abnormal accumulation of glucocerebrosides in the reticuloendothelial cells due to deficiency of glycolipid degrading enzyme (glucosylceramide beta-glucosidase) resulting in storage of these cells in the bone, lymph nodes, spleen and liver. The presentation may be:

i. Acute form in which bone lesion predominate starting in infancy with neurological anomalies and fatal by the age of three.
ii. Subacute or juvenile form which begins in childhood and presents as either Perthes' disease or subacute osteomyelitis.
iii. Chronic or adult form in which bony lesions are seen and is non-neuronopathic presenting at any age from infancy to old age with a progressively enlarging spleen or bony lesion involving the hip, knee and spine resulting in a pathological fracture. The femur may be typically involved showing *Erlenmeyer flask deformity* at the lower end of femur with generalized mottled appearance, increased breadth of the marrow resulting in flaring of the distal femur and thinning of the cortex. Histologically, the hallmark is **Gaucher's cell,** which is a round or polyhedral pale histiocyte with a small dark eccentric nucleus and wrinkled cytoplasm,

containing glucocerebroside which stains deeply with PAS reaction. When stained with Prussian blue, a diffuse bluish hue of Gaucher's cell is due to finally dispersed ferritin (protein-iron complex).

Treatment

It is basically aimed at

i. Splenectomy which improves the bleeding tendency and corrects thrombocytopenia, anaemia.

ii. Conservative management of bony lesions with minimal surgical intervention because of fear of infection in view of poor immune status.

iii. Avascular necrosis of the femoral head is best treated by prolonged non-weight bearing.

iv. However, enzyme therapy is currently the treatment of choice in significantly affected patients. **Cerezyme,** a recombinantly produced mannose-m terminated (macrophage-targeted) acid beta glucosidase, has proved highly efficacious and safe in diminishing the hepatosplenomegaly and improving bone marrow involvement and hematologic finding.

OSTEOCHONDRITIS

This is a disease of unknown etiology causing temporary softening of the ossific centres of a child leading to deformation under pressure and damaged growth subsequently.

i. *Perthes' disease* : Involves the ossific centre of the head of femur.

ii. *Scheuermann's disease* : Epiphysial osteonecrosis of adjacent vertebral bodies.

iii. *Köhler's disease* : Osteonecrosis of the tarsal navicular bone.

iv. *Kienböck's disease* : Osteonecrosis of the lunate bone.

v. *Freiberg's disease* : Osteonecrosis of second or third metatarsal head.

vi. *Calve's disease* : Collapse of body of one vertebra (dorsal).

vii. *Sever's disease* : Osteochondrosis of the heel.

viii. *Osgood–Schlatter disease* : Inflammation of the growth centre that forms tibial tuberosity.

ix. **Preoser's disease** : Osteochondritis of scaphoid

x. **Sinding–Larsen disease** : Osteochondritis of lower pole of patella

xi. **Panner disease** : Osteochondrosis of the capitellum

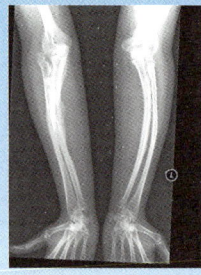

Imaging in Orthopaedics

15

MRI IN ORTHOPAEDICS

Imaging modality that utilizes the phenomenon of nuclear magnetism.

Mechanism

Nuclei of elements with odd number of protons and neutrons especially hydrogen when stimulated in strong magnetic field align themselves. The alignment is disturbed by a pulse of radio frequency, the atoms again regain their alignment and as it does, it liberates energy. This energy is assayed and converted to images. Here the sequence of procedure and imaging planes are predetermined so clinical details are must in a steady state, when a radio frequency pulse is applied, they create signals recorded in **T1** and **T2** (longitudinal and transverse) relaxation phases.

The types of images can be **T1, T2** and spin density.

The **T1** images are sharp and well defined anatomical picture, tissue with high concentration of hydrogen nuclei emit high signals producing **bright** images, e.g. fat, bone marrow, cancellous bone (Fig. 15.1a).

Tissue with low concentration of hydrogen emit low signal and hence appear **black**, e.g.

ligaments, cortical bone, air and tendons. Tissue with medium content fall in the **grey scale,** e.g. cartilage, muscle and spinal canal. In **T1** water appears **dark**, whereas in **T2** water appears **white** (**T2** water white) (Fig. 15.1b).

Proton density and short tau inversion recovery can suppress signals from fat and increase the contrast for water containing tissues.

Gadolinium is used as contrast media for early detection of infection.

Uses

For early and accurate diagnosis of:
  i. Spine and disc related disorders.
 ii. Osteonecrosis of femoral head.
iii. Assessment of tumours.
 iv. Assessment of marrow changes.
  v. Articular and periarticular structure visualization.
 vi. Internal derangement of knee, effusion.
vii. Early detection of bone and joint infections especially in the spine.

Advantages

• Non-invasive, versatile, high degree of specificity and accuracy.
• Superior soft tissue contrast resolution.

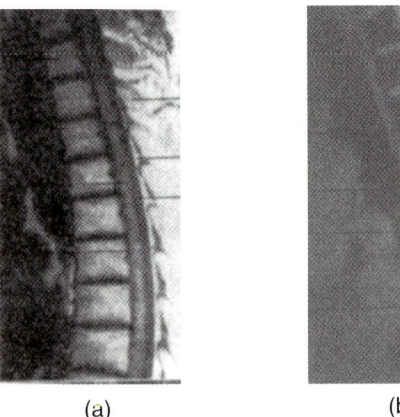

(a)   (b)

Figs 15.1a and b: (a) T1-image: Bone marrow appear–white; CSF and Disc appears–black, (b) T2-image: Bone marrow appear–black; CSF and Disc appears–white

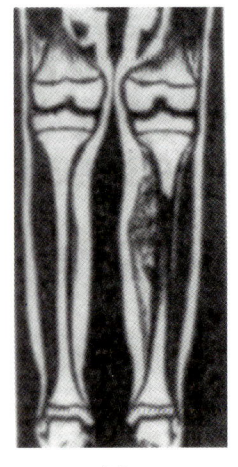
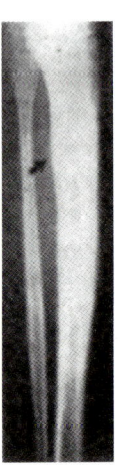

(a)   (b)

Figs 15.2a and b: (a) MRI of Ewing's sarcoma soft tissue extension in T2 image, (b) Ewing's sarcoma as seen on X-ray

- Multiplanar resolution.
- No radiation hazards.
- Better and modifiable soft tissue contrast (Fig. 15.2a).
- Ability for non-invasive vascular imaging.

Disadvantages

- Cost is high.
- Difficult in patients suffering from claustrophobia.

Contraindications for Doing MRI

- Intracranial clips, external fixators, implants.
- Cardiac pacemakers and auto defibrillators.
- Biostimulators and implanted infusion devices.
- Certain cardiac valves and internal hearing aids. Metallic orbital foreign bodies. 1st and 2nd trimester pregnancy.

CT SCAN (COMPUTED AXIAL TOMOGRAPHY)

Invented by Godfrey Hounsfield in 1973. Technique of tomography involves moving the X-ray source and receptor around the body in relation to a point in body. The resulting film has the image of structures at that point. Using a computer, the matrix of data produced can be converted to an image in a plane. The clarity of image can be enhanced by using a filter and further by setting a window. The thickness of slices produced can be decreased to enhance the clarity.

Uses

i. To assess tumour size and spread.

ii. To diagnose spinal disorders, especially inter-vertebral disc prolapse, spinal canal stenosis.

iii. Joint abnormalities and pelvic lesions.

iv. Assessment of complex fracture and fracture sites not accessible on plain X-ray, e.g. sacroiliac joints, vertebral bodies, carpal bones.

v. To assess bone density with contrast media, enhanced and accurate image can be made.

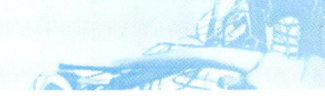

Advantages

- Axial cuts reduces problems of anatomical superimposition.
- Greater radiographic density discrimination.
- 3D images can be built up with the help of advanced software and spiral CT angiography can be done with contrast.
- CT guided biopsies can be done with precision.
- By knowing the Hounsfield unit of a shadow, we may predict the nature of a tissue involved.

Disadvantages

- Radiation is high.
- Can't do multiplanar imaging.
- Poorer soft tissue contrast.
- Prone for artifact in bony walled areas, e.g. spine.

SCINTIGRAPHY
(RADIOACTIVE ISOTOPE UPTAKE STUDY)

Tissues take up intravenously infused radioactive isotopes depending on their character and vascular status and emit protons which can be recorded by gamma camera to produce an image.

The commonly used isotopes are technetium 99m, gallium 67, etc.

Technetium 99m, is an ideal one because of its short half-life (6 hours), rapid excretion in urine, high affinity for bone tissue and sufficient emission of gamma rays.

Increased uptake indicates increased vascularity. High uptake in the delayed phase is seen in new bone formation, in fracture healing, tumours, revascularisation in osteonecrosis, heterotopic bone formation as in myositis ossification.

Uses

Early diagnosis of inflammation, metastasis, osteonecrosis, stress fracture.

USG (ULTRASONOGRAPHY)

This is based on Peizo electric effect. A disc of lead zirconate titanate is executed by means of two electrodes which causes it to resonate the beam of ultrasound which passes through the tissues. High frequency sound waves are produced by a transducer and the reflections from different tissue is recorded as echo. *Solids and fat are highly ecogenic, while cysts are low ecogenic.*

Uses

i. Diagnosis of deep seated abscess, cysts and aneurysm.

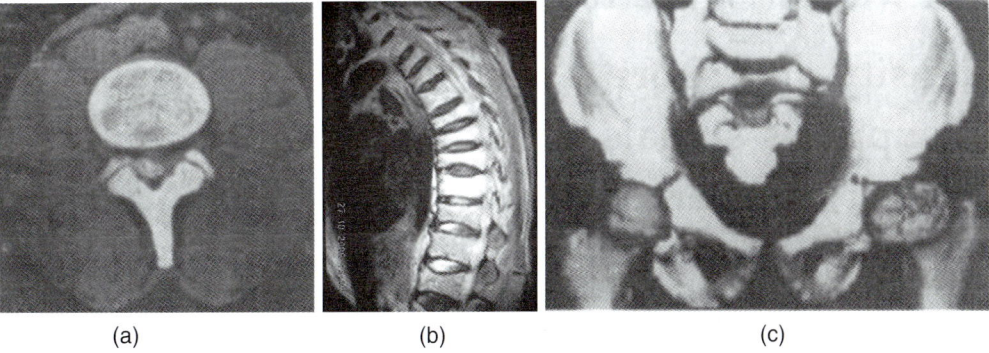

Figs 15.3a to c: (a) CT scan of spine, (b) CT scan of osteoporosis, (c) 3D image of Perthes' hip left side.

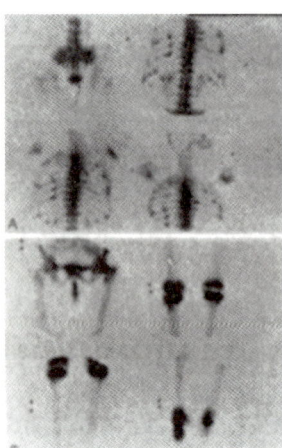

Fig. 15.4: ^{99m}Tc uptake showing multiple secondaries

ii. Imaging of hip dysplasia and infections in neonates using a 7.5-MHz probe.

Advantages

This is a non-invasive, cheap, portable and widely available diagnostic tool for an excellent guiding of percutaneous needle drainage of deep collections.

ARTHROSCOPY

Arthroscopy is an important tool for use in diagnosis and treatment of joint disorders. Arthroscopy offers distinct advantaged over open exploration of joints. The entire joint can be visualized and low morbidity of arthroscopy allows rapid rehabilitation. Common joints for arthroscopy are knee, shoulder, elbow, ankle, and wrist joint. Arthroscopy is done for diagnostic examination of joint or for therapeutic surgical interventions.

An arthroscope is an optical instrument. Fiberoptic arthroscope consist of a rod lens systems surrounded by multiple light conducting glass fibrils. These two systems are enclosed in a metal sheath. Lens is angled in the scope, usually with inclination of 25 to 90 degrees. Diameter of arthroscope varies from 1.7 to 7.0 mm one end of the scope has eyepiece for viewing. A television camera can be attached to eyepiece for viewing on television set.

Indications

- Acute haemarthrosis
- Meniscal injuries
- Loose bodies
- Selected tibial plateau fracture
- Patellar chondromalacia or mal alignment
- Chronic synovitis
- Knee instability
- Recurrent effusions
- Chondral and osteochondral fractures.

BONE DENSITOMETRY DEXA (DUAL ENERGY X-RAY ABSORPTIOMETRY)

This is a quick simple non-invasive precision technique for estimation of the status of bone density with minimal radiation exposure and can be done at multiple sites, usually two sites, the hip and wrist, are measured in combination for accurate diagnosis. It is measured in grams/cm^2 (Figs 15.5a and b).

- T-SCORE: This signifies patient's level compared to peak bone mass in normal young adults.

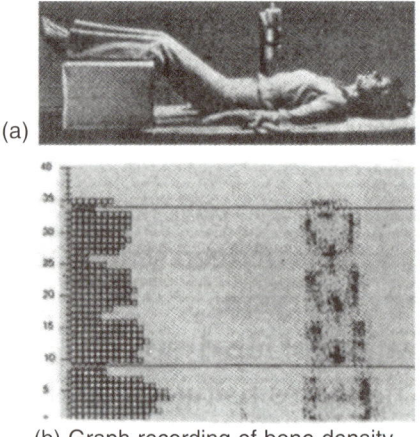

(a)

(b) Graph recording of bone density

Figs 15.5a and b

- Z-SCORE : This is patient's BMD compared to the peak bone mass in age/sex matched adults.
- The WHO criteria defines patient's bone density.
- T-SCORE : Value 1 is normal. Its value less than 1 leads to osteopenia. Between –1 and –2.5 is osteoporosis.

QUANTITATIVE COMPUTED TOMOGRAPHY

This gives excellent cortical as well as cancellous density and for deep-seated bones like the vertebra, but the radiation dose is high.

Uses

i. This is used for the detection of osteoporosis, for prediction of fractures.
ii. Confirmation of clinical diagnosis of osteoporosis.
iii. Determination of rate of bone loss for prognostic treatment of osteoporosis.
iv. For risk assessment of osteoporosis in perimenopausal women who are willing to take HRT.
v. For monitoring the response to a particular mode of treatment of osteoporosis.

LUMBAR DISC PROLAPSE AS SEEN IN DIFFERENT MODALITIES (Figs 15.6a to c)

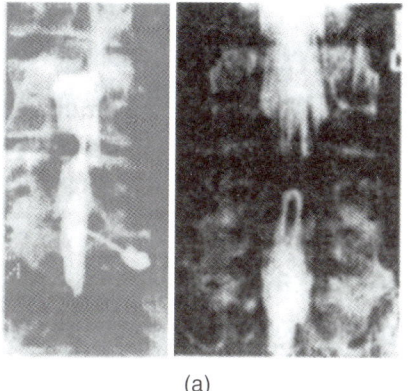

(a)

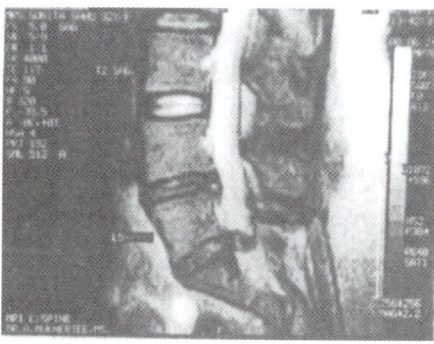

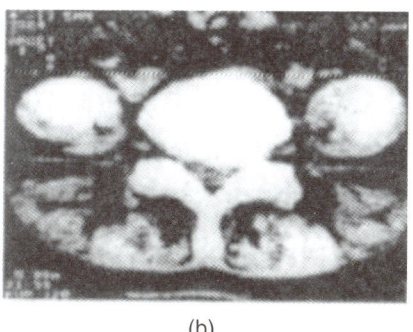

(b)

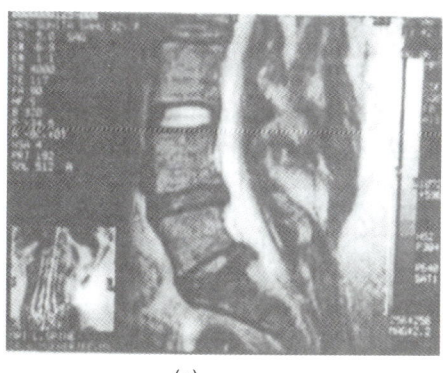

(c)

Figs 15.6a to c: (a) Myelography showing obstruction of dye, (b) Myelo CT showing disc prolapse in cross section (c) MRI showing multiple disc prolapse

16

Gait, Orthoses, Prostheses and Physical Therapy

GAIT

This is rhythmic coordinated movement of the upper and lower limb in cyclic order balancing the pelvis and spine, helping the person in forward propagation.

A normal gait must be rhythmic and soundless, having springness in the feet which work alternatively in a definite cyclic order. A normal gait cycle is divisible into two phases for each extremity.

i. The stance phase, during which the foot is on the ground (60°) (Fig. 16.1a).

ii. The swing phase, when the foot is off the ground (40°) (Fig. 16.1b).

Stance phase is further divided into heel strike, foot flat, mid stance, heel off, toe break, and push off (toe off).

Swing phase is divided into acceleration, mid swing and deacceleration phases. In rhythmic gait, while one foot is in the stance phase, other passes through the swing, touching the floor (initial contact) followed by the sole of that foot. When the whole foot is in contact with the ground, this foot is supporting the whole body weight and is in the mid-stance phase. Next follows the push off phase. After momentarily establishing the weight on the whole foot, the heel of the

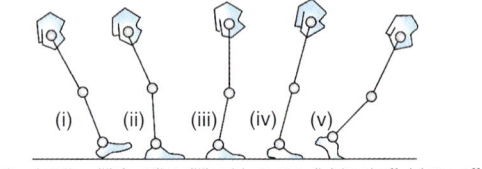

(i) heel strike (ii) foot flat (iii) mid-stance (iv) heel off (v) toe off

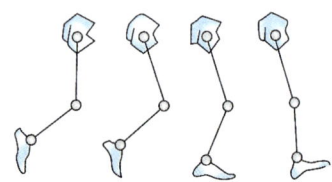

acceleration-mid swing-deacceleration

Figs 16.1a and b: (a) Stance phase, (b) Swing phase

supporting extremity rises from the floor. In succession, the balls of toes prepare to lift off from the ground. In the meantime, the strong action of gastro-soleus propels the body forward. With the toes off, the entire foot leaves the ground and enters the swing phase; the leg gets accelerated forward to get in front of the body to be prepared for the next heel strike. This is the acceleration subphase of the swing phase. While passing in this direction, at one point, the leg has to pass just beneath the body. This is the mid-swing phase. In this phase, the leg is shortened by flexing the hip and knees so that the foot completely clears the ground. Immediately after the leg goes in front of the body, the movement is restrained (deacceleration). Now the foot is prepared to go for heel strike.

During normal gait, for a moment, the two lower extremities are in simultaneous contact with the ground. This happens between push off and toe off on one side and between heel strike and foot flat on the contralateral side. During this period, both legs support the body weight and this is known as **'double support'**. The period of this double support is inversely proportional to the **cadence** (number of steps taken per minute) of the gait, i.e. if cadence of gait decrease, the period of double support increases and vice versa.

Walking can be distinguished from running by minimization of the period of double support in running. Roughly calculated, the relative period of different phases of gait are as follows: stance phase 60%, swing phase 40% and double support 10% of the cycle. With increase in the cadence, gradually the period spent in swing phase increases and vice versa.

There can be several variations in a normal gait depending upon the weight, posture, the gymnastic activities, the shape of the foot and the ground over which the individual walks. Everyone adapts the least energy consuming style of walking.

The lay description of abnormal gait can be divided into two patterns—limping and lurching.

- In limping the patient avoids weight bearing on the affected side as far as possible (*diminished stance phase*). Limping denotes a painful condition on the affected side.
- In lurch, the patient *prolongs the stance phase* to improve the stability. Lurching denotes variable failure of the abduction mechanism.

However, there are recognized patterns of gait which occur in particular conditions.

Scissor Gait

Here one leg crosses directly over the other with each step, like crossing of the blades of a scissor, e.g. cerebral palsy.

High-Steppage Gait

Here the patient flexes the hip and knee excessively in order to clear the ground for example foot drop.

Spastic Gait/Hemiplegic Gait

Here the patient muscles do not allow the hip and knee to be flexed enough for the foot to clear the ground. Therefore, the patient partially drags his weight on the spastic leg. In this attempt, there is some circumduction effect on the lower limb, example hemiplegia for ground clearance.

Lathyric Gait

In this gait there is a combination of spasticity, hyperabduction and dragging.

Waddling Gait/Duck Gait

There is increased lordosis, the body sways from side to side on a wide base. Therefore, the patient lurches on both sides while walking, e.g. bilateral congenital dislocation of hip, osteomalacia, pregnancy, myopathy.

Trendelenburg Gait

It may be unilateral or bilateral. Bilateral Trendelenburg gait is almost like the waddling gait. When unilateral, the patient lurches on the affected side. Any condition, in which there is deficit in abduction mechanism of the hip joint, e.g. CDH, polioparalysis will cause this.

Ataxic/Drunkards/Reeling Gait

Here the patient tends to walk irregularly on a wide base, swinging sideways with tendency of falling with each step (seen in cerebellar in-coordination, or in drunkard state).

Festinating/Short Shifting Gait

Here the patient with stooping body is propelled forward quickly in succession as if trying to catch up with the centre of gravity, e.g. parkinsonism. In a few cases of parkinsonism **'retropulsion'** occurs, i.e. if the patient is pushed backwards, he starts walking backward involuntarily.

Antalgic Gait

Painful gait. Due to pain, the patient avoids weight bearing on the affected limb (reduced stance phase).

Stamping Gait/Charcot's

Occurs in sensory ataxia, e.g. tabes dorsalis. The patient raises his feet abnormally high and jerks them forward to strike the ground with a stamp.

Knock Knee Gait

The gait here is also a typical one, i.e. while walking, the patient flexes the hip slightly, the knees point and oppose each other, the ankles and feet are kept apart with tendency of toe in.

Short Limb Gait

Initially the shortening is made up by equinus, with more shortening, the patient dips his pelvis on that side.

ORTHOSES

It is a mechanical device to promote stability, relieve pain, control deformity and restrict movements, e.g. axillary crutches, brace, cervical collar, calipers, surgical shoes.
  i. *Spinal paralysis:* Spinal corset brace.
  ii. *Hip weakness:* Pelvic band with hip joint.
  iii. *Knee:* Quadriceps weakness-AK with anterior knee stop.
    Hamstrings weakness: AK with posterior knee stop.
  iv. *Ankle:* Surgical shoes with caliper below knee
    a. Equinus: BK caliper with posterior knee stop.
    b. Calcaneus: BK caliper with anterior knee stop.
  v. *Subtalar*
    a. Valgus heel: Outside iron with inside T-strap.
    b. Varus heel: Inside iron, outside T-strap.
  vi. *Foot drop*
    a. Static: Ortholene foot drop splint.
    b. Dynamic: BK with toe raising device/spring.
  vii. *Cervical spondylosis and injuries:* Cervical collar (soft, hard), four poster Kumar Somi Brace.
  viii. *Taylor brace:* It is used for supporting the dorsolumbar spine following surgery or injuries.
  ix. *Cervical collar:* This is used for support-ing the cervical spine following injuries or instability as in cervical spondylosis. This may be hard or soft or modified in the form of four poster collar for a rigid support and even distraction of the cervical spine.

COMMON ORTHOSIS
UPPER LIMB

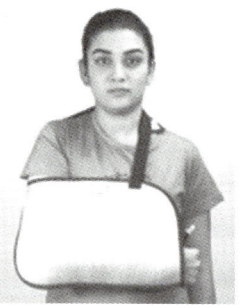 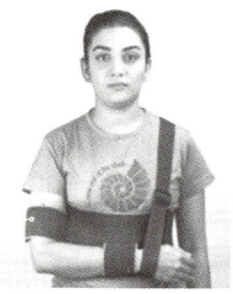

Elbow pouch   Shoulder immobilizer

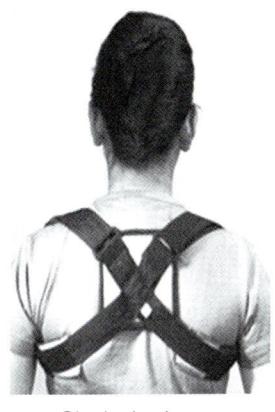

Clavicular brace

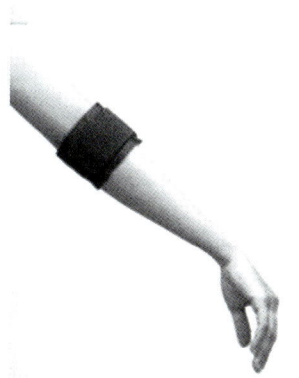

Elbow strap

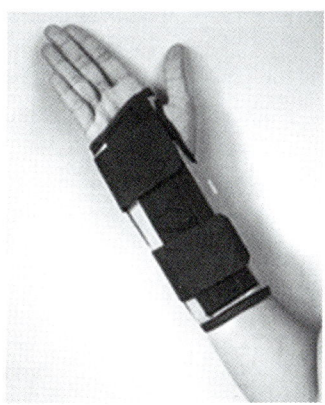

Wrist splint

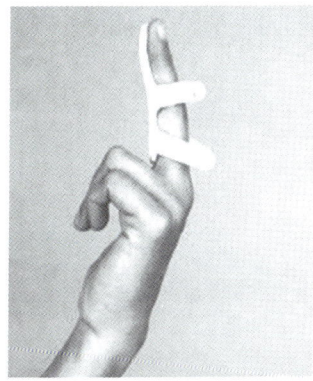

Froggy splint

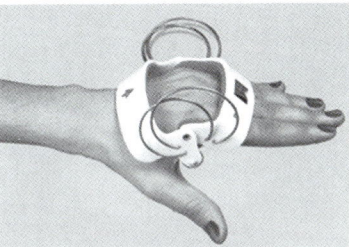

Knuckle Bender splint

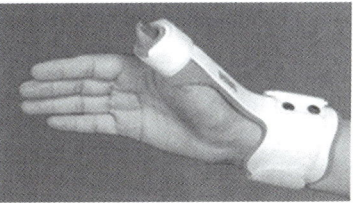

Thumb support splint

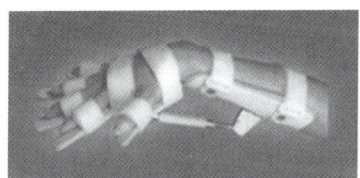

Turn buckle wrist extensor splint

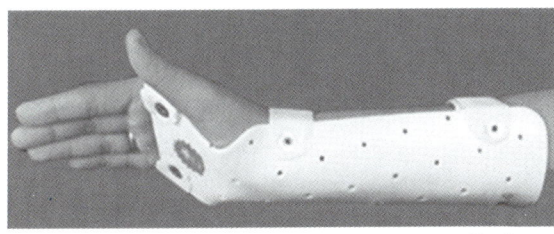

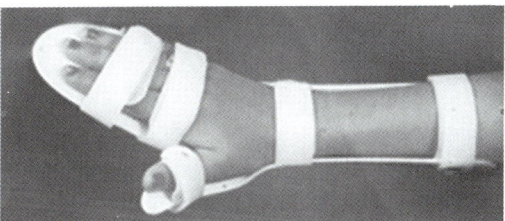

Cock-up splint

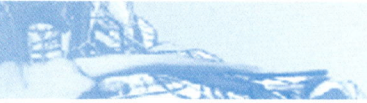

LOWER LIMB

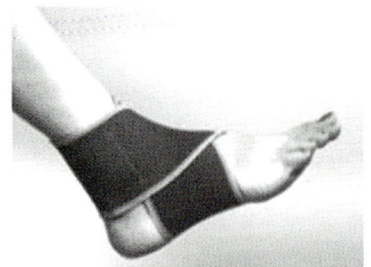

Ankle strap

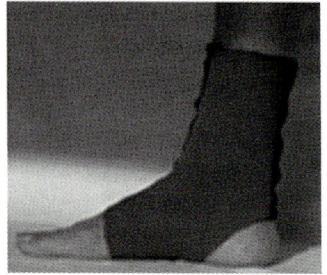

Anklet

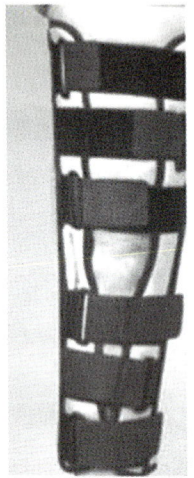

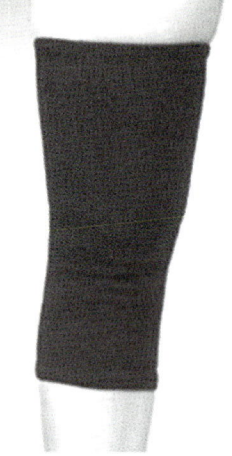

Knee extension splint   Knee cap

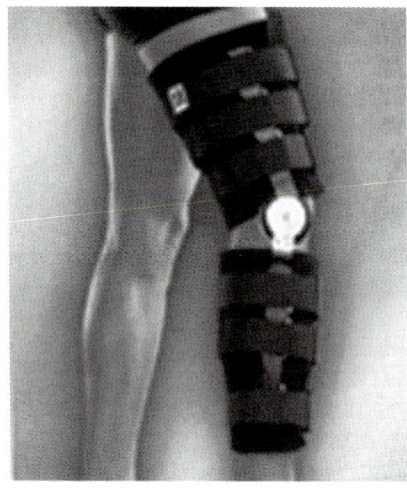

Hinged knee brace

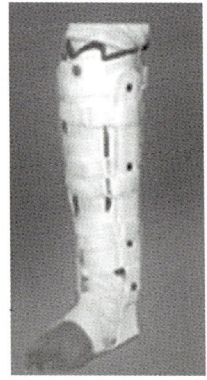

Tibial corset

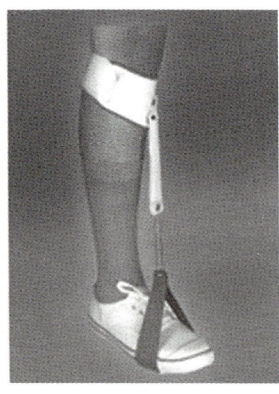

Dynamic foot drop splint

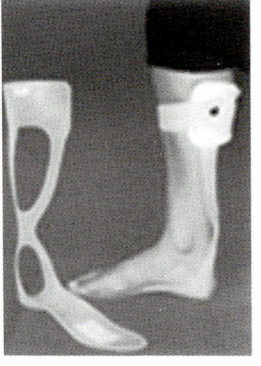

Static foot drop splint

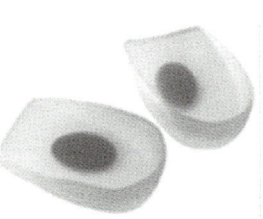

Silicon heel pad

SPINAL

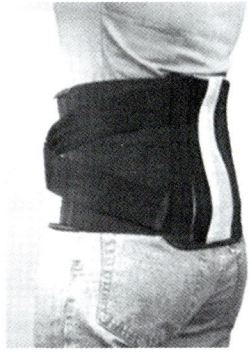

Lumbosacral

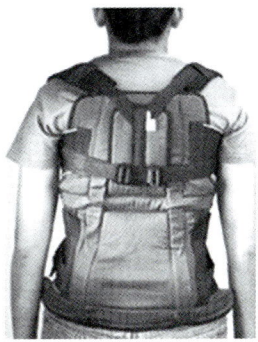

Taylor brace

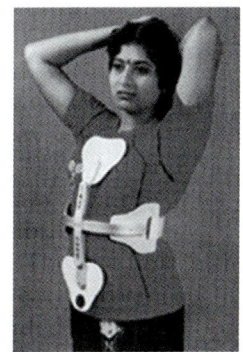

ASH brace

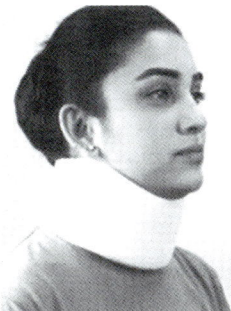

Cervical collar

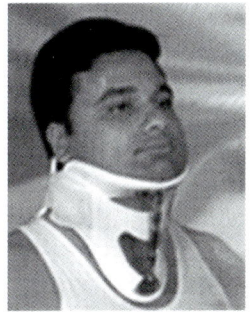

Philadelphia collar

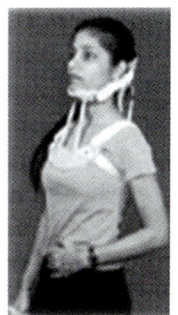

Four poster collar

WALKING AIDS AND WHEELCHAIRS

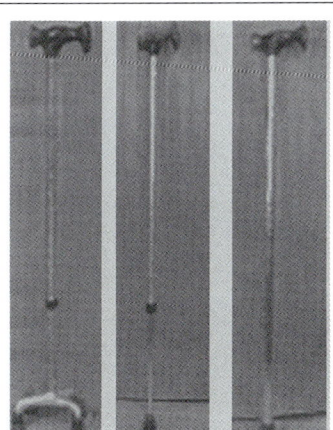

Canes

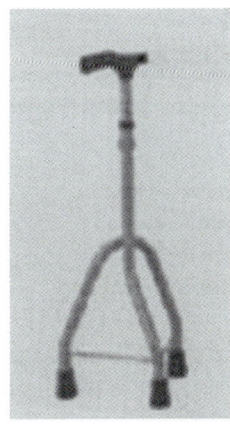

Tripoid canes

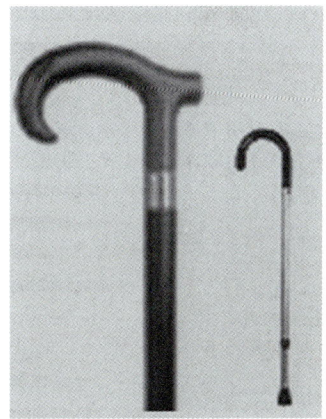

Walking stick

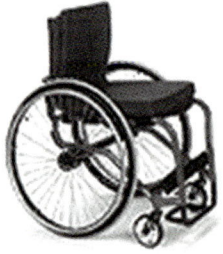

Manual wheelchair

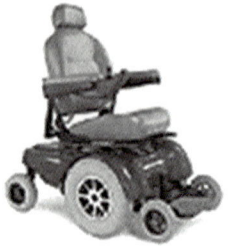

Motorized wheelchair

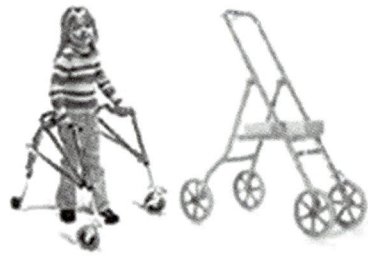

Toddler's walking aids

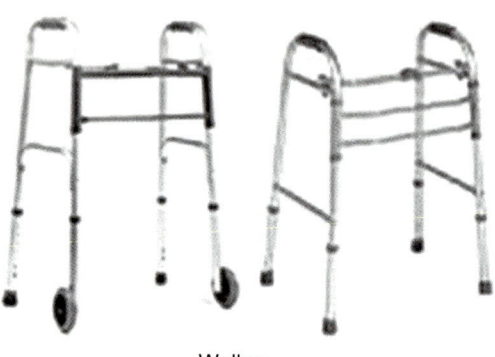

Walker

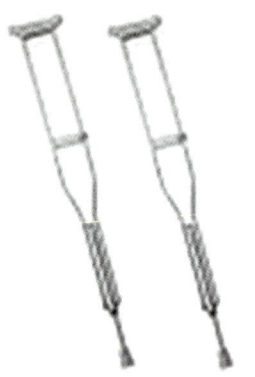

Adjustable axillary crutched

Walking Aids

These are mechanical aids to support a weak part of the body so as to help it to perform its normal function.

i. **Crutches:** This helps by aiding the lower limb during the stance phase of the locomotion by sharing the weight bearing. It may be used individually or as a pair. It consists of an axillary pad supported by two parallel bars connected by a hand grip and terminally ending in a single bar which is rubber tipped. It is measured from the anterior fold of the axilla to the heel of the foot to which 2 inches is added for the ground clearance.

The hand grip should be approximately at the level of a greater trochanter so as to keep the elbow in 30° of flexion. It may be made up of wood, aluminum, or steel.

ii. **Elbow crutch:** This is a modified walking stick which has a handgrip and a forearm cuff support to give it a wider area of contact for weight transmission through the elbow and forearm (Fig. 16.2b).

iii. **Walking stick:** It is used for elderly patients and following lower limb injuries for partial weight bearing. It is usually bent at the level of the greater trochanter for handgrip. The tip is single (Fig. 16.2c), tripod or quadripod to give it a wider base.

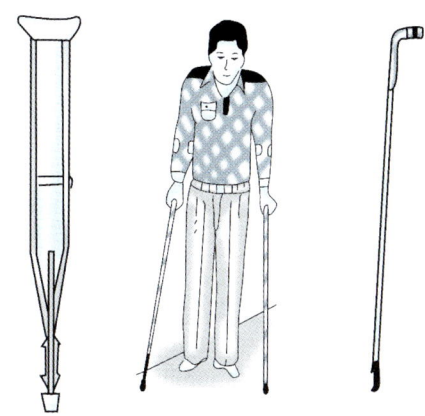

Figs 16.2a to c: (a) Crutch, (b) Elbow crutch, (c) Walking stick

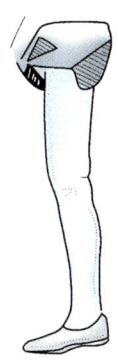

Fig. 16.3a: HKAFO

PROSTHESIS

This is an artificial device designed to replace appearance/function of the part of the body which has been removed.

i. **Upper limb:** Above/below elbow and hand, this may be cosmetic or dynamic.
ii. **Lower limb:**
   a. HKAFO (Hip knee ankle foot prosthesis) for hip disarticulation (Fig. 16.3a).
   b. Above knee prosthesis has:
      - **In young patient** need quadrilateral suction socket good.
      - **In old patient:** Total contact suction socket for old patients with pelvic band and hip joint.
        (i) suction thigh socket, (ii) knee hinge, (iii) tibial component with a distal, (iv) SACH foot (solid ankle and cushion heel) or a Jaipur foot (Fig. 16.3b).
   c. Below knee, patellar tendon bearing prosthesis has a PTB total contact socket with SACH foot (Fig. 16.3c).
   d. **Syme's prothesis:** This is total contact socket to accommodate ankle and heel pad.

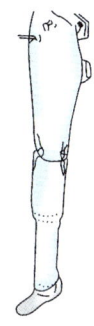

Fig. 16.3b: Above knee prosthesis

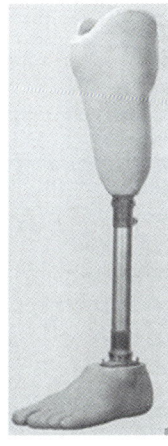

Fig. 16.3c: Below knee prosthesis

Jaipur/Madura Foot

These are fabricated out of rubber or plastic and shaped like natural bare foot with similar colour, so as to look like the normal one, ideal for rural bare-footed people.

Endolite prosthesis: This is extremely light made of carbon fibre components, highly durable but expensive.

PHYSICAL THERAPY AND REHABILITATION

Rehabilitation is defined as the whole process of restoring a disabled person to a condition in which he or she is able, as early as possible, to resume a normal life or atleast achieve his/her physical potential. Sphere of rehabilitation includes physical therapist, occupational therapist, remedial gymnast, orthotist and prosthetist.

Physiotherapy can be broadly divided into:
  i. **Passive**, i.e. directed towards the alleviation of symptoms.
  ii. **Active** physical therapy, the restoration of function by activity.

Physical Modalities
- Heat
- High frequency currents
- Ultrasonics
- Laser therapy
- Cryotherapy
- Electrical muscle stimulation (EMS)
- Transcutaneous electrical neural stimulation (TENS)
- Ionization

Heat

a. **Heating by radiation:** Radiant heat, lamps using emitters are relatively cheap source of heat using electrical pads and infrared lamps.
  Disadvantage: Takes longer time to heat up.
b. **Conductive and convective heating:** Hot water is probably the most widely used agent for conductive heating, either in the form of hot packs, hot soaks, compresses or hydrotherapy pools. Wax baths are a convenient form of heating for the extremities, particularly the hand in rheumatoid arthritis.
  Disadvantages: Impaired skin sensation, poor and fragile skin, circulatory dysfunction.

THERAPEUTIC PARAFFIN LIQUID

Benefit of hot paraffin treatment is obtained by heating a patient's body parts, particularly joints and muscles. The penetrating heat from hot paraffin helps relieves pain and stiffness in afflicted joints, relaxes muscles, reduces muscle spasms, and stimulates blood circulation to the affected area. Paraffin treatments are therefore useful before or after exercise, massage or other physical therapy. In addition, paraffin treatments are used in the symptomatic relief of pain due to arthritis, bursitis, fibrositis, tendonitis, chronic joint inflammation, muscle strains, sprains, or spasms, and additional athletic conditions in which heat therapy is recommended and beneficial. Paraffin treatment is frequently prescribed for post-fracture and post-dislocation treatment.

Infrared Rays (Fig. 16.4)

Infrared rays are electromagnetic waves, the heat energy obtained from the rays are used to relieve pain.

Where Useful?

1. Pain
2. Muscle strain and pain

Where It should not be Used?

1. Defective blood supply to the area, e.g. in case of diabetes.
2. Any blood loss
3. Defective skin sensation (nerve damage)

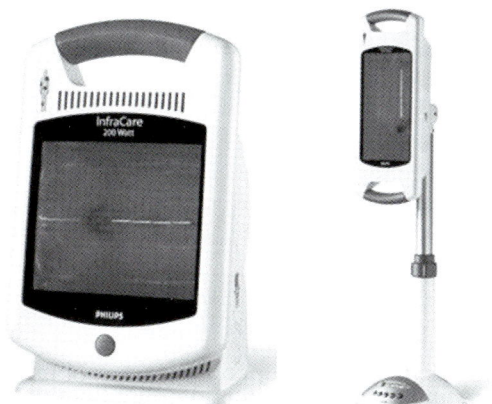

Fig. 16.4: Infrared rays generators (2 types) (1) Non-luminous generator (2) Luminous generator

High Frequency Currents

Short Wave Diathermy

The heating effects of diathermy are produced by placing the patient within an electric field created by high frequency AC current, in which the patient forms the part of the secondary circuit of a high frequency generator; good for backache and myalgia.

This deep heat modality is the therapeutic application of high radiofrequency electrical currents. The radiofrequency electromagnetic field usually is at a frequency of 27.12 MHz (l=11.06 m). Hyperemia, sedation, and analgesia are the basic physiologic effects. The reduction in muscle spasm due to muscle relaxation is a result of increased vascular supply to the treated area. A transverse technique is applied to treat a larger anatomic area with the primary concentration at the midpoint between electrodes.

The following problems can be treated with short wave diathermy, depending upon the individual condition of each patient and the desired treatment goals:

- Localized musculoskeletal pain
- Inflammation (joint or tissue)
- Pain/spasm
- Sprains/strains
- Tendinitis
- Tenosynovitis
- Bursitis
- Rheumatoid arthritis
- Periostitis
- Capsulitis

Short wave diathermy has the following precautions or contraindications:

- Malignancy
- Sensory loss
- Tuberculosis
- Metallic implants or foreign bodies
- Pregnancy
- Application over moist dressings
- Ischemic areas or arteriosclerosis
- Thromboangiitis obliterans
- Phlebitis
- Use extreme care with pediatric and geriatric patients
- Cardiac pacemakers
- Contact lenses
- Metal-containing intrauterine contraceptive devices

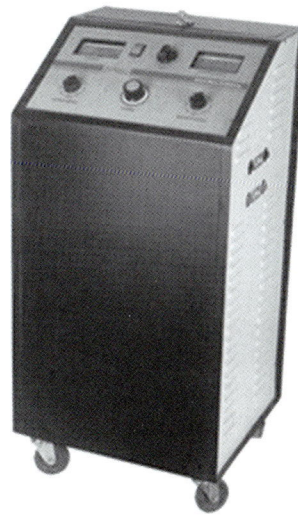

Fig. 16.5: SWD machine

- Metal in contact with skin (e.g. watches, belt buckles, jewellery)
- Use over epiphyseal areas of developing bon

Microwave Diathermy

It has a shorter wavelength than shortwave diathermy. The microwave has an antenna or director, which beams energy that is both absorbed and reflected.

Microwave diathermy, a form of electromagnetic radiation, is another deep heat modality that selectively heats tissues with high water concentration. Hyperemia, sedation, and analgesia are the physiologic effects, similar to the results of shortwave diathermy. Secondary local vascular dilatation results in increased local metabolism.

The two frequencies designated for microwave diathermy are 2456 MHz and 915 MHz, the latter being the most commonly used. Since frequencies are higher than in shortwave diathermy and wavelengths are the same size as the applicator, microwave diathermy can be focused more easily than shortwave diathermy. The lower frequency is preferred because it provides selective heat deep into muscle, and less energy is converted to heat in the subcutaneous fat. Direct contact applicators with full aperture skin contact are optimal for improved coupling and reduced stray radiation.

Pulse Electromagnetic Energy

Short waves are pulsed in packages with sufficient rest intervals that the small amount of heat generated is rapidly dissipated. This prevents cumulative rise in tissue temperature.

Ultrasonics

Therapeutic ultrasound is a physical agent with its effect being due to heating and mechanical phenomenon within the tissues. It produces ultrasound energy via the piezoelectric effect of a voltage applied to a ceramic disc or crystal for tennis elbow and painful heel.

Ultrasound is a deep heating modality that uses high-frequency acoustic vibration above the human audible spectrum, defined as frequencies greater than 17,000 Hz. Therapeutic ultrasound is in the frequency range of 0.8–1.0 MHz. Ultrasound energy is generated by the piezoelectric effect; electrical energy is applied to a crystal, causing it to vibrate at a high frequency and to produce ultrasound. Ultrasound is delivered by continuous or pulsed wave (the goal is to produce nonthermal effects such as streaming and cavitation) and provides a high heatin. Therapeutic ultrasound (Fig. 16.6) causes the following biologic effects:

- Temporary analgesia
- Increased peripheral blood flow
- Increased vascularity with associated hyperemia/inflammatory response
- Increased cell membrane permeability
- Peripheral nerve conduction changes (reversible conduction block with high-intensity ultrasound exposure)
- Relief of muscle spasms

Additional indications for ultrasound include the following:
- Joint contracture
- Joint adhesions
- Calcific bursitis
- Hematoma resolution.

Laser Therapy

Laser light is generated by the simulated emission of photons from gases, usually helium, neon or gallium arsenide. The three main characteristics of laser light are monochromaticity, coherence and minimal divergence. Laser acts by specific physiological effects at subcellular level thereby reducing oedema, increased collagen formation and increasing vascularity of wounds.

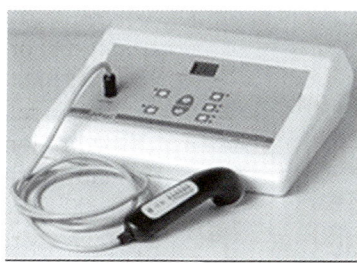

Fig. 16.6: Ultrasonotherapy

Cryotherapy

Cooling agents such as ice, gel, chemicals, freon.

Therapeutic use of ice :
a. As a first-aid measure to produce vaso-constriction.
b. To reduce pain and oedema.
c. To reduce spasticity.

Electrical Muscle Stimulation (EMS)

a. To enhance contraction when there is a reflex inhibition.
b. To supplement contraction in post-injury or post-surgical states where the limb is immobilized.
c. To reinforce contraction in strengthening programmes.

Transcutaneous Electrical Nerve Stimulation (TENS)

Based on the Gate control theory of pain, TENS produces pain relief by inhibiting the passage of sensory inflow to the cortex. TENS also decreases pain by endorphin production.

TENS currently is one of the most commonly used forms of electroanalgesia. Hundreds of clinical reports exist concerning the use of TENS for various types of conditions such as low back pain (LBP), myofascial and arthritic pain, sympathetically mediated pain, bladder incontinence, neurogenic pain, visceral pain, and postsurgical pain. Because many of these studies were uncontrolled, there has been ongoing debate about the degree to which TENS is more effective than placebo in reducing pain (Fig. 16.7).

The currently proposed mechanisms by which TENS produces neuromodulation include the following:
• Presynaptic inhibition in the dorsal horn of the spinal cord
• Endogenous pain control (via endorphins, enkephalins, and dynorphins)
• Direct inhibition of an abnormally excited nerve
• Restoration of afferent input.

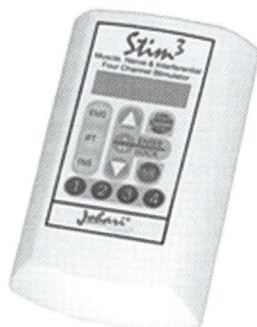

Fig. 16.7: TENS

Ionization

The process of driving ions into the tissues by an electric current is referred to as ioni-zation or iontophoresis. This technique brings about increase in blood circulation (use of hista-mine). A modified version of this technique is called **electroacupuncture**.

17

Plaster of Paris Support, Traction and Splints

This was first used by an army surgeon from Paris called Antonius Mathesen. The material used is semihydrated calcium sulphate powder finely sprayed over gauze bandages stiffened by starch or dextrose.

On immersion in water it undergoes an exothermic reaction and starts setting into a solid structure. The speed of setting depends on the material used, temperature of water and humidity.

It can be used as a slab which is a support encircling half or three-fourths of the limb or as a cast which requires a circumferential

application of the bandages around the limb and then shaped and contoured before its sets. It is always advisable to apply a fair amount of cotton padding and stockinet before applying a cast to avoid compartmental syndrome or skin damage.

Instructions to the Patients after Application of Cast

i. Elevate the limb and encourage active finger/toe movements.
ii. Immediately report to the doctor in event of
   a. Excruciating pain in the limb.
   b. Progressive oedema over the finger/toes.
   c. Numbness, tingling, pale and cynotic changes in the fingers.
   d. Paralysis or painful finger movements.

Advantages of POP Cast

This is easily available, cheap, versatile, durable, strong, simple to apply, radio translucent material requiring very little apparatus for application and can be used anywhere, anytime and in any part of the body.

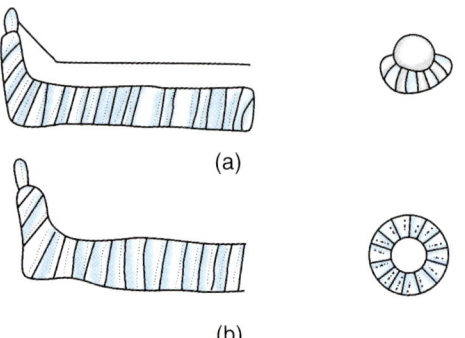

(a)

(b)

Figs 17.1a and b: (a) Slab; (b) cast

Complicalions of POP Cast

i. Pressure sores, dermatitis, skin blisters.
ii. Oedema due to tight plasters and even causing compartmental syndrome.
iii. Nerve palsy, circulatory embarrassment and deep vein thrombosis.
iv. Stiffness of joints, Sudeck's atrophy, osteoporosis.

The latest bandages which are now available are made up of fiberglass and resins, which is extremely light, strong, durable and waterproof (Figs 17.2a and b).

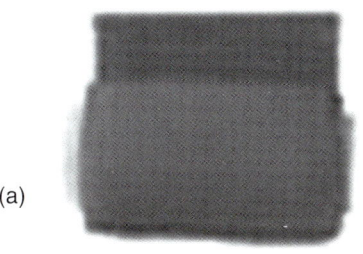

(a)

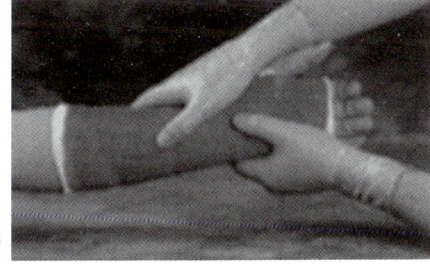

(b)

Figs 17.2a and b: Fiberglass and resins, cast bandages

Characteristics

- Lightweight and strong
- Excellent X-ray radiolucency
- Easy and simple to use
- Superior end lamination
- Moisture resistant after setting
- Superior mouldability and flexibility for patient comfort
- Good air-permeability for reduced odour and skin irritation

Alternatives

Cramer wire splint, foam padded aluminium malleable strips.

ACRYLIC BONE CEMENT

It is also known as poly methyl methacrylate (PMMA).

This is used as:
a. Space filler in bone cavities after curettage of tumours.
b. Load transferring when used along with the implants THR, TKR for cementing the implant and greater area contact at the bone/implant interphase.

It has two components:

i. **Polymer powder containing**
   a. PMMA grains 10–150 microns- 89%
   b. Radiopaque barium sulphate- 10%
   c. Polymerization initiator—1% (benzyl peroxide).

ii. **Liquid monomer containing:** Methyl methacrylate and activator 3% DMP toluidine.

When these two components are mixed there is an exothermic reaction, and within 5 to 8 minutes it forms a uniform dough, this is then filled at the desired space and if used with an implant, this is pressed for the next 10 minutes till it becomes hard. Antibiotics can be added while mixing the two components.

It is very important to lavage away all the bony debris and blood by thorough saline irrigation, before putting in the cement and hold the implant steady and well pressed while the cement is setting. Watch for hypotension during cement application.

TRACTIONS

> Traction is application of mechanical forces to counteract the deforming forces of an inflamed, injured, diseased or deformed part of the body, against countertraction.

Skin Traction

It is applied through adhesive plaster bandaged to the part distal to the deformed or injured part. The maximum of 15 pounds. can be applied. It is contraindicated in patients who are allergic to adhesive plaster, old patients with fragile skin, compound injuries with skin damage.

Technique

The adhesive strap is first applied to the skin (Fig. 17.3a) with cotton protection at the bony points and the lateral popliteal nerve, and then crepe bandage is rolled over it to give it a firm grip (Figs 17.3b and c), weights are then suspended to the wooden foot piece (Fig. 17.3d) through a hook.

Skeletal Traction

It is applied by passing a Steinmann pin or K-wire through the bone and then traction applied through it.

It is indicated when heavy traction has to be applied, the skin condition is unhealthy and needs frequent monitoring. It is best used for skull traction in cervical injuries, upper tibial for femoral fractures and calcaneal traction for injuries below the knee.

Complications associated with skeletal tractions are pin track infection, damage to neurovascular structures, arrest of epiphyseal growth in children due to prolonged traction, distraction of fracture site leading to nonunion.

Common Sites and Indications

   i. Crutchfield tongs for cervical fracture/dislocations (Fig. 17.4a).
  ii. Head halter for temporary traction to the neck as in cervical spondylosis (Fig. 17.4b).
 iii. Pelvic traction for spinal and pelvic injuries (Fig. 17.4c).
  iv. Halo pelvic traction for spinal deformities like scoliosis [pg 159, (Fig. 11.10a)].
   v. In central fracture dislocation of hip joint traction is applied through the greater trochanter by passing a cancellous screw hook into the neck of femur (Fig. 17.4d) and applying traction in the axis of the neck of femur.

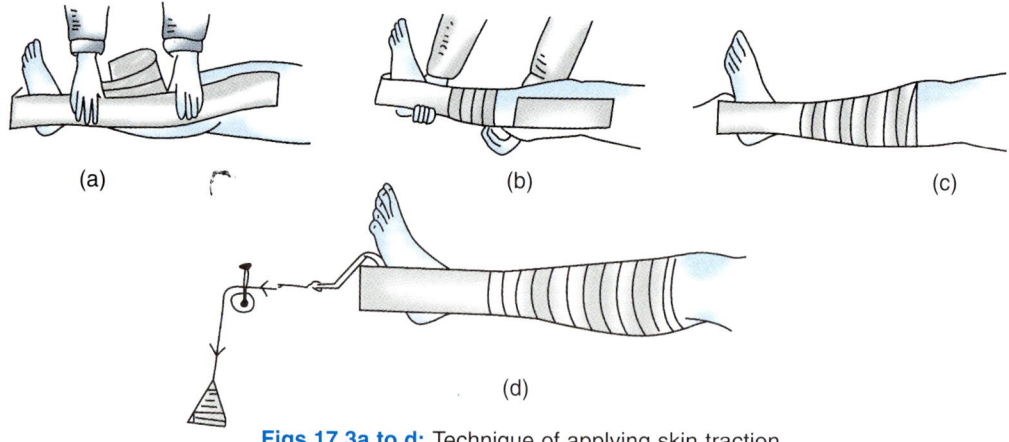

(a)   (b)   (c)

(d)

Figs 17.3a to d: Technique of applying skin traction

vi. Gallow's or Bryant's traction for shaft of femur and CDH in small children (Fig. 17.4e).

vii. Trochanteric and fracture shaft, fracture of femur by upper tibial pin (Fig. 17.4f).

viii. Fracture of tibia and ankle by calcaneal pin.

ix. In supracondylar fracture of the humerus, when there is extensive oedema blister formation, it is best to give DUNLOP traction (Fig. 17.4g) or by passing a Kirschner wire through the olecranon.

x. 90°–90° tractions in the upper limb for fracture shaft of humerus (Fig. 17.4h), lower limb for dislocation of hip and shaft femur.

Skull Traction

This is skeletal traction applied through the skull by means of Crutchfield tongs (Fig. 17.4a).

Indications

Fracture, dislocation and sprain of the cervical spine.

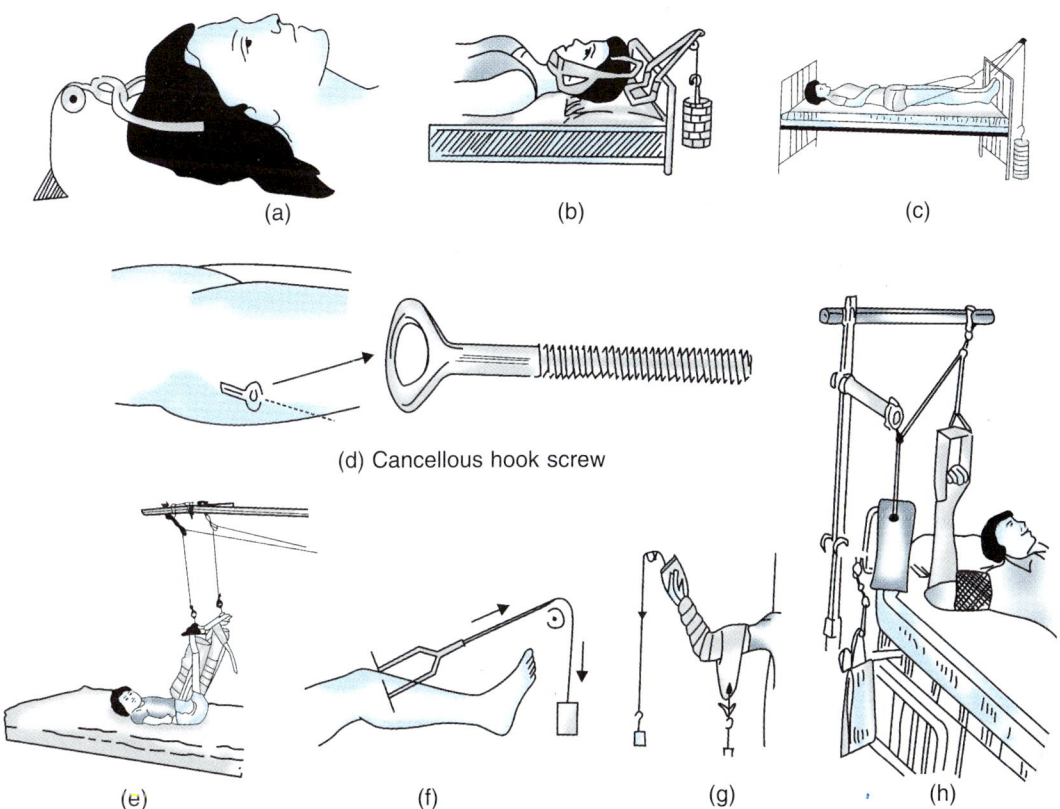

(a)   (b)   (c)

(d) Cancellous hook screw

(e)   (f)   (g)   (h)

Figs 17.4a to h: Common sites of skeletal traction

Buck's Leg Traction

Unilateral

This is the traction applied through the skin and can be either below knee or above knee and weights suspended by a pulley attached to the foot piece, and foot end of the bed elevated to provide countertraction (Fig. 17.5a).

Indications

Inflamed, injured and deformed hip and knee. Muscles spasm, sciatica and injuries involving the spine, pelvis, hip, shaft of femur and tibia.

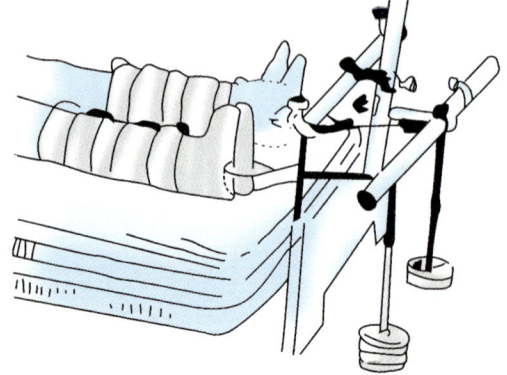

Fig. 17.5b Buck's leg traction (Bilateral)

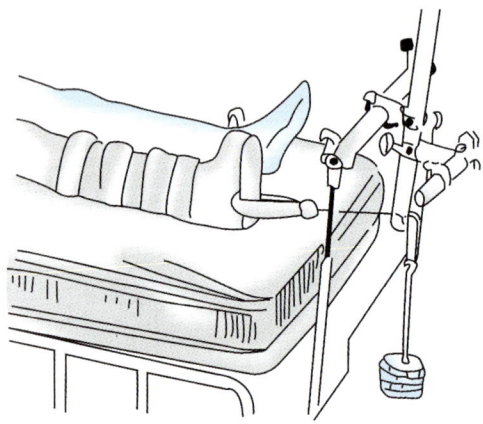

Fig. 17.5a: Buck's leg traction (Unilateral)

Bilateral Traction

In this, traction is applied to both the legs as in pelvic fracture (Fig. 17.5b).

Balanced Suspension and Traction with Thomas or Brady Leg Splint

This is indicated for fracture shaft of femur, tibia, hip and knee injuries. In this the splint is balanced and suspended. Traction is applied through a set of pulleys. A Pearson's knee attachment allows the patient to do the knee movements even with sustained traction (Fig. 17.6).

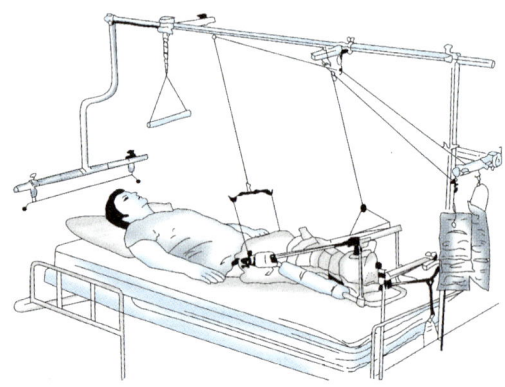

Fig. 17.6: Balanced suspensions and traction with Thomas or Brady leg splint

Hammock Traction

Fracture of the pelvis with opening of the pelvic girdle. This is a Hammock type of compression to the pelvis (Fig. 17.7).

Pelvic Traction

This is indicated for low backache, sciatica and minor injuries of the pelvis and spine. The patient is kept supine on the bed with the pelvis at a slightly lower level than the thighs which are flexed by about 15°–20° (Fig. 17.8).

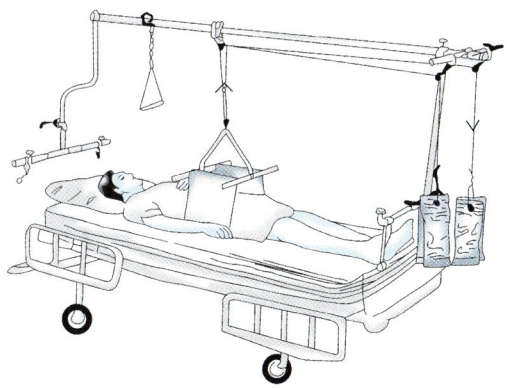

Fig. 17.7: Hammock traction

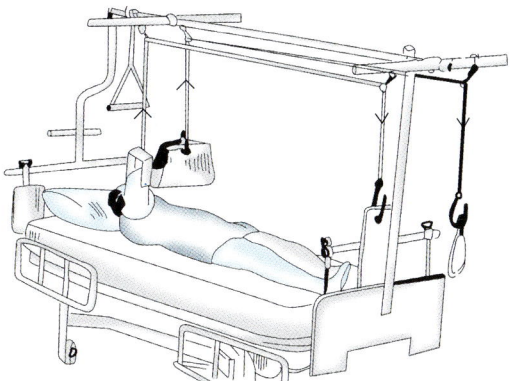

Fig. 17.9: 90–90 overhead traction

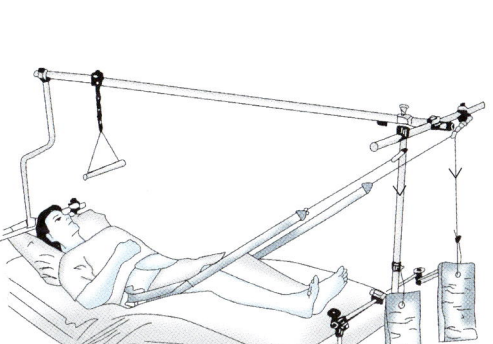

Fig. 17.8: Pelvic traction

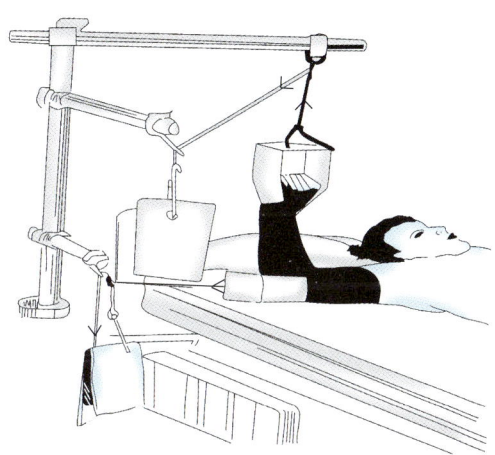

Fig. 17.10: 90–90 side traction

90–90 Overhead Traction

This is indicated for fracture, dislocation and injuries involving the shoulder and arm. Traction is applied in the long axis of the humerus vertically, while the forearm is supported in a sling horizontally over the chest (Fig. 17.9).

90–90 Side Traction

In this, traction is applied in the long axis of the humerus horizontally, while traction is applied to the forearm vertically with the elbow flexed by 90° (Fig. 17.10).

SPLINTS

Name	Use
Thomas splint	Fracture femur
Bohler–Braun splint	Fracture femur
Aluminium splint	Immobilization of fingers
Denis–Browne splint	CTEV
Toe-raising	Foot drop
Volkmann's splint	Volkmann's ischemic contracture
Aeroplane splint	Brachial plexus injury
Cock-up splint	Radial nerve palsy
Knuckle bender splint	Ulnar nerve palsy
Von Rosen splint	CDH

Thomas Splint

This is used for all types of injuries involving the lower limb, dislocation of hip, trochanteric fractures down to tibial injuries. Both skeletal as well as skin traction can be applied through this frame. The components are : (a) thigh ring and (b) two side bars, the ring is inclined at an angle of 120° to the inside bar. The splint is measured as the ring diameter equaling the thigh girth in line of the inguinal ligament plus two inches added to it for cotton padding. The length of the splint is measured from the groin to heal and six inches added to it for the traction and spreader kit. The outer bar is angled by about two inches for trochanteric clearance (Fig. 17.11a).

Pearson's knee attachment is a modified Thomas splint, which has a knee joint for flexion in traction to mobilize the knee during the period of immobilization (Fig. 17.11b).

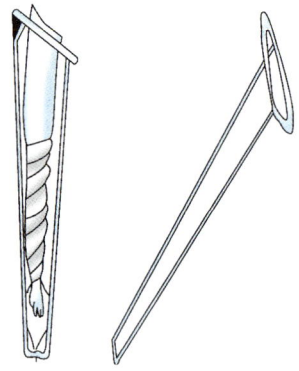

Fig. 17.11a: Thomas splint

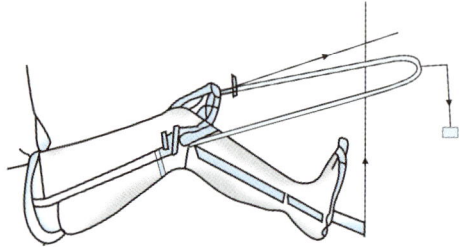

Fig. 17.11b: Modified Thomas splint with Pearson's knee attachment

Braun's Splint

This is used for injuries involving the femur and tibia including knee and ankle injuries for application of skeletal traction. It has a basic frame for support of the thigh and leg with a pulley for traction. This is an excellent splint for immobilization, elevation and traction for injuries of the lower limb (Fig. 17.12a).

Bohler's modification of Braun's splint has additional overhead three pulleys *(i)* for femoral, supracondylar traction, *(ii)* for upper tibial pin traction, *(iii)* foot drop support traction (Fig. 17.12b).

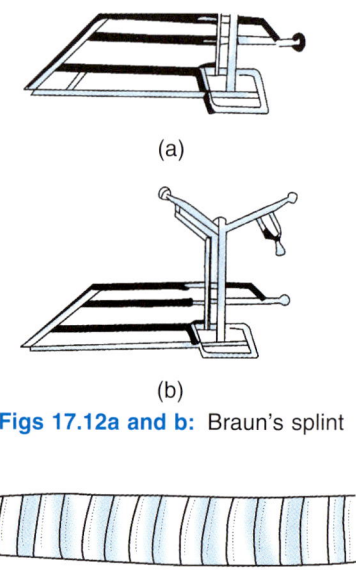

(a)

(b)

Figs 17.12a and b: Braun's splint

![Cramer wire splint illustration]

Fig. 17.13: Cramer wire splint

Cramer Wire Splint (Fig. 17.13)

This is a very light weight, versatile and malleable support and can be used for supporting injured limbs for temporary immobilization during transport of the patient pending final stabilization.

Fundamental Principles of Resuscitation in Trauma

18

The initial evaluation of a seriously injured patient is a challenging task, and mandates rapid assessment of the injuries and institution of life-preserving therapy since every minute can make the difference between life and death.

TRIMODAL DEATH DISTRIBUTION

Mortality from trauma can be grouped into:

1. Immediate (within seconds to minutes after injury)
2. Early (within minutes to several hours after injury)
3. Late (several days to weeks after injury).

The first peak of death which occurs within seconds to minutes of injury is because of fatal disruption of the great vessels, heart and lungs, lacerations of the brain or brain stem and high spinal cord injuries. This occurs at the scene of injury.

The second peak of death occurs within minutes to several hours following injury. Subdural or epidural hematomas, haemopneumothorax, lacerations of spleen, liver, pelvic fractures, and/or other multiple injuries associated with significant blood loss are a few examples of these injuries. Organized systems for trauma care focus primarily on this peak. *The first hour of care after injury "Golden hour"*

is characterized by the need for rapid assessment and resuscitation which are the fundamental principles of advanced trauma life support.

The third peak of death which occurs several days to weeks after the initial injury is most often due to sepsis and multiple organ system failure. Care provided during each of the preceding periods impacts on patient outcome during this stage. Thus the first and every subsequent person to care for the injured patient have a direct effect on long-term outcome.

GOLDEN HOUR CONCEPT

In World War I which took place in 1918, there was a real appreciation of the time factor between wounding and adequate shock treatment. If the patient was treated within one hour, the mortality was 10%. This increased markedly with time, so that after eight hours, the mortality rate was 75%. This data was subsequently used by R. Adams Cowley in his **"Golden hour"** concept.

Early Trauma Deaths Result

1. Failed oxygenation of the vital organs
2. Massive central nervous system injury
   OR
3. Both the above factors.

The mechanisms of failed tissue oxygenation include inadequate ventilation, impaired oxygenation, circulatory collapse and impaired end organ perfusion.

Injuries that cause trauma mortality occur in predictable patterns based on the mechanism of injury, the patient's age, sex, body habitus and environmental conditions. Recognition of these patterns led to the development of the advanced trauma life support (ATLS) approach by the American College of Surgeons. The ATLS is the standard of care for these patients and it is built around a standard protocol for patient evaluation. This protocol ensures that the most immediate life-threatening conditions are actively identified and addressed in the order of their risk potential.

The objectives of the initial evaluation of the trauma patient are:

1. To stabilize the trauma patient.
2. To identify life-threatening injuries and to initiate adequate supportive therapy.
3. To efficiently and rapidly organize either definitive therapy or transfer to a facility that provides definitive therapy.

TRIAGE: Triage is the sorting of patients based on the need for treatment and the available resources to provide that treatment. Treatment is rendered based on the ABC priorities (Airway with cervical spine protection, breathing and circulation with haemorrhage control).

The objective of triage is to prioritize patients with a high likelihood of early clinical deterioration. A triage of trauma patients considers:

1. Vital signs
2. Prehospital clinical course
3. Mechanism of injury
4. Patients age
5. Comorbid conditions.

Findings that lead to an accelerated work up include:

1. Multiple injuries
2. Extremes of age
3. Evidence of severe neurologic injury
4. Unstable vital signs
5. Pre-existing cardiac or pulmonary disease.

Multiple casualities: The number of patients and the severity of their injuries **do not exceed** the ability of the facility to render care. In this situation, patients with life-threatening problems and those sustaining multiple system injuries are treated first.

Mass casualities: The number of patients and the severity of their injuries **exceed** the capability of the facility and staff. In this situation those patients with the greatest chance of survival with the least expenditure of time, equipment, supplies and personnel are managed first.

ORGANIZATION OF CARE

Regardless of the clinical setting, organize the care team prior to patient's arrival. Leadership and unity of command are essential for directing a rapid and efficient workup.

Ideally a resuscitation area should be available for trauma patients.

Proper airway equipment (laryngoscopes, endotracheal tubes) should be organized, tested and placed where it is immediately accessible.

Warmed intravenous crystalloid solutions (e.g. Ringer's lactate) should be available and ready to infuse as soon as the patient arrives.

TRAUMA TEAM

The Core Trauma Team is that group of professionals that receives and treats the patient. This includes:

• Team leader
• Anaesthesiologist
• Nurse anaesthestist
• General surgeon

- Orthopaedic surgeon
- Emergency room physician
- Two nurses (three if no anesthetic assistant)
- Radiographer
- Scribe (nurse or doctor).

INITIAL ASSESSMENT

The initial evaluation follows the protocol of:
1. Primary survey
2. Resuscitation
3. Secondary survey
4. *Definitive treatment or transfer to an appropriate trauma centre for definitive care.*
   This approach is the heart of the ATLS system which is designed to identify life-threatening injuries and to initiate stabilizing treatment in a rapidly efficient manner.

PRIMARY SURVEY

The steps of the primary survey are encapsulated in the mnemonic ABCDE
A Airway maintenance with cervical spine protection
B Breathing and ventilation
C Circulation with haemorrhage control
D Disability: Neurologic status
E Exposure/Environment control: Completely undress the patient, but prevent hypothermia

AIRWAY MAINTENANCE WITH CERVICAL SPINE PROTECTION

The airway is the first priority; it should be assessed first to ascertain patency. The rapid assessment for signs of airway obstruction should include inspection for foreign bodies and facial, mandibular, or tracheal / laryngeal fractures that may result in airway obstruction.

Measures to establish a patent airway should be instituted while protecting the cervical spine. Initially the chin lift or jaw thrust manoeuvres are recommended to achieve this task. If the patient is able to communicate verbally, the airway is not likely to be in immediate jeopardy.

Severe head injury patients with an altered LOC or a GCS score of 8 or less usually require the placement of a definitive airway. The finding of nonpurposeful motor responses strongly suggests the need for definitive airway management. Neurologic examination alone does not exclude a cervical spine injury.

While assessing and managing the patient's airway great care should be taken to prevent excessive movement of the cervical spine.

The patients head and neck should not be hyperextended, hyperflexed or rotated to establish and maintain the airway.

It is based on the history of the trauma incident, the loss of stability of cervical spine should be suspected. Protection of the patient's spinal cord with appropriate immobilization devices (Philadelphia collar) should be accomplished and maintained. If immobilization devices must be removed temporarily, the head and neck should be stabilized with manual in-line immobilization by one member of the trauma team.

Stabilization equipment used to protect the patient's spinal cord should be left in place until cervical spine injury is excluded. **Protection of the spine and spinal cord is an important management principle.** Cervical spine X-rays may be obtained to confirm or exclude injury once immediate or potentially life-threatening conditions have been addressed.

Remember: Assume a cervical spine injury in any patient with multi-system trauma, especially with an altered level of consciousness or a blunt injury above the clavicle.

BREATHING AND VENTILATION

Airway patency alone does not assure adequate ventilation. Adequate gas exchange is required to maximize oxygenation and carbon dioxide elimination. Ventilation requires adequate function of the lungs, chest wall, and diaphragm. Each component must be examined and evaluated rapidly. The patient's chest should be exposed to adequately assess chest wall excursion. Auscultation should be performed to assure gas flow in the lungs. Percussion may demonstrate the presence of air or blood in the chest. Visual inspection and palpation may detect injuries to the chest wall that may compromise ventilation.

Injuries that may acutely impair ventilation are:

1. Tension pneuomothorax.
2. Flail chest with pulmonary contusion.
3. Massive haemothorax.
4. Open pneumothorax.

These injuries should be identified in the primary survey.

CIRCULATION WITH HAEMORRHAGE CONTROL

Haemorrhage is the predominant cause of post-injury deaths that are preventable by rapid treatment in the hospital setting. Hypotension following injury should be considered to be hypovolemic in origin until proved otherwise. Rapid and accurate assessment of the injured patient's haemodynamic status is therefore essential. The elements of clinical observation that yield important information within seconds are:

1. Level of consciousness
2. Skin colour
3. Pulse

External haemorrhage is identified and controlled in the primary survey. Rapid, external blood loss is managed by direct manual pressure on the wound. Pneumatic splinting devices may also help control haemorrhage. These devices should be transparent to allow monitoring of underlying bleeding.

Tourniquets should **not** be used (except in unusual circumstances such as traumatic amputation of an extremity) because they crush tissues and cause distal ischaemia.

Haemorrhage into the thoracic or abdominal cavities, into soft tissue surrounding a major long bone fracture, into the retroperitoneal space from a pelvic fracture or penetrating torso injury are major sources of occult blood loss.

DISABILITY (NEUROLOGIC EVALUATION)

A brief neurologic evaluation is performed at the end of the primary survey. This establishes the patient's level of consciousness, as well as the pupillary size and reaction. A simple mnemonic to describe the level of consciousness is the **AVPU** method.

A Alert
V Responds to vocal stimuli
P Responds only to painful stimuli
U Unresponsive to all stimuli

The Glasgow Coma Scale (GCS) is a more detailed neurologic evaluation that also is quick, simple, and predictive of patient outcome. This should be performed as part of the more detailed secondary survey. If hypoxia and hypovolemia are excluded changes in the level of consciousness should be considered to be of traumatic central nervous system origin until proved otherwise.

EXPOSURE/ENVIRONMENTAL CONTROL

The final step in the primary survey includes patient exposure and control of the immediate environment. The patient should be completely undressed, usually by cutting off the garments to facilitate thorough examination and assessment. After the patient's clothing is removed and assessment is completed, it is imperative to cover the patient with warm blankets or an external warming device to prevent hypothermia. Intravenous fluids should be warmed before infusion, and a warm environment (room temperature) should be maintained. It is the patient's body temperature that is most important, not the comfort of health care providers.

RESUSCITATION

Aggressive resuscitation and the management of life-threatening injuries, as they are identified, are essential to maximize patient survival.

The airway should be protected in all patients and secured when the potential for airway compromise exists. A nasopharyngeal airway may initially establish and maintain airway patency in the conscious patient. If the patient is unconscious and has no gag reflex, an oropharyngeal airway may be helpful temporarily.

A definitive airway should be established if there is any doubt about the patient ability to maintain airway integrity. Definitive control of the airway should be accomplished with continuous protection of the cervical spine.

A surgical airway should be performed if oral or nasal intubation is contraindicated or cannot be accomplished.

A tension pneumothorax compromises ventilation and circulation dramatically and acutely and if suspected chest decompression should be accomplished immediately.

Every injured patient should receive supplemental oxygen. If not intubated, the patient should have oxygen delivered by mask/reservoir device to achieve optimal oxygenation.

Control bleeding by direct pressure or operative intervention.

A minimum of two large caliber intravenous catheters should be established. The maximum rate of fluid administration is determined by the internal diameter of the catheter and inversely by its length, not by the size of the vein in which the catheter is placed.

When establishing the intravenous lines, blood should be drawn for type and crossmatch and for baseline hematologic studies, including a pregnancy test for all females of childbearing age.

Intravenous fluid therapy should be initiated with a balanced salt solution. Ringer's lactate solution is preferred as the initial crystalloid solution and should be administered rapidly. Such bolus intravenous therapy may require the administration of 2 to 3 liters of solution to achieve an appropriate response in the adult patient. All intravenous solutions should be warmed.

The shock state associated with trauma is most often hypovolemic in origin. If the patient remains unresponsive to bolus intravenous therapy, type-specific blood may be administered.

Hypovolemic shock should not be treated by vasopressors, steroids, or sodium bicarbonate, or by continued crystalloid/blood infusion. If blood loss continues it should be controlled by operative intervention.

The endpoints of resuscitation are:
1. Normal vital signs.
2. Absence of blood loss.
3. Adequate urine output (0.5–1.0 cc/kg/hr).
4. No evidence of end organ dysfunction.

Parameters such as blood lactate levels and base deficit on an arterial blood gas may be helpful in patients who are severely injured.

ADJUNCTS TO PRIMARY SURVEY AND RESUSCITATION

ECG Monitoring

Unexplained tachycardia, PVCs, AF and ST segment changes indicate blunt cardiac injury.

Pulseless electrical activity or electromechanical dissociation indicates cardiac tamponade, tension pneumothorax, and/or severe hypovolemia.

Bradycardia, aberrant conduction and premature beats indicate hypoxia, hypoperfusion or hypothermia.

X-Rays and Diagnostic Studies

X-rays should be used judiciously and should not delay patient resuscitation.

AP chest film and AP pelvis may provide information that can guide resuscitation efforts of the patient with blunt trauma.

A lateral cervical spine X-ray that demonstrates injury is an important finding whereas a negative film does not exclude a cervical spine injury.

Diagnostic peritoneal lavage (DPL) and Focused abdominal sonogram for trauma (FAST) are useful tools for the quick detection of occult intra-abdominal bleeding.

URINARY OUTPUT

Is a sensitive indicator of the volume status of the patient and reflects renal perfusion. Monitoring of urinary output is best accomplished by insertion of an indwelling bladder catheter. Transurethral bladder catheterization is contraindicated in patients in whom urethral transection is suspected. Urethral injury should be suspected if there is:

1. Blood at the penile meatus
2. Perineal ecchymosis
3. Blood in the scrotum
4. A high-riding or non-palpable prostate
5. A pelvic fracture.

MONITORING

1. Ventilatory rate and arterial blood gases should be used to monitor the adequacy of respirations.
2. Pulse oximetry measures the oxygen saturation of Hb colorimetrically.
3. The blood pressure should be measured, realizing that it may be a poor measure of actual tissue perfusion.

Secondary Survey

The secondary survey does not begin until the primary survey (ABCDE) is completed, resuscitative efforts are well established, and the patient is demonstrating normalization of vital functions.

The secondary survey is a head-to-toe evaluation of the trauma patient, i.e. a complete history and physical examination, including a reassessment of all vital signs (Tables 18.1 and 18.2).

In this survey a complete neurologic examination is performed, including a GCS score determination, if not done during the primary survey.

During this evaluation indicated X-rays are obtained. Specific radiological evaluations and laboratory studies are also obtained at this time.

The secondary assessment might well be summarized as tubes and fingers in every orifice.

PATIENT TRANSFER

During the primary survey and resuscitation phase, the evaluating doctor frequently has enough (Table 18.3) information to indicate the need for transfer of the patient to another facility. Once the decision to transfer is made, referring doctor-to-receiving doctor communication is essential. Remember, life-saving measures are initiated when the problem is identified, rather than after the primary survey.

FIRST SUCCESSFUL TRAUMA RESUSCITATION
(July 16, 1774)

The Humane Society, London was founded originally as 'The Institute for Affording Immediate Relief for Persons Apparently Dead from Drowning'. Only 3 months after the society was founded a member of the society was called to attend a 3-year-old child

Table 18.1: Revised trauma score

	Variables	Score	Start of transport	End of transport
A. Respiratory rate	10–29	4		
(breaths/minute)	> 29	3		
	6–9	3		
	1–5	2		
	0	0	—	—
B. Systolic rate	>89	4		
(mmHg)	76–89	3		
	50–75	2		
	1–49	1		
	0	0		
C. GCS score	13–15	4		
conversion	9–12	3		
$C = D + E^1 + F$		6–8	2	
(adult)	4–5	1		
$C = D + E2$	<4	0	—	—
D. Eye opening	Sponaneous	4		
	To voice	3		
	None	1		
E^1 Verbal response,	Oriented	5		
Adult	Concused	4		
	Inappropriate words	3		
	Incomprehensible words	2		
	None	1	—	—
E^2 Verbal response,	Appropriate	5		
Pediatric	Cries, consolable	4		
	Persistently irritable	3		
	Restless, agitated	2		
	None	1	—	—
F. Motor response	Obeys commands	6		
	Localizes pain	5		
	Withdras (pain)	4		
	Flexion (pain)	3		
	Extension (pain)	2		
	None	1	—	—
Glasgow Coma Score (Total = D + E^{10} + F)			—	—
Revised trauma Score + A + B + C			—	—

Table 18.2: Pediatric trauma score			
Assessment component	Score		
	+2	+1	–1
Weight	> 20 kg (>44 lb)	10–20 kg (20–44 lb)	< 10 kg (22 lb)
Airway	Normal	Oral or nasal airway; O_2	Intubated; cricothyroidotomy; or tracheostomy
Systolic blood pressure	> 90 mmHg; good peripheral pulses, perfusion	50-90 mmHg; carotid /femoral pulses palpable	< 50 mmHg; weak or no pulses
Level of consciousness	Awake	Obtunded or any LOC	Coma; unresponsive
fracture	None seen os suspected	Single, closed	Open or multiple
Cutanoues	None visible	Contusion, abrasion; laceration < 7 cm; not through fascia	Tissue loss; any GSW/SW; through fascia
Total:			

*Loss of consciousness

named Catherine Sophie Greenhill, who had fallen from an upper storey window onto flagstones in nearby Pudding Lane, and been pronounced dead. The society member, an apothecary named Squires, was on the scene within twenty minutes, and revived her by giving several electric shocks through a portable electrostatic generator.

Basic life support comprises the elements:
1. Initial assessment
2. Airway maintenance
3. Expired air ventilation (rescue breathing)
4. Chest compressions.

Basic life support implies that no equipment is employed and no drugs are given. When a simple airway or facemask for mouth-to-mouth ventilation is used, this is defined as "basic life support with airway adjunct".

CHAIN OF SURVIVAL

In 1990, the American Heart Association developed the chain of survival. This protocol addresses the fact that most sudden cardiac arrest episodes occur outside of a hospital, with death occurring within minutes of onset. For the chain to be effective, quick execution of each and every link is critical. With each minute that passes, the likelihood of survival decreases 7–10%.

To provide the best opportunity for survival, each of these four links must be put into motion within the first few minutes of the onset of sudden cardiac arrest.

1. **Early access:** When an emergency is recognized, the first link in the chain of survival is early access. This means activating the emergency medical services, or EMS, system by calling 911. (911 does not work in every community. Be sure to check

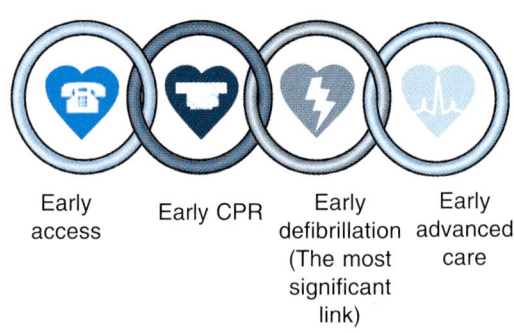

Early access   Early CPR   Early defibrillation (The most significant link)   Early advanced care

Table 18.3: Triage decision scheme

Measure vital signs and level of consciousness

STEP 1

- GCS<14 or
- RR<10 or >29 or
- Systolic BP <90 or
- RTS<11 or
- PTS<9

YES, take to trauma center; alert trauma team

NO, assess anatomy of injury

STEP 2

- Flail chest
- Two or more proximal long bone fractures
- Amputation proximal to wrist/ankle
- All penetrating trauma to head, neck, torso and extremities proximal to elbow and knee
- Limb paralysis
- Pelvic fracture
- Combination trauma with burns

Yes, take to trauma center; alert trauma team

NO, Evaluate for mechanism of injury and evidence of high energy impact

STEP 3

- Ejection from auto
- Death in same passenger compartment
- Roll over
- Auto pedestrian injury with > 5 mph (8 kph) impact
- Motorcycle crash >20 mph (32 kph) or with separation of rider and bike
- High speed auto crush:
  – Initial speed > 40 mph
  – Major auto deformity >20 inches
  – Intrusion into passenger compartment>12 inch

- Extrication time >20 minutes
- Falls>20 ft   • Pedestrian thrown or run over

YES, take to trauma center; alert trauma team

NO

STEP 4

- Age< 5 or 55 years
- Pregnancy
- Immunosuppresed patients
- Cardiac disease; respiratory disease
- Insulin dependent diabetes; cirrhosis; morbid obesity; coagulopathy

YES, take to trauma center; alert trauma team

NO, Re-evaluate with medical control

your local directory, and know the correct emergency telephone number in your community.)

2. **Early CPR:** The second link in the Chain of Survival is to perform CPR until a defibrillator becomes available.

3. **Early defibrillation:** The third and most critical link in the Chain of Survival for a victim of ventricular fibrillation.

4. **Early advanced care:** The last link in the Chain of Survival is early advanced life support. This is provided by experienced medical personnel such as paramedics, nurses, and doctors. Advanced life support includes giving medications and using advanced oxygen delivery techniques to resuscitate a person.

PURPOSE OF BASIC LIFE SUPPORT

To maintain adequate ventilation and circulation until means can be obtained to reverse the underlying cause of the arrest. It is therefore a **"holding operation"** although on occasions, particularly when the primary pathology is respiratory failure, it may itself reverse the cause and allow full recovery. Failure of the circulation for three to four minutes (less if the victim is initially hypoxemic) will lead to irreversible cerebral damage. Delay, even within that time, will reduce the eventual chances of a successful outcome.

Adult BLS Healthcare Provider Algorithm

1. Ensure safety of rescuer and victim
2. Check responsiveness
   Check the victim and see if he responds: Gently shake his shoulders and ask loudly:
   "Are you OK?"
3. If he does not respond:
   Phone 108 or emergency number
   Get Automatic External Defibrillator

Or send second rescuer (if available) to do this

4. Open airway, check breathing.
   Look, listen and feel for no more than 10 seconds
   If not breathing normally, pinch nose and cover the mouth with yours and blow until you see the chest rise. Give 2 breaths. Each breath should take 1 second.
5. If no response, check pulse:
   Do you definitely feel pulse within 10 seconds?
6. *If definite pulse present*
   Give 1 breath every 5 to 6 seconds.
   Recheck pulse every 2 minutes.
7. *If no pulse present*
   Give cycles of 30 compressions and 2 breaths until AED/defibrillator arrives, ALS providers take over, or victim starts to move.
   - Push hard and fast (100/min) and release completely.
   - *Minimize interruptions in compressions.*

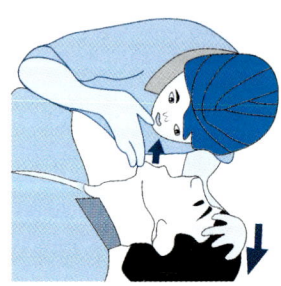

8. AED/defibrillator arrives
   Check Rhythm
   Rhythm Shockable or Not
9. *Rhythm shockable:*
   Give 1 shock of 360 joules
   Resume CPR immediately for 5 cycles
10. *Rhythm not shockable:*
    Resume CPR immediately for 5 cycles
    Check Rhythm every 5 cycles, continue until ALS providers take over or victim starts to move.

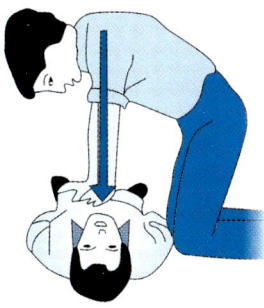

The five major changes in the 2005 emergency cardiovascular care guidelines:

1. Emphasis on and recommendation to improve delivery of effective chest compressions.

2. A single compression to ventilation ratio (30 : 2) for all single rescuers for all victims (except neonates).

3. Recommendation that each rescue breath be given over 1 second and should produce a visible chest rise.

4. A new recommendation that single shock, followed by immediate CPR, be used to attempt defibrillation for ventricular fibrillation cardiac arrests. Rhythm checks should be performed every 2 minutes.

5. Endorsement of the 2003 ILCOR recommendation for use of AED'S in children 1 to 8 years old (and older) Use a child dose—reduction system if available.

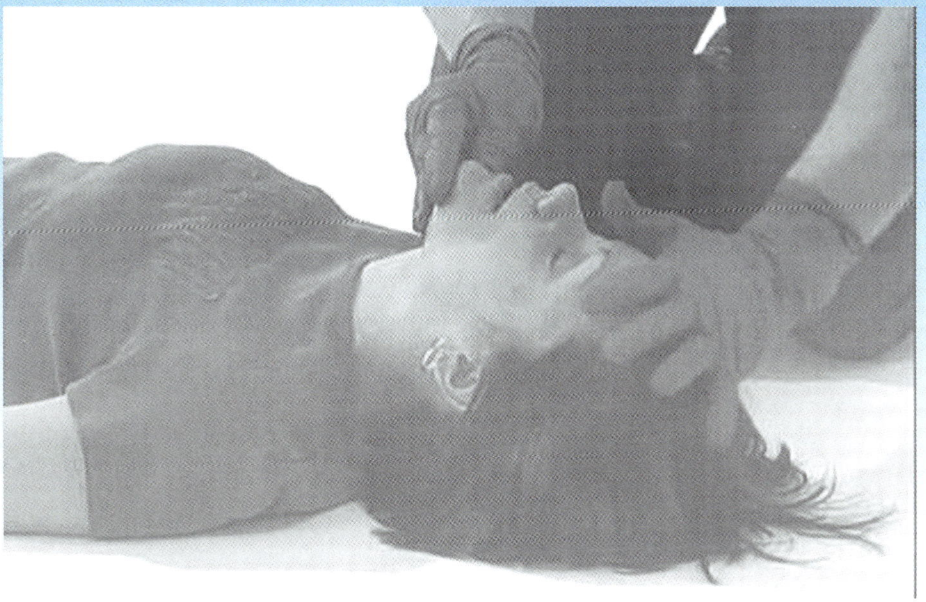

19

Instruments, Implants, Sutures and Sterilization

CLASSIFICATION

Implants in orthopaedics can be classified as:
• Prosthetic devices
• Fixation devices
• Artificial tendons and ligaments
• Segmental bone replacement.
  Material used in making implants can be divided into:
• Metallic
• Non-metallic.

Metals

They are strong, ductile and biocompatible. Metals used in making implants are generally alloys of various metals.

Purpose of using alloys: Carbon decreases corrosion and lowers freezing point. Nickel is a stabilizer, chromium increases corrosion resistance, molybdenum being antichloride increases corrosion resistance, iron increases fatigue strength and toughness.

i. *Steel:* Steel is iron and carbon. If to this, chromium, nickel, and molybdenum are added, it becomes stainless steel. The modulus of elasticity of stainless steel is 12 times that of cortical bone.

ii. *Cobalt based alloys*
  • *Cast vitallium:* Co, Cr, Ni, Mo.

• Superior corrosion resistance, bio-compatible, tough and strong but very expensive.
• *Wrought vitallium:* Co, Cr, Ni, tungsten.
  – Extremely strong, can be machined but very expensive and high local disintegration.

iii. *Titanium based alloys:* Ti (90%), Al (6%), vanadium (4%) are excellent corrosion resistant but not so strong.

  Advantages: MRI and CT compatible.

  Disadvantages: High coefficient of friction and low wear resistance makes it a poor material for joint surface. Most common alloy combinations used are:
  a. Ti-6Al-4V.
  b. Co-Cr-Mo.
  c. 316L stainless steel.

Non-Metallic Materials

i. Polymeric materials can avoid corrosion, but ductility is doubtful.
ii. Biodegradable polymeric materials-avoids removal of implant but tissue clearance is a problem.
iii. Ceramic materials, hydroxy apatite and tricalcium phosphate, gives improvement on bone growth but brittleness and

limited strength restricts their use as material for internal fixation.
iv. Carbon used for making artificial ligaments.
v. Silicon used for making artificial tendons and joint lubricant.

Future Trends

Bioabsorbable Implants

Polyglycolic acid (PGA) was the first totally synthetic bioabsorbable suture and was introduced in 1970 as dexon. This was followed in 1975 by vicryl, a copolymer of 92% PGA and 8% polylactic acid (PLA) and polydioxanone (PDS) in 1981. PDS was the first bioabsorbable material to be made into screws. Currently, PGA, PDS, polylevolactic acid (PLLA), and racemic poly D, L- lactic acid (PDLLA) are the alpha polyesters used for bioabsorbable materials.

The most common orthopaedics use of bioabsorbable implants is for the attachment of soft tissue to bone, as in the shoulder and knee surgeries.

Bioabsorbable implants offer the advantages of gradual load transfer to the healing tissue, reduced need for hardware removal, and radiolucency, which facilitates post-operative roentgenographic evaluation.

Due to limited mechanical properties they are of interest for implants which must resist only minor loading and where surgical removal is a major undertaking. An ideal sterilization process is not yet available. Some cautions is advised in situations susceptible to infection, as degradable material seems to exhibit a reduced resistance to infection if compared to the best metal implants.

High Strength Alloys

We have seen many materials being proposed to solve problems, such as avoiding implant failure under extreme mechanical load.

Improved strength may be achieved by using alloy component for titanium (e.g. vanadium) which is less biocompatible than nickel. The good overall corrosion resistance of titanium alloys neutralizes part of this potential disadvantage.

The choice of an implant material depends on the priority given to mechanical advantages over biological tolerance.

ORTHOPAEDIC INSTRUMENTS

Periosteal Elevators

Farabeuf Periosteal Elevator

This has a flat handle, a narrow neck and a wide blade. The proximal part of the blade is serrated at the top for the thumb grip, while the tip is straight, bevelled and sharp. Its tip may be straight or curved.

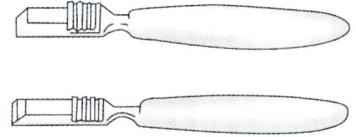

Fig. 19.1a: Farabeuf periosteal elevator

This is used for stripping off the periosteum before application of bone levers/forceps, so as to avoid damage to muscles/vessels and nerves overlying the bone.

Bristow's Periosteal Elevator

This has small oval fenestrated handle and a long shaft, which is gently curved and sharp at the tip.

This is used for stripping off the periosteum cum bone lever.

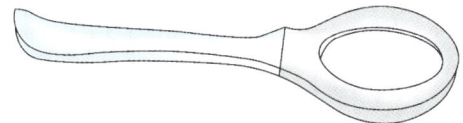

Fig. 19.1b: Bristow's periosteal elevator

Mitchell's Periosteal Elevator

This has a round handle for a good grip, elevated and serrated thumb rest and a straight sharp tipped blade.

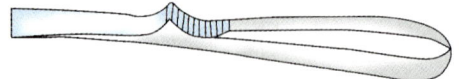

Fig. 19.1c: Mitchell's periosteal elevator

BONE LEVERS

Lane's Bone Lever (Plain)

This has a fenestrated oval handle for a finger grip, a long shank and a narrow blade, which is smooth and conical at the tip, which is gently curved.

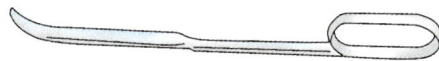

Fig. 19.2a: Lane's bone lever (plain)

This is used for long bones of the upper and lower extremities. The periosteum is first stripped from the bone by periosteum elevator and while the periosteum elevator is still in place the lever is introduced so that the soft tissues are separated along with the periosteum from the bone allowing room for the bone forceps to hold the bone.

Lane's Bone Lever (Serrated Tip)

This has a round thumb grip, a long shank and a serrated curved blade at the terminal end.

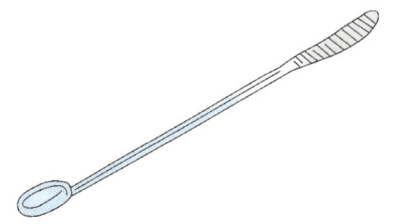

Fig. 19.2b: Lane's bone lever (serrated tip)

This is used for femur and tibia. The serrated blade prevents it from slipping while the bone is being levered out.

Narrow Blade Bone Lever

This bone retractor has a fenestrated handle, a narrow shank, and a blade, which is conical and pointed at the tip, which is gently curved.

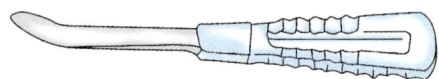

Fig. 19.2c: Narrow blade bone lever

Broad Blade Bone Lever

This is used for retraction of soft tissue especially around joints. The broad blade and narrow tip gives it an excellent and minimal engagement on the bone, all the same, a wide area of soft tissue retraction giving freedom of instrumentation. It is available as straight and angled shank.

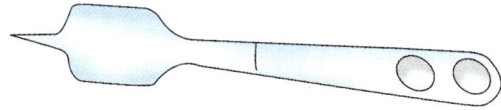

Fig. 19.2d: Hohmann's retractor

SKIN HOOKS

Single Hook Skin Retractor

This has a small, thin and flat handle, serrated in between, a long shank which is tapered and shaped into a fine hook at the tip.

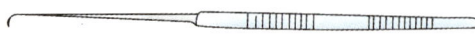

Fig. 19.3a: Single hook skin retractor

This is used for retraction of soft tissue while doing micro-dissection as in the cases of neonates and neurovascular surgery.

Double Hook Skin Retractor

This has two prongs for a better grip in the skin.

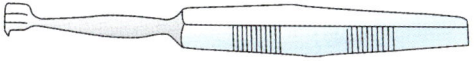

Fig. 19.3b: Double hook skin retractor

Four Prong Skin Retractor

This is used for paediatric surgery.

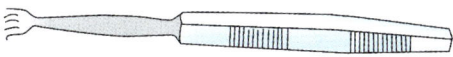

Fig. 19.3c: Four prong skin retractor

Retractors

Paton's Retractor

This is used for the retraction of sub-cutaneous tissue, muscles and vessels.

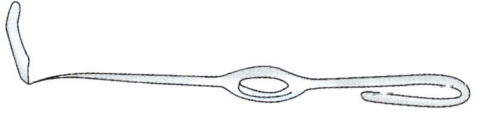

Fig. 19.4a: Paton's retractor

LANGENBECK RETRACTOR

This has a long shank, serrated triangular, fenestrated handle. The blade is angled at 90° and bent at the tip with long and short lengths.

This is very useful for retraction of deep tissues and muscles during surgery.

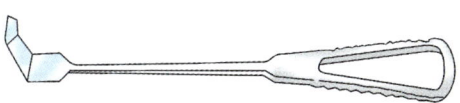

Fig. 19.4b: Langenbeck retractor

Volkmann's Retractor

This has a long shank with a triangular serrated fenestrated handle at one end and four hooked prong sharp retractor at the other. This is also known as **cat's paw retractor**.

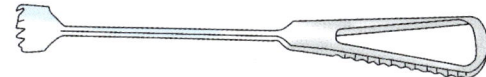

Fig. 19.4c: Volkmann's retractor

This is an excellent soft tissue retractor as the hooks bite into the subcutaneous tissue and prevents slippage of the skin during surgery.

Kocher's Hook Retractor

This has a handle and a long shank that is conical, tapered and the tip is bent to form a hook, which is smooth tipped.

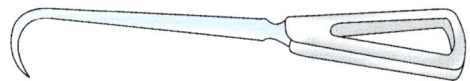

Fig. 19.4d: Kocher's hook retractor

This is used for hooking/retraction of the bone during surgery.

Beckmann–Adson Self-Retaining Retractor

This has an outfaced hook multiprong retraction tip, long-curved arms which are hinged to be bent at a suitable angle, a handle with a rachet lock.

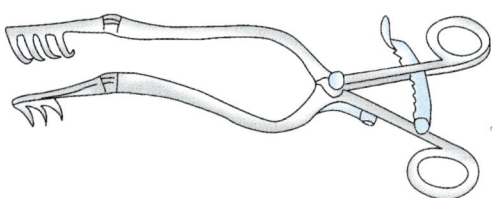

Fig. 19.4e: Beckmann-Adson self-retaining retractor

This is used for retraction of muscles especially in posterior spinal surgery. The muscles are first retracted by a Langenbeck's retractor on both sides of the spinous process, the prongs are then introduced, the jaws are then opened up and are held automatically at the desired retraction by the rachet lock. The blades can be bent at a suitable angle so that deep retraction can be achieved. To release the retraction, the rachet lock is pressed and the jaws close by themselves. Two retractors are invariably used, one for the proximal and other for the distal soft tissue retraction so that the wide area of laminae and spine is visible and does not require help of an assistant to do the same.

Smith-Peterson's Osteotomes

This has a smooth, round handle, a narrow neck, a long blade and a flat top for hammering.

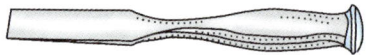

Fig. 19.5

This is used for cutting the bone for correction of deformities and making a window into the bone. It is available in blade sizes varying from 5 to 35 mm

Stille's Chisel

This has a flat top for hammering, a narrow cylindrical handle which is ribbed and a blade which is bevelled at the tip.

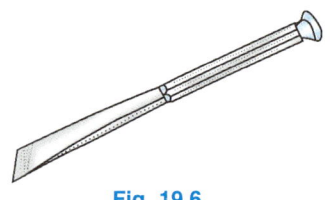

Fig. 19.6

This is used for chiselling out a bony growth, cutting wedge into the bone and removal of bone grafts. This is either straight or curved. The latter is more convenient while removing bone grafts from the iliac crest or while cutting through a curved surface. This is available in blade sizes 5 to 30 mm.

Stille's Bone Gouge

This has a flat top, ribbed handle and a blade which is semitubular in shape and has a cutting edge.

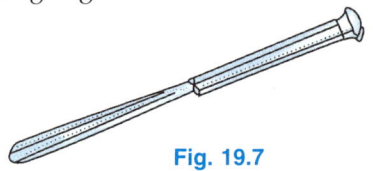

Fig. 19.7

This is used to gouge out bone cavities and removal of bone grafts. This is available in blade sizes 5 to 30 mm.

Gigli's Wire Saw With Hook Handle

This Gigli's wire is a useful device for sawing the bone as in the cases of amputation and correction of deformities. The periosteum is elevated from all around the bone, the soft tissue retracted by Lane's lever and then the wire is passed around the bone. The tips are then held in T-hook handles and by sea-saw movement the bone is cut through by the spiked wire. *One must always take precautions to protect the soft tissues adequately while sawing through the bone.* The wire is available in lengths of 30 to 70 cm.

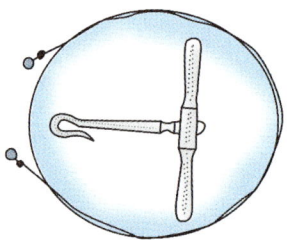

Fig. 19.8

Doyan's Periosteal Elevator

This has a smooth round handle, a conical shank and a U-curved cutting blade.

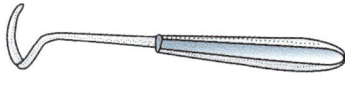

Fig. 19.9

It is curved in right and left direction and is exclusively used as a rib raspatory for stripping of the periosteum from the rib, while protecting the intercostal vessel and nerve.

Volkmann's Curette

This has a flat handle serrated in between and has two scoops at either end.

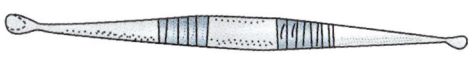

Fig. 19.10

This is used for curetting out bone cavities in cases of bone tumour, osteomyelitis, etc. It is available in cup sizes of 2 to 12 mm. It usually has a small cup on one side and a large cup on the other.

Heath Mallet

This is a stainless steel hammer with serrated handle.

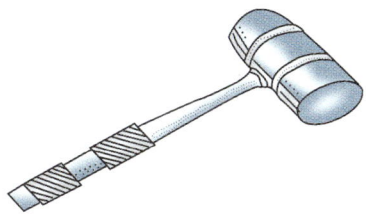

Fig. 19.11

This is used for hammering during introduction of nails for intramedullary fixation of fractures, cutting the bone while using a chisel or osteotome. In cases of prosthetic use, one end of the head of the hammer is tufnol tipped to avoid any indentation or damage to the surface of the prostheses. It is available in different weights of 1 to 2 pounds with a standard handle length of 8 inches.

Fibre Mallet

This is made up of fibre with a tufnol head.

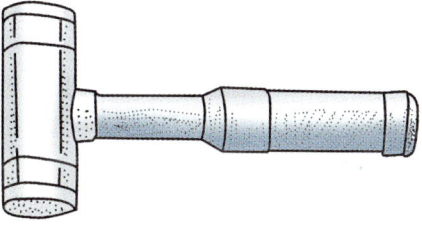

Fig. 19.12

It has the same strength as that of a brass hammer and has an excellent advantage of not marring chisel or other cutting tools or the head of prostheses during introduction. This mallet is perfectly balanced, sympathetic to touch, non-spark and can be autoclaved or boiled in a routine way.

Air Powered Drill

This has a handle with inlet and outlet nozzles for pressurized air and a Jacob's chuck positioned at right angled to it. This utilizes pressurized air to rotate the Jacob's chuck to which different attachments can be fitted, it is versatile and powerful equipment and can be used for drilling holes through the bone, intramedullary and acetabular reaming, cutting through the bone with a saw, etc.

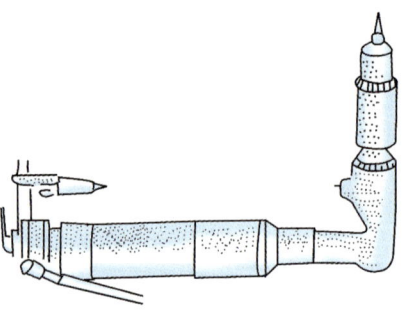

Fig. 19.13

Twin Saw Attachment

This is used for cutting through the bone, for correction of deformities and for cutting through the cortex to open up windows in the bone.

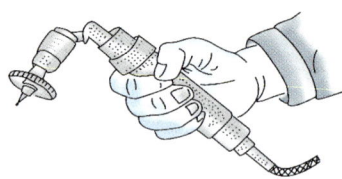

Fig. 19.14

Cannulated Drill bit

It is used for drilling holes directly into the diaphyseal area or through a guide wire into the neck of femur/condylar zone of femur and tibia, the speed of the drill can be controlled by the air entry.

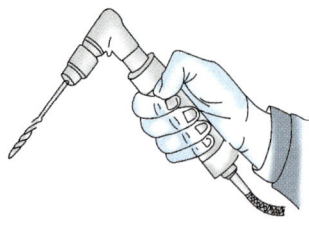

Fig. 19.15

Small Air Drill

This has a handle, a short shaft and a quick coupling chuck. The handle has an inlet nozzle, the air can be utilized to rotate the chuck in both directions, i.e. clockwise/anticlockwise by pressing the two finger button jets by choice.

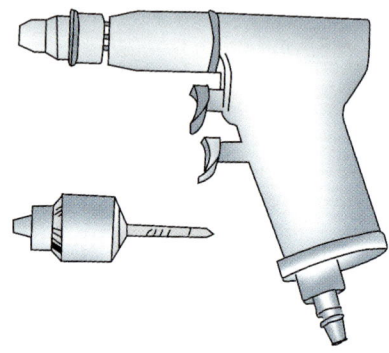

Fig. 19.16

This is a very useful instrument, driven by compressed air/oxygen power and can be used to drill holes, tapping and above all it is used for insertion as well as extraction of screws. One push of the upper trigger rotates the chuck clockwise while the second push turns it anticlockwise. The lower trigger controls the speed of air flow. This machine has a speed of 0 to 600 rpm. with an air consumption of approximately 250 litres per min and can be autoclaved at 140 °C.

It is unsuitable for intramedullary reaming and oxygen should never be used in place of compressed air for the fear of spark and fire.

Universal Bone Drill

This has a manual rotational gear, which is connected to the shaft by cog wheel. It has a Jacob's chuck for loading K-wire and drill bit which is tightened by a key. The shaft is cannulated for the long K-wire to pass through from front to back.

This is a very useful instrument for drilling in K-wire, Steinmann pin and making holes with drill bit for introduction of screws. The drill bit is loaded into the triple jawed chuck, which are in turn tightened for a firm grip by a key which is supplied along with the drill. It is available in various small and large sizes and can hold 1 mm K-wire to 6.5 mm Shanz pin. Clockwise rotation of the handle rotates the chuck in a similar direction.

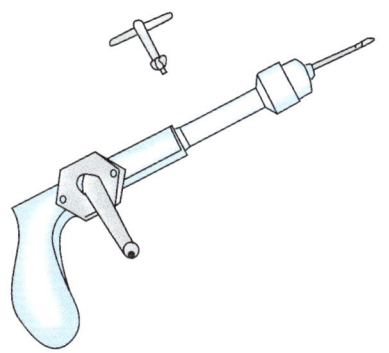

Fig. 19.17

Steinmann Pin Introducer

This has a long T-handle, the shaft of which is cannulated throughout its length with Jacob's chuck at the end.

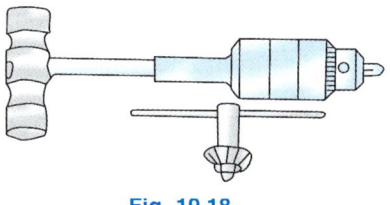

Fig. 19.18

This is used for introduction of K-wire, guide wire, Steinmann pin and Shanz pin into the bone. The wire is first introduced into the shaft and while a desired length is allowed to remain outside. The chuck is tightened with the key.

Watson–Jones Handle For Guide Wire

This has a short 'T' handle which is cannulated for holding a guide wire and a butterfly sleeve which is tightened over the shaft thereby compressing the grip.

This is used for holding the guide wire during introduction into the neck of femur, by gentle oscillating movements.

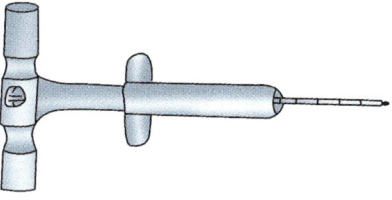

Fig. 19.19

Stille Horsley Bone Cutting Forceps

This has sharp cutting jaws which are bent at right angle and double-hinged lever arms which are separated by a tension strip.

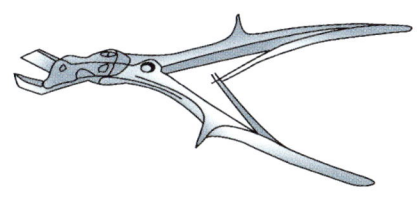

Fig. 19.20

This is used for cutting the spinous process during laminectomy. The right angled bent cutting tip is an advantage in cutting deep lying bone and can also be used to cut bone spikes and edges to give it a uniform edge, the double hinges give it an extra mechanical advantage while cutting strong cortical bone.

Ruskin Bone Cutting Forceps

This is a straight double-hinged bone cutting forceps.

This is used for cutting bone spikes.

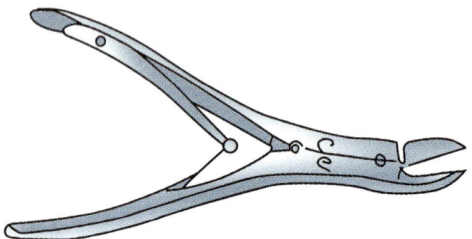

Fig. 19.21

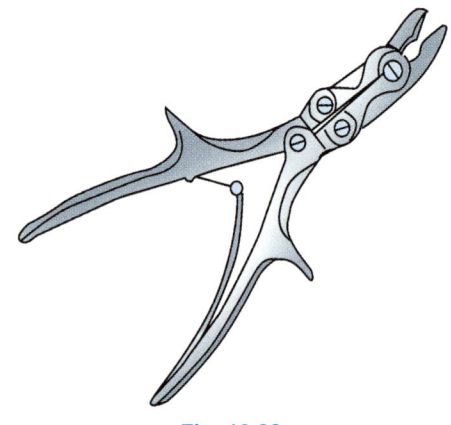

Fig. 19.23

Bone Nibbler Single Action Straight

This is a straight bone nibbler with a single hinge and a tension strip in between the handles.

This is used for nibbling away the bone margins in a piece meal style to give it a uniform edge or desired contour.

This is used for nibbling cortical bone, the angled tip gives it an extra advantage for in depth working and the strong jaws can cut out bone with ease.

Northfield's Rongeur Heavy Double Action

This is a straight double-hinged bone nibbler.

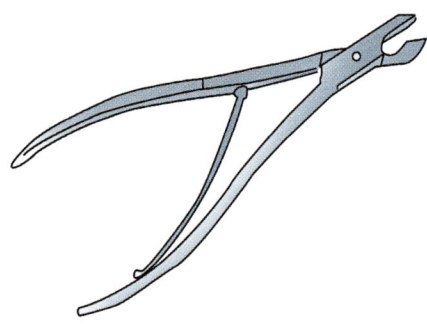

Fig. 19.22

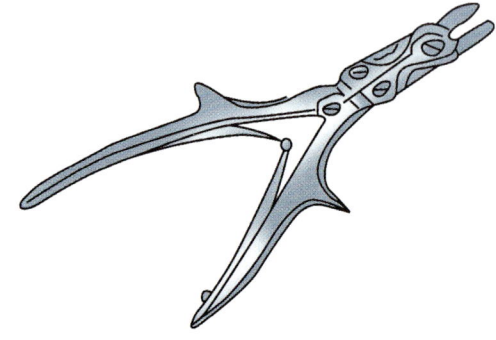

Fig. 19.24

Sargent Rongeur

This is a strong double-hinged nibbler with an angled jaws.

Kerrison's Punch (Heyjack Rongeur)

This has a handle which on grip closing causes the long twin shafts to slide over one another and close the cutting tips.

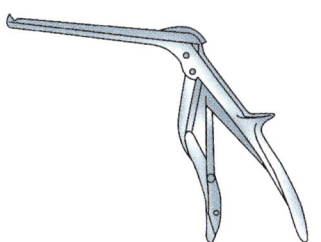

Fig. 19.25

This is used for holding the long bones. The bone is held and the butterfly nut is tightened for a fixed grip so as to avoid slippage during reduction of fractures.

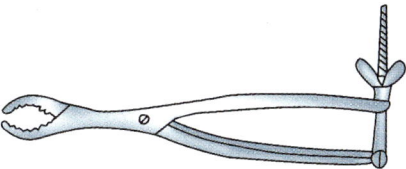

Fig. 19.27

Burn's Bone Holding Forceps

This has a rachet lock handle and fenestrated jaws.

This is a very useful instrument for holding the forearm bones during reduction and fixation, the fenestrated jaws are a great advantage as it allows to drill and pass a screw through it while holding the plate on the bone.

This is used for cutting/nibbling the laminae and pedicles while doing a spinal decompression, the long shaft is a great advantage to cut the deeply placed bone; it is also used as a sphenoid punch. It is available in up cutting as well as down cutting tips.

Straight Disc Punch

This is a scissor type of instrument with a long shaft and small terminal jaws.

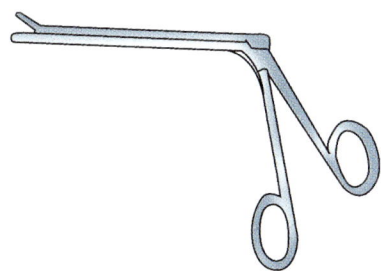

Fig. 19.26

This is used for catching and pulling out disc material in between the vertebral bodies in cases of disc prolapse, the small narrow shaft allows the instrument to enter a narrow space and the small jaws can open up in a limited space and can tightly grip the tissue in between, while it is being pulled out.

Heygrove's Bone Holding Forceps

This has long handles with a butterfly nut and bolt at the base to lock the griped bone, a long shaft and curved serrated jaws.

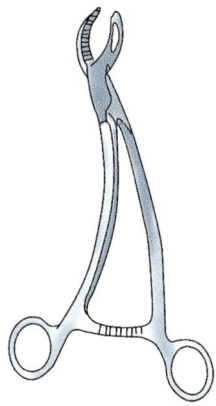

Fig. 19.28

Lanes Fagg's Bone Holding Forceps

This is a long, large bone holding forcep. It has two serrated arms, one of which is curved to avoid slipping of grip while manipulating the bone during reduction of fracture, the thick lion toothed jaws give a firm grip on the bone.

This is used for holding the femur and tibia. It is about 12 inches long. It should be used with caution in osteoporotic bones for the fear of crushing the bones.

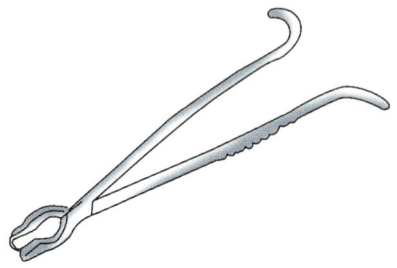

Fig. 19.29

Lowman's Bone Holding Clamp

This has two intersliding jaws, which are serrated and controlled by a chuck nut.

This is a useful instrument for holding the plate on the bone while it is being fixed by screws. It is available in sizes varying from 4–8 inches.

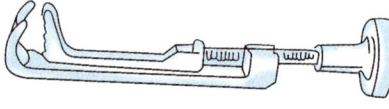

Fig. 19.30

Self-Centering Bone Holding Forceps

This forcep has a beaked jaw, the grip of which is variable by the use of eccentric hinge in the shank. The handle has a butterfly-nut to fix the grip on the bone.

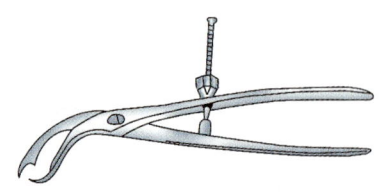

Fig. 19.31

This instrument is used for holding the bone of variable dimension. The conical beaked tips hold the bone with minimal stripping of periosteum and the grip is self-adjusting because of its peculiar hinge. It can also be used for holding the plate after reduction of fracture. Once the plate and the bone are firmly gripped, the handles are locked using the nut and bolt. This ensures that the forceps will not allow the bone or the plate to slip off during reduction and fixation. It is available in sizes varying from 150 mm for small bones to 280 mm for femur and tibia.

Reduction Forceps

This has a sharp serrated pointed jaw, and handles with a locking device.

This is used for holding long bones during manipulation and reduction of fractures. The sharp teeth give it a firm bite in the bone and prevent the slipping of forceps. This should be used with caution in osteoporotic bones since it may cause crushing of the bones. It is available in sizes varying from 140 to 170 mm in length.

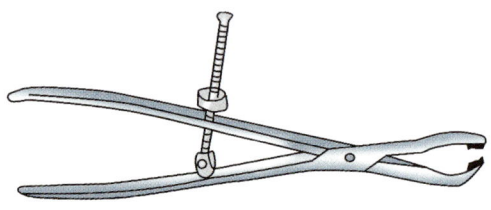

Fig. 19.32

Patella Forceps

This is shaped like a large towel clip with sharp pointed prongs and a bolt lock in the handle.

This is used for holding the reduction of patellar fragments during fixation by screws or tension band wiring. The sharp pointed prongs bite deep into the proximal and distal fragments to give desired reduction. It is available in single and double prongs in each jaw and is about 175 mm.

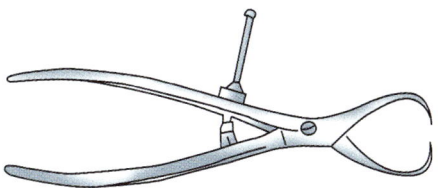

Fig. 19.33

Reduction Forceps With Points

This is a modified towel clip with bolt lock in the handles.

This is used for reduction of small fragments like medial malleolus, olecranon butterfly fragments, etc. and the spiked jaws bite into the bone and give it a good grip. It is available in sizes 130 to 200 mm.

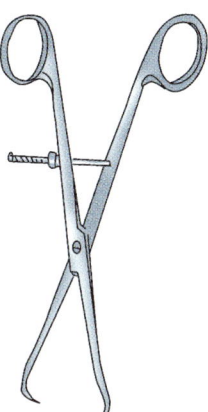

Fig. 19.34

Charnley's Compression Clamp

This has a self-collapsing shaft with two pairs of clamps to hold the Steinmann pin. The clamps are loaded over a butterfly nut bolt.

This is used extensively for arthrodesis of the knee and ankle. It can also be used for controlling and compressing osteotomies around the knee. First, the joint is excised and Steinmann pin are passed in each fragment. The Steinmann pins are then passed through the hole in the clamp on each side of the joint. The butterfly-nut on tightening causes compression of the joint thereby causing an early bony ankylosis. These clamps are available in single and double pin option.

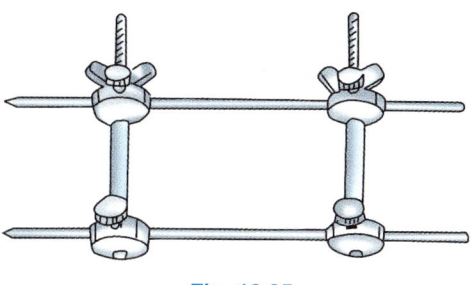

Fig. 19.35

K-Nail Extractor With Two Hooks

This has a long smooth shaft threaded at both ends. The proximal end is for the hook extractor and the distal end is for fixing the handle. A sledge hammer freely moves along the shaft. All the components can be dismantled.

This is a very useful instrument required for the extraction of intramedullary ordinary nails (K. nail and V. nail). The hook is first passed through the eye of the nail and then the shaft is threaded into it. The sledge hammer is then loaded onto the shaft after which the handle is tightened into the tail end. Once this unit is assembled, the sledge hammer is moved to and fro, hammering onto the handle. This gives pulling force in the axis of the shaft, thereby extracting the nail. This is available with a set of three hooks which are sharp, round and acute tipped. *One must always keep spare hooks whenever extraction of the femoral nail has been planned*. The sledge hammer weighs 1 to 3 pounds.

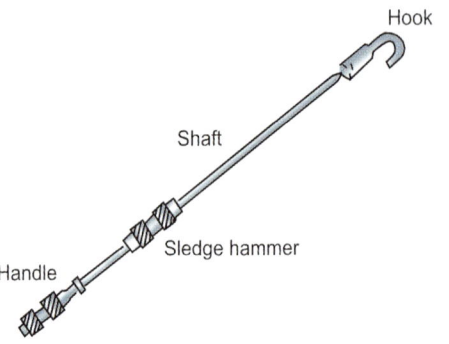

Fig. 19.36

Kuntscher's Diamond Pointed Awl

This has a U-shaped handle, an angled shaft and a diamond pointed tip.

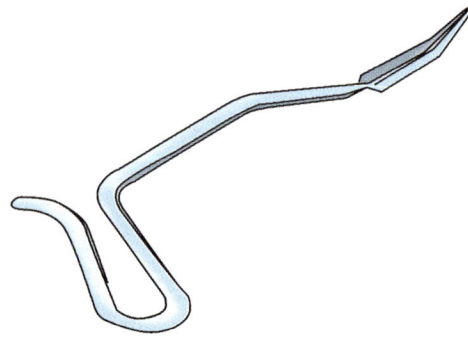

Fig. 19.37

This is used for making an opening hole in the trochanter and tibial condyles for introduction of intramedullary nails. The starting hole is made along the medial surface of the greater trochanter preferably the piriform fossa for a femoral nail or the proximal end of the tibial tuberosity of tibia. The sharp point is thrust into the bone and then subsequently directed into the line of the medullary canal by twisting movements.

Always direct the awl in the long axis of the bone to prevent perforation of the posterior cortex.

Bone Awl With Eye

This has a smooth and oval-shaped handle, a narrow straight shaft, and diamond tipped cutting edge with a small eye.

This is a useful instrument for making entry holes in the radius and ulna for intramedullary nailing. The eye in the tip can be used to pull out stainless steel wire or suture material through the bone.

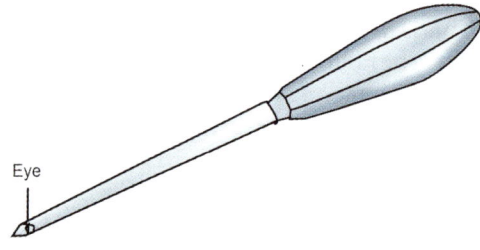

Fig. 19.38

Smith-Peterson Impactor

This has a bell-shaped tip, a hollow shaft and a top for hammering.

This is used for impaction of the neck of femur following fixation by SP-nail or parallel pins. The impactor is placed on the lateral surface of the greater trochanter and hammered in the axis of the neck of femur. The hollow bell-shaped tip gives room for the protruding tip of the implant.

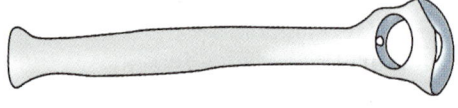

Fig. 19.39

Cannulated Sterling Holder Punch

To hammer the bone after the pins have been passed through the fracture site.

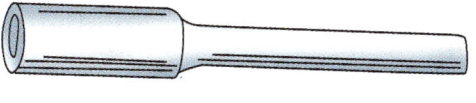

Fig. 19.40

Kuntscher's Nail Driver

This is a solid rod with a hollow tip, which is slotted. The grip is serrated.

This is used for impaction of K-nail into the femur. The hollow tip allows the eye of the nail to remain out of the trochanteric bone so that the hook can be fitted into it whenever it is necessary to extract the nail.

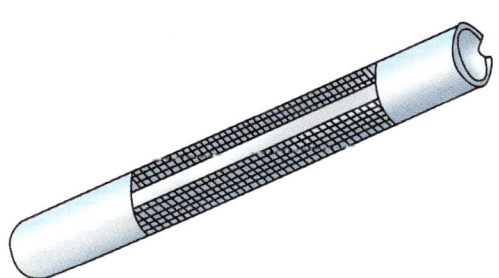

Fig. 19.41

K-Nail Punch

This is a solid rod with a small stud at the tip.

This is used for hammering the K-nail into the femur. The stud enters into the hollow of the nail and hence does not allow the punch to wander during hammering, and keeps the eye of nail out of the bone for easy extraction.

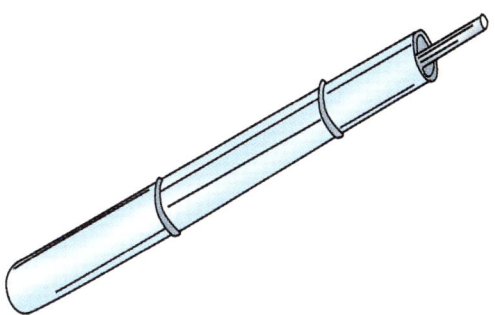

Fig. 19.42

Intramedullary Reamer

This is a long T-shaped instrument with a spiral cutting flute.

This is used for reaming of the medullary cavity so as to make a uniform canal for the intramedullary nail. The reamer is introduced into the bone after making an entry hole by an awl or directly through the fracture site while doing open reduction, the self cutting and reaming tip makes a bore along the medullary canal so that the nail is not jammed at the isthmus of the bone. It is available in sizes varying from 1.5 to 15 mm and can be used for practically all long bones requiring intra-medullary fixation. The modified reamers are now available which can be motor driven and are flexible in cases of closed interlocking nail fixation of long bones.

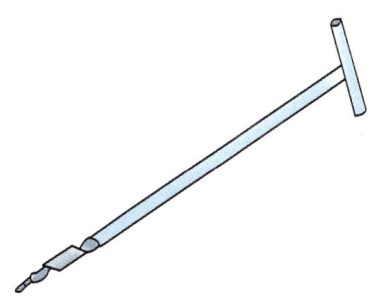

Fig. 19.43

Bending Plier For Small Plates

This has powerful jaws utilizing the power of two lever handles.

This is used to bend plates of 3.5 mm and 2.7 mm.

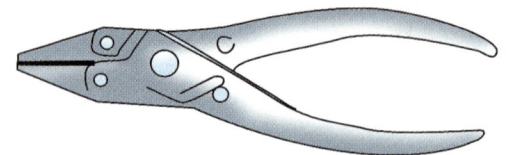

Fig. 19.46

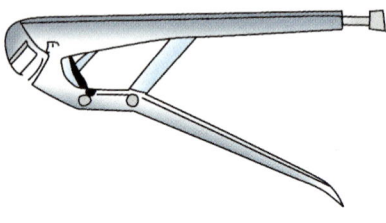

Fig. 19.44

Amputation Saw

This has a small handle and a long stainless steel blade.

This is used for cutting the long bones during amputation.

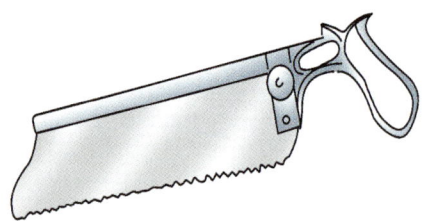

Fig. 19.47

Plate Bender Pair

This has a long-tempered shaft with oval terminal ends, which are slotted to accommodate the plate.

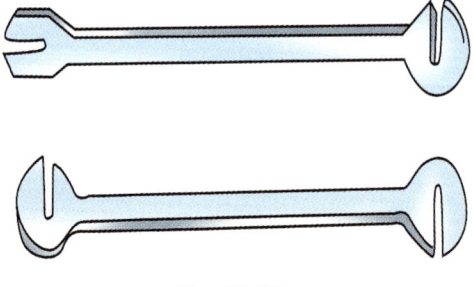

Fig. 19.45

Plaster Saw With Aluminium Handle

This has an aluminium handle with a semilunar stainless steel cutting blade attached to it.

This is used for bending of plates, both narrow as well as broad. The plate is held in between two bending irons at the desired junction and while one bender holds the plate the other bender contours it.

Flat-Nosed Parallel Plier

This is used for twisting the circlage wire and holding K-wires during extraction. This is available in sizes varying from 4 to 12 inches.

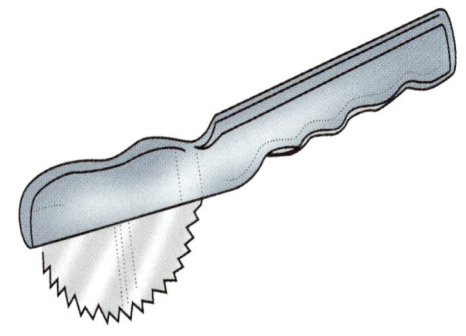

Fig. 19.48

This is used to saw the plaster for removal or to make a window into the POP cast for inspection of wounds.

Bohler's Plaster Cutting Scissor

This is a strong large scissor with the upper blade a little shorter than the lower, which is extended blunt tipped.

This is used for cutting the plaster casts, cotton and bandage. The lower blade is introduced inside the cast; the blunt tip protects the skin. While cutting, the scissor cuts through the hard POP material and avoids any entrapment of the soft tissue.

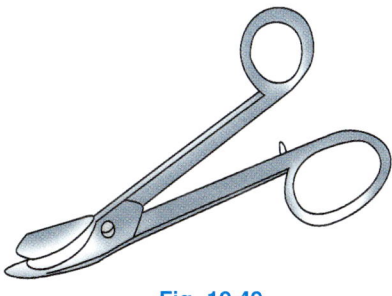

Fig. 19.49

Lorenz Plaster Shear

This has two strong handles, hinged to one other, the lower handle is fixed to the slotted jaw, through which the upper blade moves in a lever fashion, shearing through the hard POP cast.

This is used for cutting open small forearm cast as well as heavy hip spica.

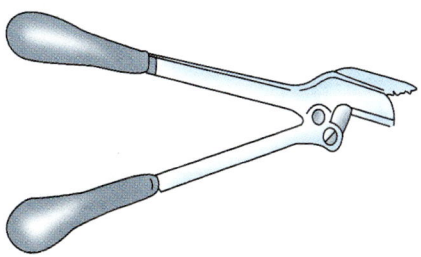

Fig. 19.50

Henning's Plaster Cast Spreader

This has two long handles, a narrow hinged shank and wide blades which are serrated on the outer side.

This has a peculiar function, i.e. on closing the handles the blades open out. The plaster cast is first cut, opened by saw or shear and then the spreader is introduced into the gap, the handles are then pressed thereby opening up the cast, the serrated blades prevent the slippage of the spreader.

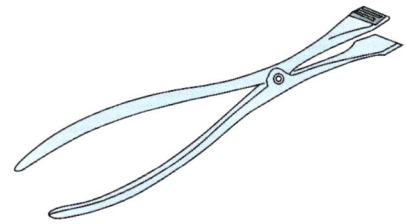

Fig. 19.51

Bohler's Stirrup Steinmann Pin Holder

This is a U-shaped steel rod twisted at the base to form a loop for traction, to the ends of this rod is attached small clamps to hold a Steinmann pin which can be tightened by the help of small bolts.

This is used for application of skeletal traction through the lower femoral, upper tibial or lower tibial sites. The stirrup helps in transferring the traction from the weights hanged through the pulley to the pin.

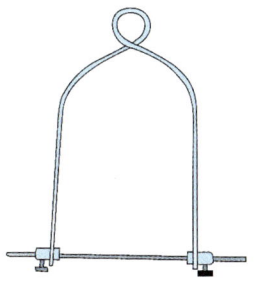

Fig. 19.52

Drill Bit

This is a stainless steel or carbon tempered rod which has a twisted cutting tip.

This is used for drilling holes in the bone for introduction of screws, pins and nails. It is available in short and long shapes from 1.0 to 4.5 mm and the base may be ordinary to fit into a manual drill or designed for quick coupling in powered instruments. It is important to protect the soft tissues adequately while using the drill bit, by using the drill sleeve, as its rotatory movement can entangle soft tissue fascia, muscle and vital tissues extensively.

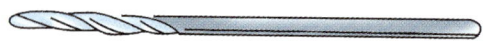

Fig. 19.53

Twin DCP Drill Guide

This has a handle with eccentric drill guide on one end and neutral on the other.

This is used for drilling holes in the bone for cortical screws. The guide on one side has a central/neutral hole while the other has an eccentric/loaded hole for compression screw. The dynamic compression plate is fixed on the bone and the hole drilled with neutral guide on the one side, and eccentric (with arrow towards fracture) on the other side of the fracture. For compression greater than 1 mm at the fracture site, the holes on both the sides of the fracture can be drilled using an eccentric drill guide. The tip of the guide is flattened on the sides to exactly fit into the plate holes down to the bone. The guides are mounted on the rings of the handle end so that they can be conveniently rotated. They are used for 2.0 mm as well as 3.2 mm drill bits (Fig. 19.54).

Mini Drill Sleeve (3.5/2 mm)

This has a small handle with two sleeves attached on each handle.

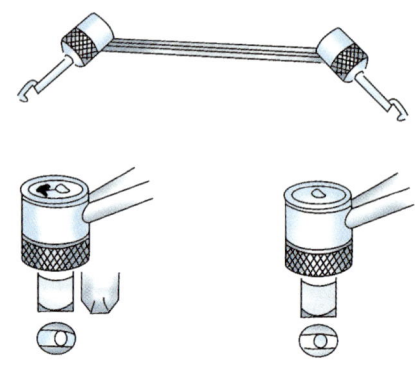

Fig. 19.54

The sleeves are to accommodate drill bits inside and prevent the entanglement of soft tissues while the drill is being rotated.

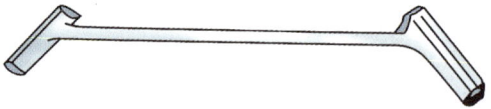

Fig. 19.55

Countersink

This is a T-handle with a small cutting tip of 4.5 mm.

This is used for making room for the head of the screw in the proximal cortex, when used as a lag screw, so that the head sinks into the bone and does not protude out especially if the screw is introduced along the subcutaneous surface of the bone.

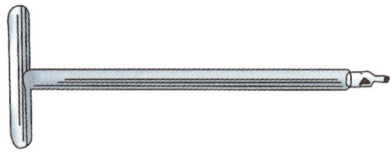

Fig. 19.56

Depth Gauge

This has a flat scale to which is attached measuring rod which is bent at the tip. It moves inside a tubular sleeve.

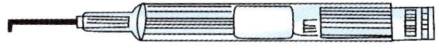

Fig. 19.57

This is used for measuring the depth of the hole in the bone for selecting appropriate length of the screw to be used. The hole is first drilled by a twist drill bit and then the rod of depth gauge is passed through the plate hole and the bone bypassing the opposite cortex. The outer sleeve is fixed to the plate, while the rod tipped scale is pulled up, the bent end of the rod engages the outer cortex at the far end. The depth of the hole is then read directly looking at the scale. Separate depth gauges are available for 2.5 mm, 3.5 mm and 4.5 mm screws.

Tap

This is a quick coupling tap for making threads in the holes drilled in the bone for introduction of screws.

This is used for making threads for non-self tapping cortical screws, cancellous screws and malleolar screws. It is available in sizes varying from 2.7 to 6.5 mm. It is used in power driven instruments.

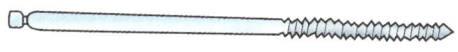

Fig. 19.58

Tap With Fixed Handle

This is a T-shaped tempered rod with cutting threads and flutes.

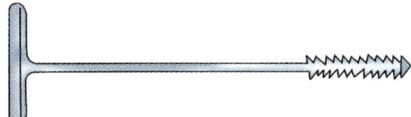

Fig. 19.59

This is used for manual threading of holes in cortico-cancellous bone for screws and is available in sizes from 2.7 to 6.5 mm. The flutes allow the bone debris to come out while the hole is being tapped.

Screwdriver

This is an ordinary screwdriver, flat tipped with a fibre handle.

This is used for screws with ordinary heads, which are now obsolete.

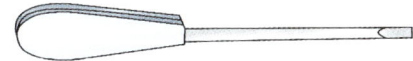

Fig. 19.60

Hexagonal Screwdriver With Fibre Blade

This has a flat fibre handle and a smooth shaft which has a high tempered hexagonal shaft at the tip (as shown in insert).

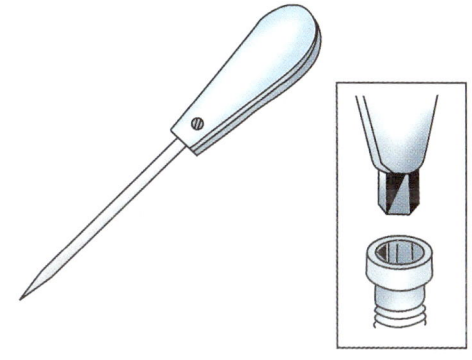

Fig. 19.61

This is used for introduction of dynamic compression screws for plate fixation and directly on the bone also. The flat handle is a great advantage during tightening of the screw and the hexagonal tip gives it a mechanical grip on the head of the screw, which does not require the need of applying vertical pressure during rotational tightening. It is available in 3.5 and 4.5 mm. The latter can also be used for malleolar as well as 6.5 mm cancellous screws.

William's Screwdriver

This is a screwdriver with a lever that can lock the screw grip by moving the sleeve at the tip of the screwdriver.

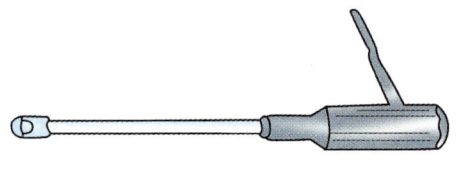

Fig. 19.62

This has an aluminium handle with a lever in it, which moves the sleeve at the tip of the screwdriver. The screw is fixed to the tip of the handle and then the lever is pressed, which locks the head of the screw and the sleeve so that the hold does not slip while the screw has been tightened. Once the screw is finally seated the lever is pulled up to unlock the hold on the screw head. The disadvantage of this screwdriver is that the final tightening has to be done after removal of the screwdriver.

Guide Wire

This is a tempered stainless steel wire with alternate dark and light marks along its smooth round shaft, which is pointed at one end and blunt at the other.

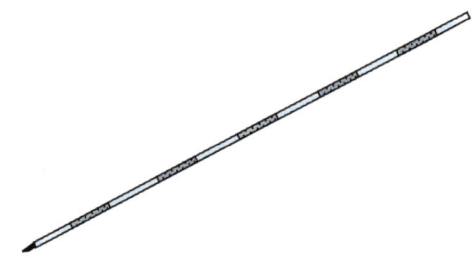

Fig. 19.63

This is used for deciding the length of the implant (SP-nail, cancellous screw, etc.) in cases of fracture neck of femur. After reduction of the fracture, the guide wire is passed using an angle guide so that the wire enters at an appropriate depth and at a desired angle. The position is further checked by X-ray. It is available in a standard 9 inches length and 2.5 mm diameter. The part of the wire, which remains outside the bone, is deducted from the total length thereby giving an exact intramedullary distance.

Angle Guide (Fixed)

This is a T-shaped instrument with a fenestrated tube connecting the horizontal with the vertical bar.

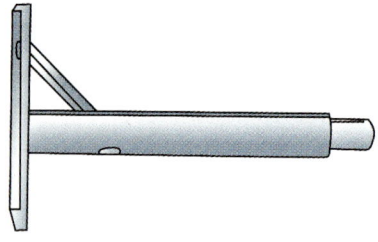

Fig. 19.64

This is used as a fixed angle guide for introduction of the guide wire in the neck of femur. It is available in a wide range of angles of 120°–170° and allows a guide wire of 2.5 mm to pass through.

Adjustable angle guides are also available.

Cancellous Tap (6.5 mm)

This has a smooth cannulated shaft, which has cancellous threads at one end and a flat base for quick coupling.

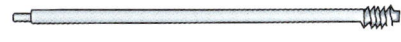

Fig. 19.65

This is used for making threads in healthy adult cancellous bone for introduction of 6.5 mm screws as in cases of fracture neck of femur or condylar fractures where dynamic compression system is going to be used. It is used with power instruments.

Triple Reamer

This has a cannulated drill bit combined with a slotted shank for the screw and a tapering collar for the barrel of the plate.

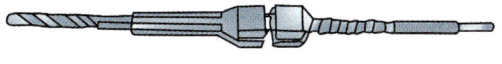

Fig. 19.66

This is used for 3-in-1 functions, i.e. to make a drill hole along the guide wire for the shaft of the screw as well as a larger hole in the proximal cortex for the barrel of the DHS to fit in. The length of the drill bit and the collar shaft can be conveniently adjusted. This is used with powered instrumentation. It is used for fracture neck of femur, trochanteric fracture in the proximal end of femur and also intercondylar/ supracondylar fracture at the distal end of femur.

CHS Wrench (Cannulated Hip Screw)

This is a T-handle with a hollow tip for introduction of cannulated hip screw in cases of fracture neck of femur. It has a vertical plate in the tip to fit into the slot of cancellous screw.

This is used for the introduction and extraction of 6.5 mm compression hip screws in the neck of femur and condyles. A guide wire is first passed, the hole is then drilled and tapped. An adequately sized screw is loaded into the wrench and then tightened.

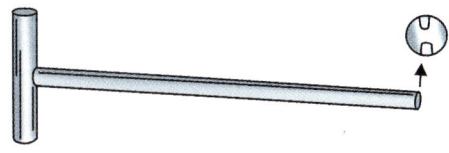

Fig. 19.67

Impactor

This has a smooth solid shaft, a round head and a blunt tip at the end.

This is used for impaction of the plate barrel assembly onto the compression screw in the trochanteric area and can also be used for impaction of bipolar prosthesis in cases of fracture neck of femur.

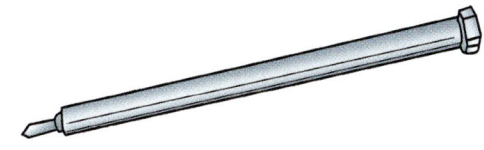

Fig. 19.68

Judet Femoral Head Extractor

This is a long T-shaped handle, with the tip of the shaft conical in shape and threaded like a cancellous screw.

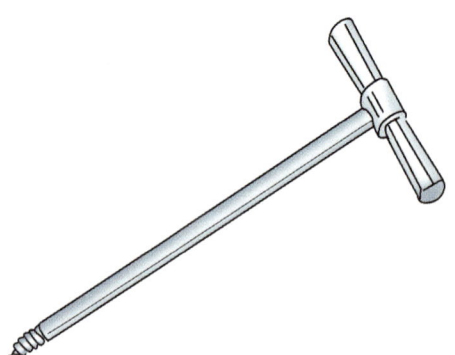

Fig. 19.69

It is used for extraction of the femoral head from the acetabular cavity in fracture neck of femur.

ORTHOPAEDIC IMPLANTS

SMITH-PETERSEN NAIL

This is a triflanged nail, the shaft is cannulated, the core is threaded with serrated base and sharp pointed tip.

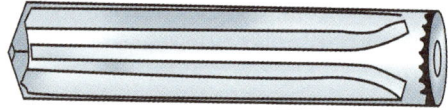

Fig. 19.70

This triflanged cannulated nail is used for fracture neck of femur (not used these days) and as a part of McLaughlin plate for cervicotrochanteric fractures. It has a cannulated core for the insertion. First a guide wire is introduced into the neck of femur and after satisfactory localization, the length of SP nail is decided and the nail is hammered into the neck of femur over the guide wire. It has a threaded, serrated base for fixation of introducer and extractor. It can be fixed to the McLaughlin plate with a bolt in case of cervicotrochanteric fractures. It also has a triflanged shaft, for three point fixation in the neck of femur which prevents rotation, and sharp pointed tip for easy penetration. It is available in a wide range of length of 2.5" to 5".

McLaughlin Plate With Washer and Bolt

This has three components a plate, washer and bolt.

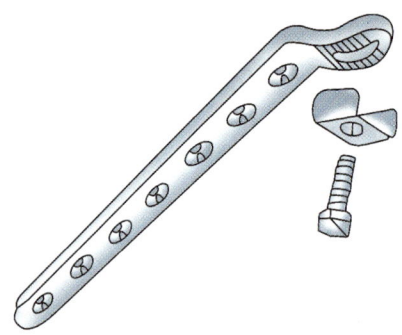

Fig. 19.71

The plate is rigid with 3 to 8 holes with the proximal end contoured like a spoon to adapt to the base of the SP nail and is serrated both on the medial and lateral surface to provide better fixation. It has a washer and bolt which helps to fix the SP nail to the plate. This is used in combination with SP nail for fixation of cervicotrochanteric fractures and has the advantage of fixation that can be done at a wide range of neck shaft angle. The SP nail is introduced into the neck of femur and then the plate is fixed to the shaft of femur to stabilize the neck shaft angle. The disadvantage of this device is its inherent weakness of the junction of nail, plate and the bolt which invariably gives away and is an insecure fixation.

Jewett Nail Plate

The components are triflanged cannulated nail in the proximal end and a plate in the distal end.

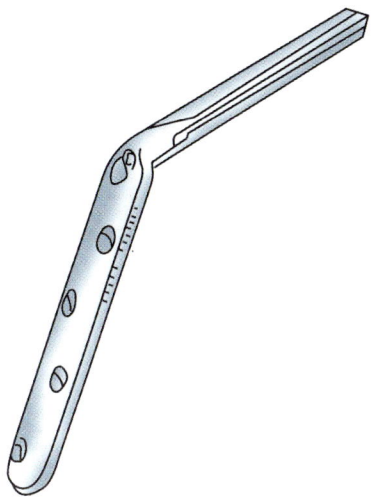

Fig. 19.72

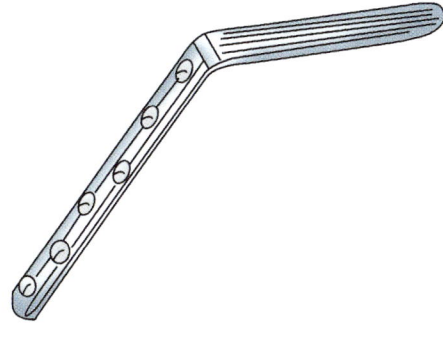

Fig. 19.73

Austin Moore's Pin

This has a smooth shaft with diamond pointed tip and a threaded base with 2 nuts.

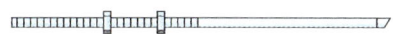

Fig. 19.74

A guide wire is first introduced into the neck and after deciding the exact length and the neck shaft angle, an appropriate nail plate is selected. The triflanged proximal end is guided and hammered into the neck threaded over the guide wire and the plate is subsequently fixed to the shaft by screws. This is a rigid nail plate fixation implant with fixed nail plate angle available with 130° to 145° angle. It has 6 to 8 hole plate, a rigid SP nail fixed to it as a single unit and scores over McLaughlin plate because of its fixed nail plate angle which gives it the advantage of a strong cervicotrochanteric stabilization system.

Moore Blount Blade Plate

The upper part is shaped like a blade while the distal part is like a plate.

This is used for fixation of subtrochanteric fractures and osteotomies. The blade is hammered into the neck and the plate is fixed to the shaft with screws. It is available in a wide range of angles from 90° to 135° and can be used for proximal as well as distal femoral fractures.

This is used for fixation of fracture neck of femur in children. After reduction of the fracture 3 to 4 parallel pins are introduced into the neck and 2 nuts are threaded over the base of the pin and are interlocked to prevent proximal migration of the pin. It is available in a wide range of sizes varying from 2.5" to 7". The disadvantage of this pin is frequent loosening of the nuts, proximal migration of the pin and bending.

Knowle's Pin

This is a tempered pin with a threaded diamond pointed tip, a smooth shaft with a broad nut base and a breakable proximal shaft.

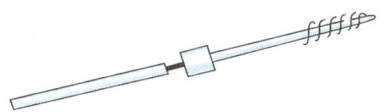

Fig. 19.75

This is used for fixation of neck of femur in children and adults and because of its threaded tip, it has a secure fixation in the head of femur which prevents its proximal migration which is further aided by the nut-shaped base. Because of its tempered steel the chances of bending are less. After introduction of the pin the tail end of the nail is broken off. It is available in 4 mm diameter ranging from 2" to 5" in length.

Garden's Screw

This is a cannulated cancellous screw.

It is used for fixation of fracture neck of femur in adults. The fracture is reduced and guided wire is passed into the head and neck of femur, over which the screw is tightened. Minimum of 3 screws are used for securing fixation. The cancellous threads of the screw give a secure grip in the head of the femur and should never be across the fracture site.

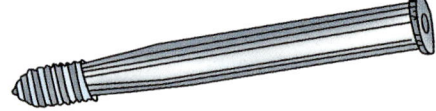

Fig. 19.76

Cannulated Bolts

This has a cannulated shaft with cancellous thread at the tip, a washer over the shaft and base is nut-shaped.

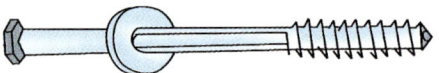

Fig. 19.77

This is used for fixation of intercondylar fractures of femur and tibia. A guide wire is passed after reduction of the fracture and the bolt is tightened over it, the washer prevents the sinking in of the bolt.

Thompson's Hip Prosthesis

This has a smooth polished head, neck and shaft.

This is used for replacement of the head of femur following fracture neck in elderly patients where the calcar is less than 2.5 cm. The neck of this prosthesis compensates for the absorbed neck of femur. After extraction of the head and shaping the remaining neck, the medullary canal is rasped. The size of the prosthesis is selected depending on the head of the femur, which is extracted, and measured by a gauge. The prosthesis is then hammered into the medullary cavity, if necessary in osteoporotic patients. Bone cement may be used, the bevelled tip of the shaft prevents perforation of the lateral cortex during introduction of the prosthesis. It is available in a wide range of sizes from 35 to 55 mm of head size.

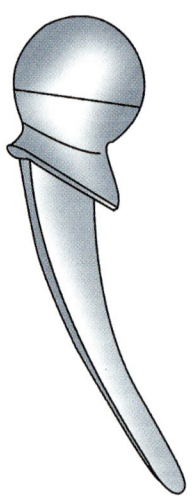

Fig. 19.78

Austin Moore's Prosthesis

This has a smooth polished head, short neck with hole for extraction, shank with sharp lateral ridge and fenestrated shaft with bevelled tip.

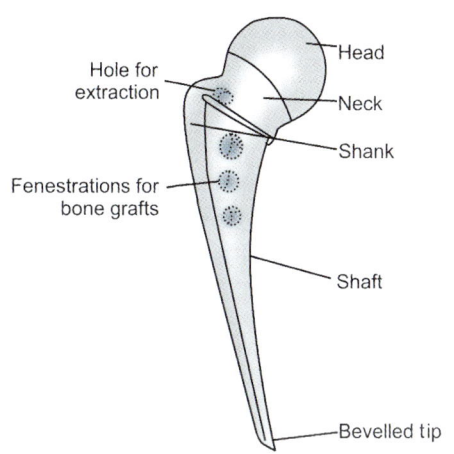

Head
Hole for extraction
Neck
Shank
Fenestrations for bone grafts
Shaft
Bevelled tip

Fig. 19.79

This is used for replacement of head and neck of femur in patients with fracture neck of femur, beyond the age of 60, with a calcar of atleast 2.5 cm and have a good articular cartilage lining, the acetabular cavity. The fenestrations in the shaft make it light and give room for introduction of bone grafts, the rigid shank gives a good hold in the trochanter and the bevelled tip prevents lateral perforation during introduction. Bone cement can be used where there is a risk of loosening in osteoporotic patients available in size 39–55 mm.

Bipolar Hip Prosthesis

The components are an acetabular cup with an outer polished surface and an inner polyethylene core, the metallic stem with a small head which fits into this cup.

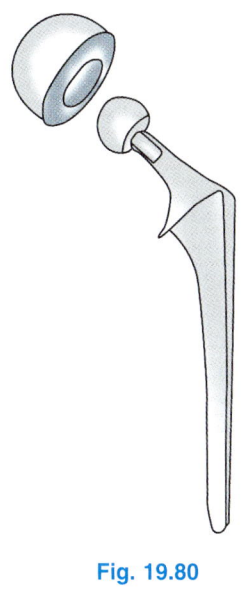

Fig. 19.80

The modern bipolar prosthesis has two articulations, both of which contribute to total hip motion (i) The outer joint, the large bipolar head against the acetabular cartilage, (ii) the inner articulation is formed by the small femoral head that fits into the large head cup. The stem is either press fit inserted into the medullary canal or in elderly patients bone cement is used. In younger patients revision is very easy and in old patients conversion to total hip can be conveniently done by changing the acetabular cup. This hemi-arthroplasty is more conservative than total hip replacement since the articular cartilage is not removed. It is indicated when degeneration is limited to the femoral side of the hip joint as in cases of osteonecrosis, tumour invasion or displaced fracture neck of femur in elderly patients. It is not indicated in patients who have developed advanced osteoarthritis of the hip with acetabular erosion. Modular orus are now available with variable head and neck lengths.

Total Hip Prosthesis

It has a metallic stem, head and high density polyethylene cup. The femoral stem is made up of titanium alloy which has high stress transfer quality and the head is made up of cobalt-chrome alloy which has superior wear resistance. The acetabular cup is made up of ultra highmolecular weight polyethylene, many components are now covered with metal shell to improve stress transfer to underline cement bone junction, can be coated with hydroxyapatite which encourages bone in growth.

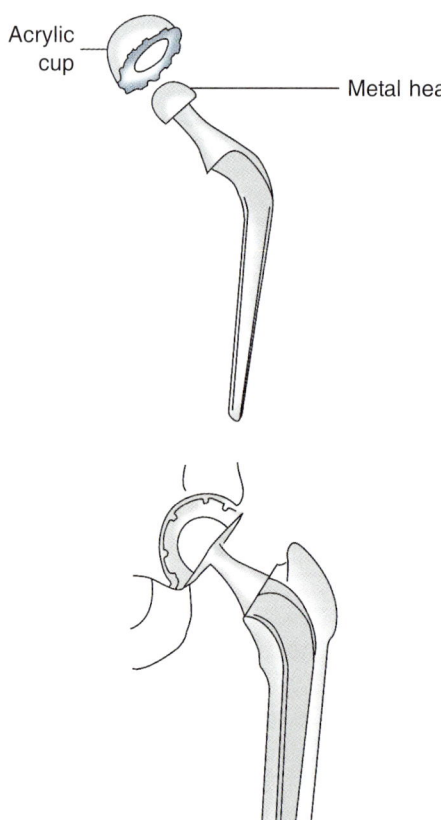

Acrylic cup

Metal head

Fig. 19.81

The total hip replacement is designed to enable the implant to support the loads which reach three times the body weight during walking. Femoral components with large cross section are stronger, proper neck length selection helps in restoration of the hip motion, accurate femoral offset decrease the bending stress with each step. The femoral component is either press fit in young patients or cemented in elderly. The acetabular cup is used with cement or screw fixed. Occasionally bone grafts are packed in the acetabular floor if it is deficient. Indications for THR are primary/secondary osteoarthritis, inflammatory diseases, avascular necrosis, displaced fracture neck of femur and non-union in elderly, bone tumours, metabolic and dysplastic involvement of hip, rheumatoid arthritis, ankylosing spondylitis and gout, congenital dislocation of hip, Perthes' disease and slipped capital femoral epiphysis.

Modular variety is also available with different sizes of head, neck length and shaft diameter.

Total Knee Prosthesis

Femoral and tibial component is made up of cobalt and chromium alloy, the tibial insert and patellar component is made up of UHDMP. Both are cemented onto the prepared precut bone surface.

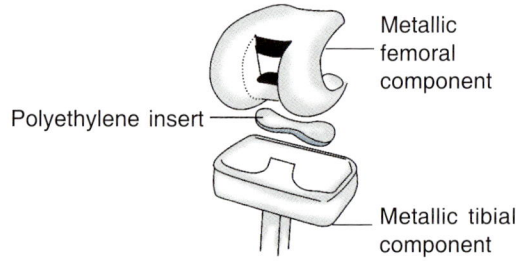

Metallic femoral component

Polyethylene insert

Metallic tibial component

Fig. 19.82

Indication: Advanced osteoarthritis of the knee, rheumatoid arthritis, ankylosed knee following trauma or infection; the short come of this implant is that it allows only 110° of free flexion and no room for rotation which is very much required in Indian lifestyle.

Murphy's Skid

This has a wide and narrow spoon-shaped ends, smooth on one side and serrated on the other side.

It is used for reposing and levering the head of the femoral component of the prosthesis into the acetabulum.

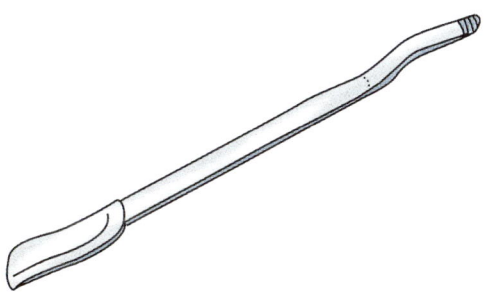

Fig. 19.83

Austin Moore's Rasp

This has a long curved shaft with serrated tapering tip, a fenestrated handle, square top and a tommy bar.

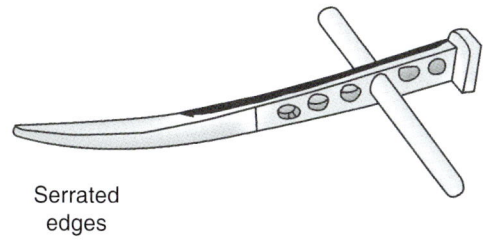

Serrated edges

Fig. 19.84

This is passed into the medullary canal of the neck of femur after accurate positioning which is helped by the tommy bar and is hammered into the shaft to make room for the stem of the prosthesis. The tommy bar helps in guiding the rotational adjustment of the rasp and in extraction too.

Prosthesis Impactor/Punch

This is made of aluminium or steel handle and has teflon tip on one end.

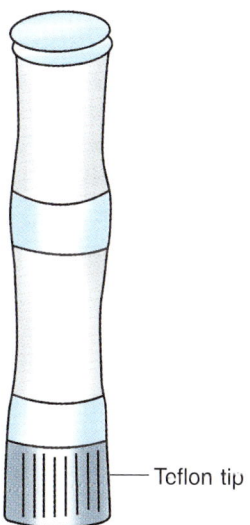

Teflon tip

Fig. 19.85

It is used for impaction of the femoral component of the prosthesis in the medullary canal. While it is hammered at one end, the tuflon tip prevents any damage to the surface of the prosthesis.

Kuntscher's Clover Leaf Nail For Femur

This is a long sheet moulded into clover leaf shape as seen in cross-section, there are two eyes at each end for extraction of the nail (Fig. 19.86a).

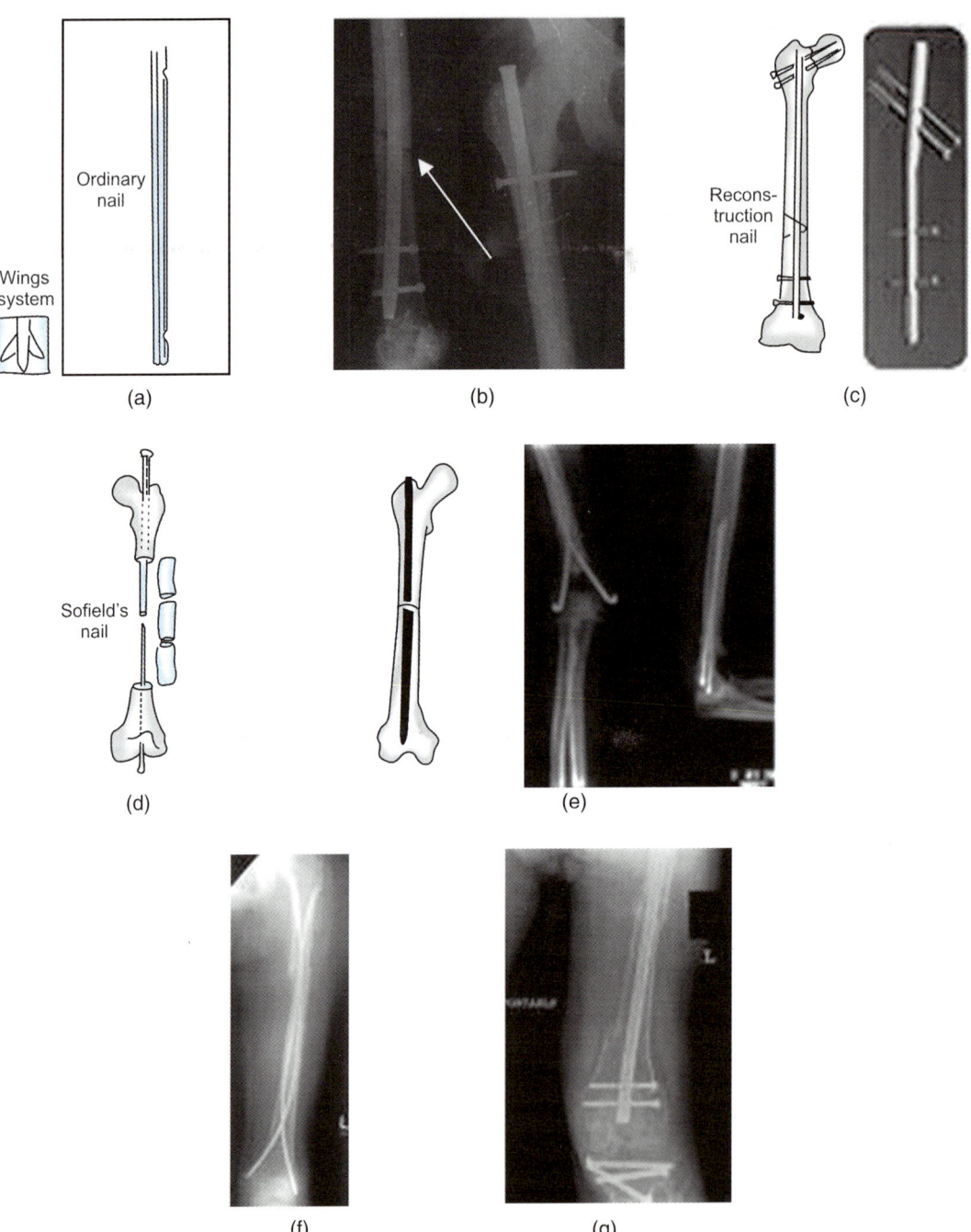

Figs 19.86a to g: (a) Ordinary 'K' nail; (b) interlocking nails; (c) reconstruction nails; (d) Sofield's nail for imperfecta; (e) and (f) ender nails; (g) supracondylar nail

The shape gives it the strength to resist bending force, it is used for intramedullary fixation of the upper two-thirds of femur shaft. The straight nail inside a twin curved medullary canal gives it a three-point fixation. After exposure of the fracture site, the length of the nail and diameter is assessed by reaming the canal to the maximum diameter and then using a guide wire, adding at least 2" to the intramedullary length for the nail eye to protrude above the tip of the trochanter for easy extraction (Fig. 19.86d).

This can be inserted **prograde,** i.e. from the piriform fossa in the distal direction entering the proximal fragment first and then across the fracture site into the distal fragment as is done in closed intramedullary nailing. It can also be introduced **retrograde** by first exposing the fracture site, introducing the nail in the proximal fragment out through the trochanter and then back into the distal fragment after reduction of the fracture, the nail is in this case hammered over the punch from the greater trochanter. The disadvantage of intramedullary nailing is that it disrupts the medullary vessel network and because of the wide medullary canal it is not suitable for the lower third femoral shaft fractures, this has now been modified and is available as **interlocked nail** (Fig. 19.86b) with two screw holes in the proximal and distal ends for interlocking which overcomes the short-coming of the simple nail in its inability to give a good hold in the lower third fractures of femur and also in comminuted and segmental fracture. It also helps in early dynamization of fracture and early weight bearing. It is available in length from 20 to 44 cm and 7 to 15 mm in diameter. The distal locking can be done with the help of Cotter pins or by **wings system** of nails (insert, Fig. 19.86a). Reconstruction nail for fracture neck and shaft (Fig. 19.86c) is also available.

Bailey and Dubow's, **Sofield's** telescoping rods (Fig. 19.86d) are also available for use in cases of osteogenesis imperfecta and **Peter William's** rods for pseudo-arthrosis of tibia. In this set of nails, the outer nail is hollow like a pipe and the inner one is solid like a rod, the inner one slides in and out and hence it lengthens as the bone of the child grows, thereby maintaining internal support to the growing bone and preventing it from deforming.

Rush Nail

This is a malleable nail, one end is hook-shaped while the other is bevelled.

It is used for intramedullary fixation of fracture of long bones in children as it can be bent to a desirable shape, the bevelled tip prevents penetration of the cortex while negotiating it through a curve, the hooked tip prevents sinking in of the nail and helps during extraction.

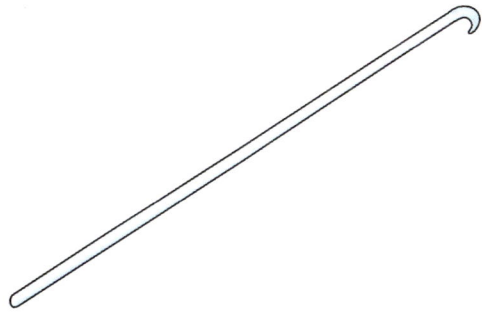

Fig. 19.87: Rush nail

Kuntscher's "V" Straight Nail For Humerus

This is a straight nail with an eye at one end for extraction, the tip is pointed and bevelled.

This is used for intramedullary fixation of humerus, the nail is inserted from the greater tuberosity across the fracture site into the

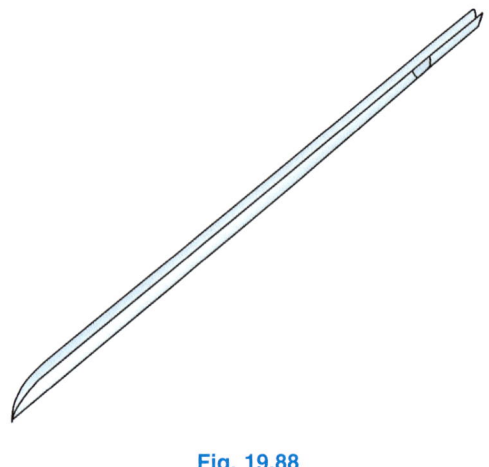

Fig. 19.88

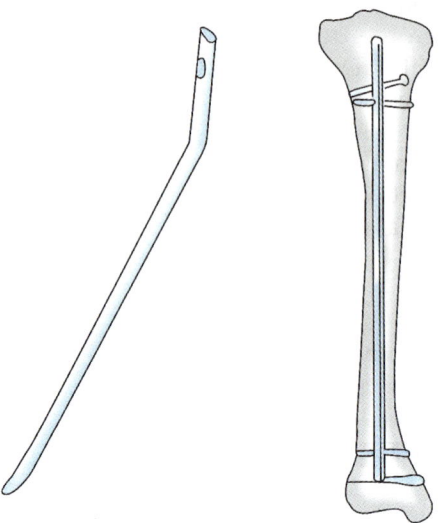

Fig. 19.89

distal fragment and the bevelled tip prevents the perforation of the cortex during insertion. It can be introduced in the retrograde direction through the roof of the olecranon fossa. The nail has a triangular cross section, which gives it three-point fixation, but the disadvantage is that it cannot provide compression at the fracture site and hence distraction often occurs. It has now been modified and has a hole above and below for transfixation screws so that the nail can be interlocked for early mobilization of the elbow. It is available in 5 to 8 mm diameter and 20 to 30 cm in length.

Kuntscher's "V" Angled Nail For Tibia

This is a proximally angled at the junction of upper one-fourth and lower three-fourths, has an eye in the proximal end, the tip is pointed and bevelled.

This is used for intramedullary fixation of lower two-thirds of fracture tibia. It is inserted in prograde direction medial to the tibial tuberosity or from above it. Because of wide medullary cavity in the upper part of the tibia it has a poor hold. It has now been modified with two screw holes above and below for interlocking and can be used for a large variety

of fracture of the tibia. The angulation in the upper one-third, helps it for a better localization in the medullary canal and is an advantage during extraction. It is available in 6 to 11 mm diameter and 20 to 36 cm in length. For early mobilization, modified interlocked nails have holes in the proximal as well as distal ends for interlocking screws, using Cotter pins.

Talwalkar's Square Nail For Ulna

This is straight nail square in cross-section with a pointed tip and a threaded base.

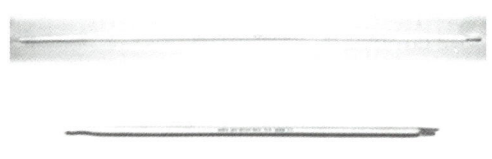

Fig. 19.90

This is used for intramedullary fixation of the lower half of ulna, because the medullary canal of ulna is wide in the proximal third, this is unsuitable for fixation here. It is introduced through the tip of the olecranon into the proximal fragment through the fracture site into the distal fragment. Due to its square cross section it has a multipoint fixation here. The threads in the base are used for attachment of the extractor device. It is available in 2 to 4 mm diameter and 17 to 30 cm in length.

Talwalkar's Square Nail For Radius

This is a straight nail, square in cross section with a notch and bevelled tip. The tail end is threaded.

Fig. 19.91

This is a nail used for intramedullary fixation of upper half of radius, because of wide medullary cavity in the lower third, it is unsuitable for fixation. The nail is introduced, held in a T-handle and the point of entry is either the styloid process or lateral to the Lister's tubercle into the distal fragment across the fracture site into the proximal fragment up to the head of radius. The bevelled tip prevents perforation of cortex while negotiating the curved medullary canal. The threads in the base are used for attachment of the extractor device. It is available in 2 to 4 mm diameter and 17 to 30 cm in length.

Ordinary Staple

This staple has equal pointed prongs and is square cut in shape.

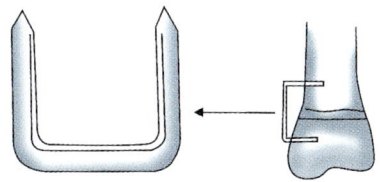

Fig. 19.92: Staple used for lower end of femur

This is used for stabilization of osteotomy for correction of deformities, for stapling epiphyseal plate for controlling growth in limb length discrepancies and metaphyseal deformities.

Coventary Staple

This is a staple with one limb straight and the other lazy S-shaped in the upper part.

This is used for stabilization of the bone after high tibial osteotomy. This peculiar shape helps in an accurate sitting of the staple on the proximal and distal fragment.

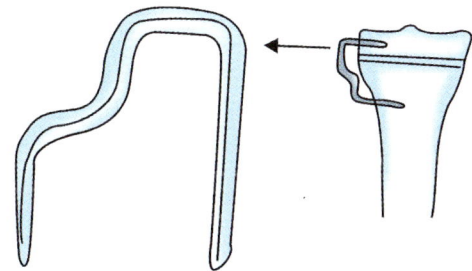

Fig. 19.93: Staple used for upper end of tibia

Cancellous Hook Screw

This is a cancellous screw with a long thread and a hooked head.

This is used for skeletal traction in cases of central fracture dislocation of hip and pelvic injuries, it is introduced into the head and neck of femur through the trochanter for application of traction. The hooked head is used for applying traction through weights, the cancellous threads give an excellent purchase in the head and neck of femur.

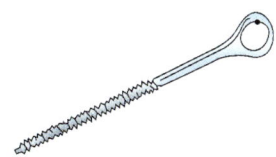

Fig. 19.94

Sherman's Screw (Machine screw)

This has an ordinary head, a full length symmetric threads and fluted tip.

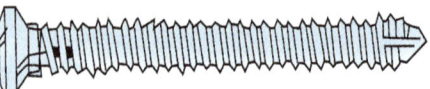

Fig. 19.95

This screw was used for cortical fixation. The fluted tip did not require the screw hole to be tapped and was hence known as self-tapping screw. Because of the fact that the flutes were not wide enough for bone debris, hence a larger bone drill had to be made. Due to symmetric threads, the purchase in the cortex was poor, hence for these reasons the screw is now obsolete.

Cortical Screw (4.5 mm)

It has spherical head of 8 mm diameter and hexagonal socket for screwdriver with asymmetric full-length threads and a non-tapping tip. The thread diameter is 4.5 mm the core diameter is 3 mm and requires a drill bit of 3.2 mm for the threaded hole and of 4.5 mm for gliding hole and a tap of 4.5 mm diameter.

This is used for diaphyseal fractures and plate screw fixation of femur, tibia and humerus, the thread profile is suitable for hard cortical bones and requires predrilled hole in which the threads are precut by a tap. It can be used as a bicortical fixation alone or with a plate and can also be used as a lag screw if the near hole is overdrilled by a 4.5 mm drill bit. The spherical head gives it a maximum contact with the plate even if it is introduced at an angle. The hexagonal socket gives it an advantage over an ordinary screw head and does not require axial pressure during introduction or extraction. Asymmetric thread gives an excellent bone contact. It is available in a wide range of length from 12 to 70 mm.

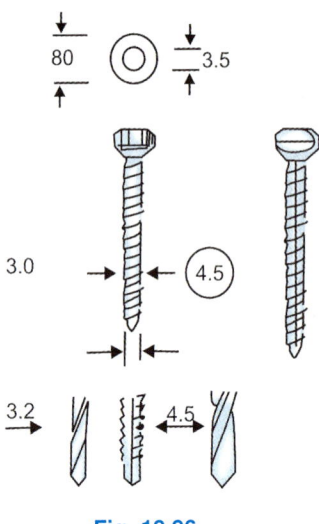

Fig. 19.96

Smaller screws with 1.5 to 3.5 mm diameters are also available for use in thin and small bones like radius, ulna and metacarpals.

Cancellous Screw (6.5 mm)

This has a partial or full-threaded shaft, spherical head with hexagonal socket and has a self-tapping tip. The thread dimension is 6.5 mm, shaft is 4.5 mm, while the core is 3 mm.

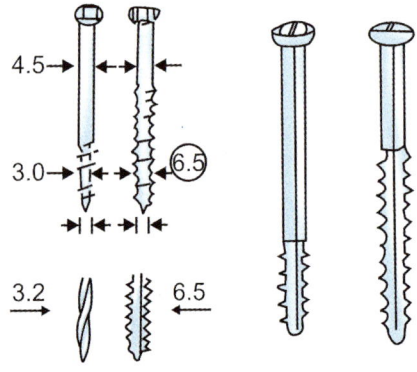

Fig. 19.97

This is used in epiphyseal and metaphyseal injuries for intercondylar and supracondylar fractures. It can be used alone or at the end hole of a plate in cancellous area. The deep threads and coarse pitch ensures a good hold in the compressed cancellous trabeculae. After the hole is predrilled only the cortex needs to be tapped, the screw tip is capable of cutting its own path through the cancellous bone. It is available in a wide range of length from 25 to 110 mm. Smaller cancellous screws of 4.5 mm and 4 mm diameters and lengths ranging from 10 to 70 mm are also available.

Epiphyseal Screws

This is a screw with cancellous threads at the tip and smooth shaft. The head is tall and bolt like.

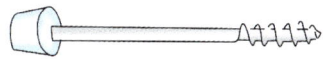

Fig. 19.98

This is used for the fixation of slipped epiphysis in children, the extra tall head prevents in growth of bone over it.

Malleolar Screw

This has a spherical head, a smooth shaft, cortical threads in the distal half.

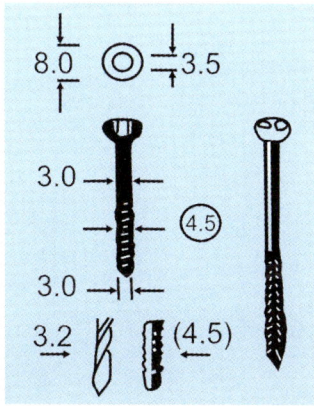

Fig. 19.99

These screws are used as lag screw for fixation of epiphyseal and metaphyseal injuries, e.g. fracture of medial malleolus. The thread profile is like a cortical screw and the tip can cut its own thread, hence tapping is seldom necessary, the thread diameter is 4.5 mm, while the core and shaft diameter is 3 mm and requires a 3.2 mm drill bit to make a hole. It is available in lengths of 25 to 70 mm.

Dynamic Compression Plate

This is a flat rigid plate with multiple spherical gliding holes on each side the middle zone.

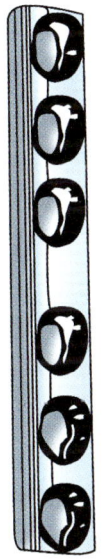

Fig. 19.100

This is used for diaphyseal fracture stabilization of long bones. It is an improvement over traditional round hole plates with several additional advantages due to its special hole geometry. When the screw is inserted through these holes, it moves in a downward and horizontal direction because of its slanting cylindrical shape of the hole which causes the 'e' underlying bone to move horizontally thereby creating intefragmentary compression. The oval screw holes allow screws to be inserted at an angle to the plate. An eccentrically loaded screw can cause compression of 1 mm at the fracture site on either side even in segmental fractures, thereby eliminating the use of compression device. Nevertheless, it can still be used at the end hole which has a slot cut-in for the hook of the compression device for additional compression. The plate can be prebent to give compression at the far cortex and can be contoured to a desirable shape to suit the underlying bone. This is available as broad, narrow, and mini sizes varying from 39 mm (2 holes) to 295 mm (18 holes). The end holes are large enough to allow the passage of 6.5 mm cancellous screws (Table 19.1).

Newer low contact plates are available which are contoured in the inter hole area to reduce area of bone contact.

Use of Dynamic Compression Plate

A selected plate is placed after the reduction of fracture and the first hole near the fracture site is drilled with 3.2 mm drill bit and tapped with 3.5 mm. The plate is slightly overbent and contoured. The necessary screw length is then inserted after measuring it with a depth gauge in neutral position. The next screw hole on the other side of the fracture site is drilled using an eccentric drill guide. The other screws are then inserted and the last screw is kept short, cutting through only the near cortex to avoid stress.

Table 19.1: Screw-Drill Bit-Tap								
Screw type	*Small cortical*				*Small cancellous*	*Cortical*	*Malleolar*	*Cancellous*
1. Diameter (mm)	1.5	2.0	2.7	3.5	4.0, 3.5	4.5	4.5	6.5
2. Tap	1.5	2.0	2.7	3.5 cortex	3.5 Cancellous	4.5	4.5	6.5
3. Drill for gliding hole	1.5.	2.0	2.7	3.5 new	None 3.5	4.5	None	In hard bone 4.5
4. Drill bit for threaded hole corresponding to core diameter	1.1	1.5	2.0	2.0	2.0	3.2	3.2	3.2

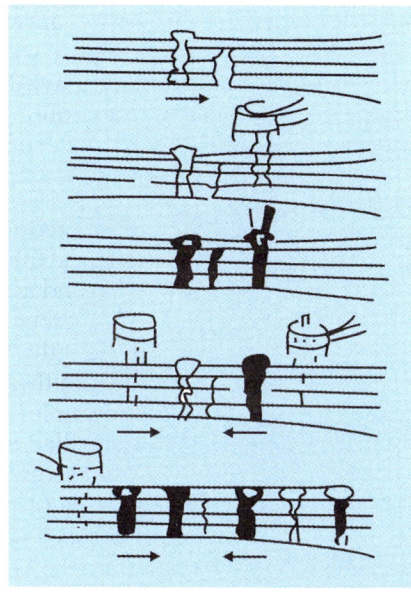

Fig. 19.101

The near hole is then over drilled with 4.5 mm drill and then the appropriate screw is tightened to get compression at the fracture site. The screw is placed perpendicular to the fracture line. In such situations, it is mandatory to first fix the screw on the obtuse angle side (Fig. 19.103). Chapter 15 under orthopaedic implants

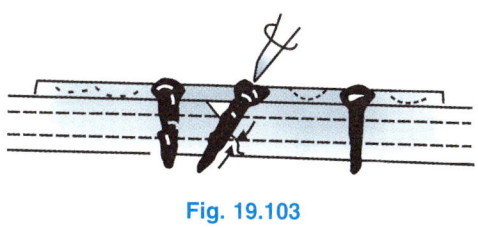

Fig. 19.103

DCP Used As Compression Device

If the holes on either side of the fracture site are eccentrically drilled then a compression of 2 mm can be achieved at the fracture site.

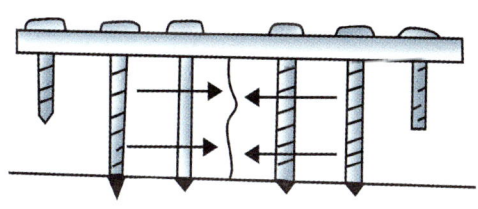

Fig. 19.102

Compression Device

The fracture is reduced and appropriate sized, contoured and prebent plate is placed across the fracture site, one screw near the fracture is inserted and the hook of the compression device is attached to the slot in the last hole of the DCP, the device is fixed to the bone with a screw inserted in only one cortex, the compression bolt is then tightened to achieve the desired compression and the screw in the near hole is fixed (Fig. 19.104).

Lag Screw Through DCP

In dealing with oblique fractures an oblique lag screw is a great advantage (while using a DCP). All the screws are inserted as usual, the inter fragmentary screw hole is first drilled using a 3.2 mm drill bit, the screw length gauged and the hole tapped with 4.5 mm tap.

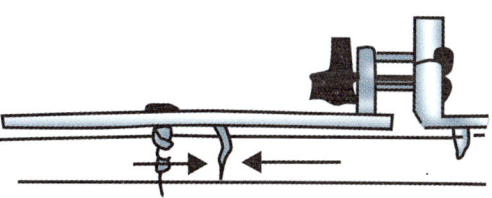

Fig. 19.104

Newer Plate are as under

1. **Limited Contact DCP (LC-DCP):** The newly designed LC-DCP stands for a new approach to plate fixation: reduced trauma to bone, preservation of blood supply, avoidance of producing stress risers at implant removal, and excellent tissue tolerance were the goals to be realized. The contact of the plate with the bone is limited and the plate-induced remodelling is small. Grooves on the under surface of the LC-DCP serve three purposes:

   1. They improve blood circulation by minimizing the damage due to contact between plate and bone.

   2. They allow for a small bone bridge beneath the plate at a place which is otherwise weak due to stress concentration effect of non-healed fracture gap at the periosteal surface.

   3. They result in more evenly distribution of stiffness of the plate than in conventional plate, where the cross-section at the screw holes is softer and weaker, while the full rectangular cross-section between the screw holes is markedly stiffer, i.e. more resistant to bending and torque. The difference in stiffness results in a relatively increased load within the weak spot at the screw holes.

2. **Locking compression plate:** The newly designed LC-DCP stands for a new approach to plate fixation: providing both dynamic compression and locking. Locking plates are ideal for fractures in osteoporotic bone. The screw head and the hole in the plate are both threaded to snuggly fit into each other for a better stable screw head and plate hole stability thereby preventing any toggle of the screw in osteoporotic bones.

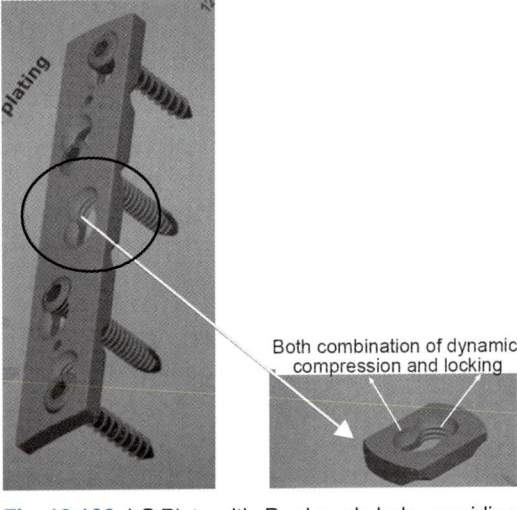

Both combination of dynamic compression and locking

Fig. 19.106: LC Plate with Dual mode hole providing both dynamic compression and locking

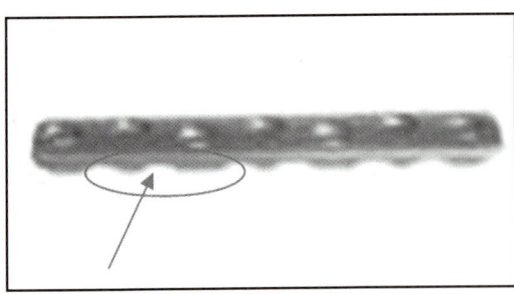

Fig. 19.105: LC-DCP with grooves on the under surface (arrow)

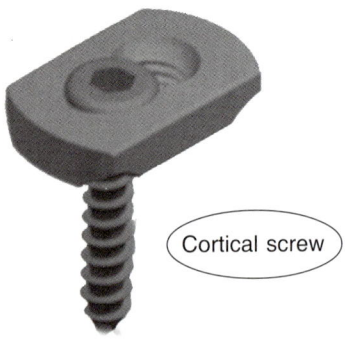

Cortical screw

Fig. 19.107: Locking compression plate with a cortical screw

Reconstruction Plates

This plate has lateral notches making it possible to bend the plate in three dimensions. The oval holes permit self-compression.

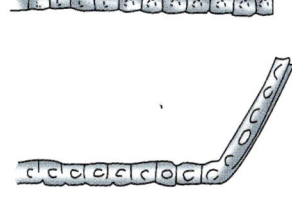

Fig. 19.108

This is used for mandibular fixation and reconstruction; the screws used are of size 3.5 mm. It is available in 5 holes (58 mm) to 12 holes (142 mm).

T-Mini Plate

These small 2 mm buttress plates are available in various shapes and are used for fixation of small bones of the hand and feet. 2 mm drill bit and 2.7 mm tap is used for insertion of 2.7 mm mini screws, which have a spherical head and hexagonal socket. These have 3 to 6 holes. Smaller plates (mini) for 2 and 1.5 mm cortical screws are also available.

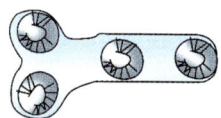

Fig. 19.109

Y-Reconstruction Plate

This plate is used for reconstruction of inter- and supracondylar fracture of the humerus. Because of its peculiar shape it can be moulded in three dimensions which can be contoured to suit the distal flare of the humerus. The arms of this plate can support the medial and lateral pillars of the supracondylar area and can be bent and cut short using pliers, stem of the Y-segment of the plate is screwed onto the shaft of the humerus by 3.5 mm screw. It is available in a standard 10 mm size.

Bending more than 15° must be avoided.

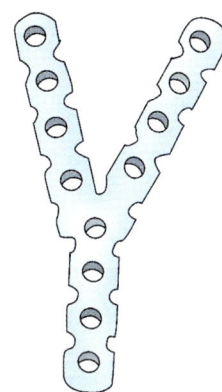

Fig. 19.110

T-Buttress Plate

This is T-shaped with 2 holes in the upper part and several compression holes in the vertical part.

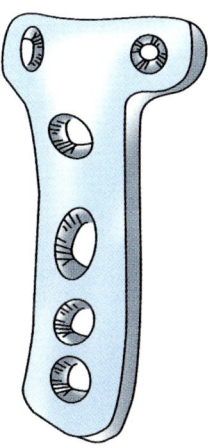

Fig. 19.111

This is used for stabilization of metaphyseal fractures as in intercondylar fractures of the tibia and prevents the collapse of fracture fragments held by screws. It is also used for the fractures of the upper end of the humerus. The oval middle hole meant for temporary cortical screw fixation of the plate while final positioning and compression is done, it also allows a lag screw to be inserted at a wide range of angle. It is available in the sizes ranging from 84 mm (4 holes) to 116 mm (6 holes). The upper end of the plate is bent to adjust to the flare of the tibial condyles.

Condylar Plate

This has a blade, which is 'U' shaped in cross-section, giving it high strength with minimal bone displacement, fixed at an angle of 95° to 130° with the plate, the upper two holes in this plate can take cancellous screws of 6.5 mm, while the other holes take cortical screws at various angles.

This is used for proximal and distal femoral fractures and available in a wide range of sizes, the blade is 50 to 80 mm in length and 6.5 mm thick, plate has 5 to 10 holes and is 92 to 204 mm in length.

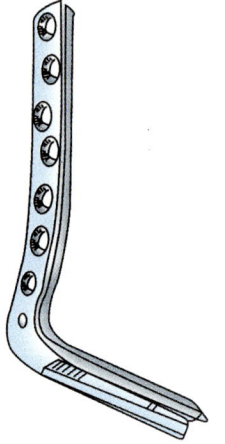

Fig. 19.112

Richard's Compression Hip Assembly

Compression Hip Screw

This has a rectangular cannulated shaft, slotted at one end for the wrench for introduction and extraction, the tip has 6.5 mm cancellous threads. The cannulation is meant for the guide wire.

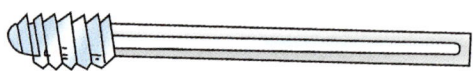

Fig. 19.113a

This is used as a part of the dynamic compression hip system as a lag screw, in cases of fracture neck of femur and trochanteric fractures. The guide wire is first passed into the antero-inferior quadrant of the head and neck of femur over which the hole is drilled and tapped by a triple reamer. The screw length is gauged and then an adequate sized screw is loaded on the T-wrench and then introduced into the head. Following which the guide wire is withdrawn and the barrel plate is then loaded over the slotted end of the screw. It is available in sizes ranging from 50 to 115 mm.

Compressing Screw/Top Screw

This is a screw with hexagonal head and machine threads, it is basically a bolt. This is part of the DHS assembly.

This is used for compression of fracture neck of femur. After insertion of the cancellous screw and loading the barrel plate over it, this screw is passed through the barrel into the threaded, slotted distal end of the cancellous hip screw. On tightening, it causes compression between the cancellous screw which grips the head on one side and the barrel plate which holds the shaft of femur on the other.

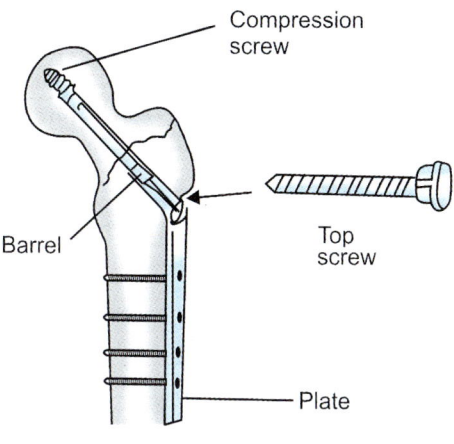

Fig. 19.113b

Barrel Plate

This has a short barrel circular in shape and the inner core rectangular in cross-section to match the shaft of the cancellous screw inclined at and angle of 130–150° to the plate which has 4–6 compression holes for cortical screws.

The barrel slides over the compression hip screw and then the plate is fixed to the shaft of femur by cortical screws. The first hole is meant for the cancellous screw and the compressing screw is finally tightened through this hole, thereby creating compression at the fracture site. The last hole is slotted for attachment of compression device. This is used for fracture neck, cervicotrochanteric and subtrochanteric fractures. It is available in barrel size of 38 mm in an angle of 130°–150° and the plate of 4–6 holes.

External Fixator Assembly

This is an AO type of external fixator system used for temporary stabilization of compound fractures, load bearing splints, interfragmental compression, arthrodesis, corrective osteotomies and stabilization of pelvic fractures. The components are the basic frame made up of tubular rods, the Schanz's pins hold the bone. The clamps connect the Schanz's pins to the tubular rods. The rods are interconnected to give three point stability. The assembly can be uni, bi, or triplanar (Fig. 19.114a).

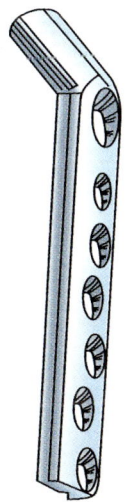

Fig. 19.113c

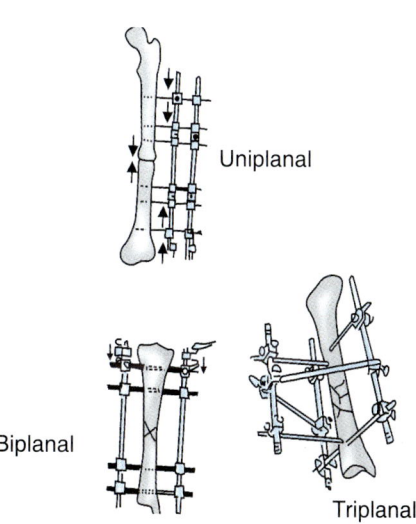

Fig. 19.114a

Tubular Rod

These are longitudinal stress bearing hollow, tubular rods used as columns in 1 to 3 planes for stabilizing the skeletal system, available in standard 11 mm and 8 mm diameter and lengths varying from 10 to 45 cm (Fig. 19.114 b).

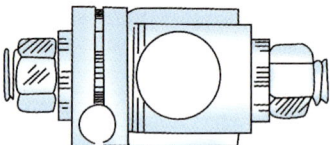

Fig. 19.114c

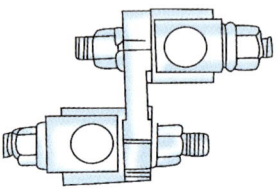

Fig. 19.114d

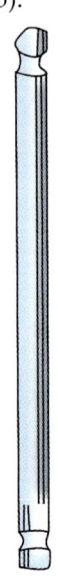

Fig. 19.114b

Transverse Pin Adjusting Clamps

This is a long plate with a central hole for fixation of the tube and two side rectangular sockets for pin holding clamps. This is used for the stabilization of condylar fractures of the tibia.

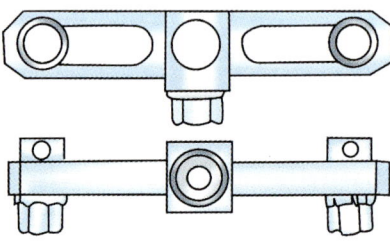

Fig. 19.114e

Standard Adjustable Clamp

This is a versatile device which connects the Schanz's pins, holding the bone to the tubular rods. It permits over 15° adjustment in the frontal plane. It has a 5 mm space for the Schanz's pin on one side and 11 mm on the other side for the tubular rod. Both of these holes can be compressed by nuts on the either side by an 11 mm spanner. Specially designed clamps for holding 2 parallel Schanz's pins are also available.

Universal Joint For Two Tubes

This is a coupled AO clamp hinged together for holding and stabilizing two rods together. The hinge allows adjustment in one plane.

Schanz's Pin

This is a modified Steinmann pin with a smooth shaft having cortico/cancellous threads at the tip which is self-cutting. The tail end is triangular for holding in a T-handle or drill. It is available in a wide range of diameter of 1.8 to 6.5 mm and 10 to 25 cm in length. The threads at the tip may be short or long. Cortical threads are used for fixation in diaphyseal part of the bone, while cancellous long threads are used for condylar fixation and the neck of femur.

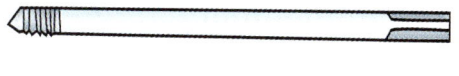

Fig. 19.114f

Asculab Clamp

This is a modified clamp in which Schanz's pin can be placed at a variable rotational position connected with two parallel 8 mm rods. A single nut fixes both the components. It is ideal for fixation of humerus and forearm bones.

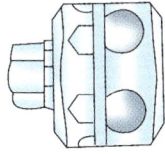

Fig. 19.115

'T' Handle

This 'T' shaped handle has a triangular socket for holding and quick coupling of Steinmann's/Schanz's pin for introduction in the bone.

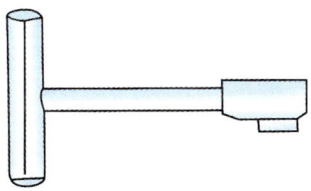

Fig. 19.116

Steinmann' Pin

This is the most commonly used implant in the wards. It has a smooth shaft with a diamond pointed tip and a triangular tail end. This is used for application of skeletal traction. The diamond pointed tip makes it easy for the pin to enter the hard cortical bone, while the triangular base gives it a three-point grip and prevents slipping during introduction using a drill. There are certain modifications of this pin which are described as under. It is available in diameter ranging from 1.8 to 6.5 mm and length of 12.5 to 30 cm.

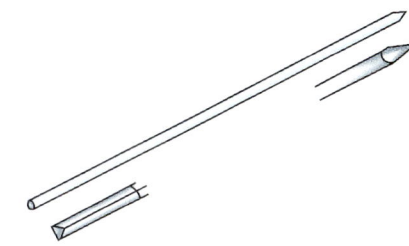

Fig. 19.117

Denham's Pin

This is a modified Steinmann pin in the sense that the middle of the pin has a cutting flute and is threaded, cortical for young adults and cancellous threads for osteoporotic old patients. Threads give it a hold in the bone, thereby preventing its migration or slipping.

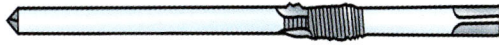

Fig. 19.118

Trocar

This is used along with a drill sleeve for making a bone entry for introduction of drill bit and Steinmann's/Schanz's pin, the trocar is first loaded into the sleeve of 5 mm which is in turn loaded into a 6.5 mm sleeve.

A subcutaneous cut is made and the triple guide penetrates down to the bone, it is then gently tapped with a hammer so that the trocar tip penetrates the bone, the trocar is then withdrawn and a 3.2 mm drill bit is introduced to make a hole in the cortex. The drill bit and the inner drill sleeve of 5 mm is now withdrawn. The pin is now introduced through the 6 mm sleeve which is removed after the pin penetrates through the opposite cortex. This triple guide helps in smooth entry of the pin through the soft tissue preventing any entanglement of the soft tissue while the pin is being rotated.

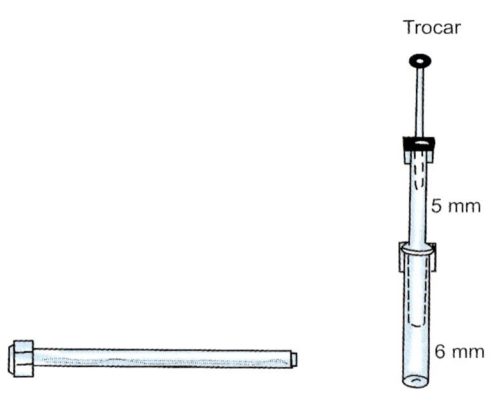

Fig. 19.121

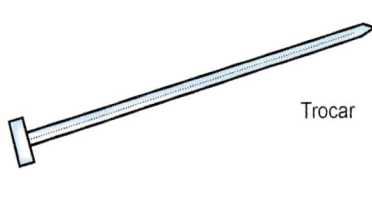

Fig. 19.119

Drill Sleeve (5 mm)

This is a cannulated sleeve to accommodate a 3.5 mm trocar.

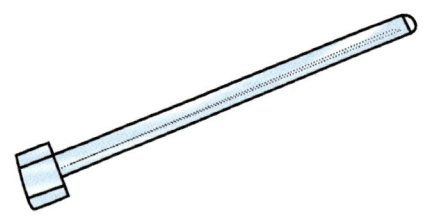

Fig. 19.120

Drill Sleeve (6 mm)

This is a cannulated sleeve to accommodate the trocar and 3.5 mm drill sleeve.

ILLIZAROV FIXATOR

Ring fixator was developed by Professor Garvil A Illizarov.

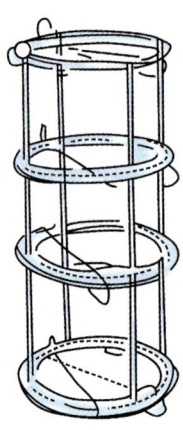

Fig. 19.122a

Illizarov ring system is a highly versatile simple assembly made up of an external skeleton comprising of rings which are interconnected by several long-threaded rods spanning the length of the limb, this is then connected to the bone through fine wires which pass through the bone and are tightened to the rings with the help of small wire fixation bolts. This can be used for a wide range of conditions varying from stabilization of fractures, correction of deformities, limb lengthening, management of non-union, malunion and arthrodesis.

The components are as follows :

a. **Primary components:** Half rings, threaded rods, K-wires, fixation bolts.

b. **Secondary components:** Used to construct the frame of apparatus e.g. bolts, nuts, rancho cubes.

Rings

This contains two and a half rings in sizes varying from 80 to 240 mm in diameter with 18 to 28 holes for introduction of bolts or threaded rods, each hole is 8 mm in diameter and spaced 4 mm from the next hole, the two and a half rings are connected to each other by small bolts converting into a full-ring. These rings are made of stainless steel.

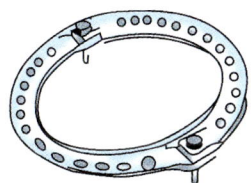

Fig. 19.122b

The newer ones are made up of carbon, which is light and radiolucent, but very expensive.

Threaded Rod

These are stainless steel threaded rods 6 mm in diameter and is used for connecting the rings together to form the external frame and is available in 60 to 400 mm in length. The distance between two threads (pitch) is precisely 1 mm so that the compression or distraction can be accurately done everyday. It is preferable to do .25 mm eight hourly. This

is controlled by twisting of the nut at a desired rate. One full circle of which moves the thread by 1 mm Usually about 4 rods at equidistance are used for connecting the rings.

Telescoping rods are available which give an automatic shift of 1 mm everyday.

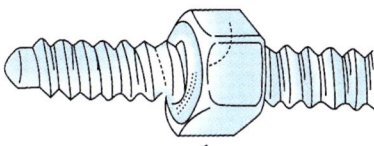

Fig. 19.122c

K-Wires

These are specially tempered K-wires of 1.5 mm for children and 1.8 mm for adults. The tip of these wires may be: (i) trocar for cancellous bone; (ii) bayonet for hard cortical bone; (iii) olive wires are used as stoppers and available in lengths of 300 to 400 mm. The wires are passed through the bone using a drill keeping in mind the safe corridor and are then transfixed to the rings by bolts. These wires, are tensioned after introduction to increase its strength. The olive wires are used to act as stopper for controlling transverse traction in a butterfly fragment or for side-to-side translation.

i. Trocar tip
ii. Bayonet tip
iii. Olive wire

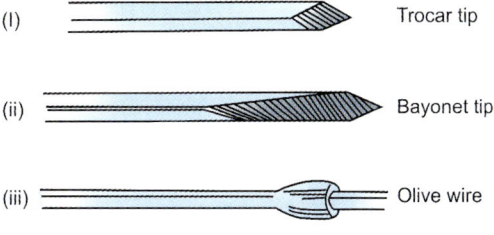

Fig. 19.122d

Dynamometric Wire Tensioner

The wire is first firmly fixed to the ring by bolts at one end while the other end is tensioned using a dynamometer so as to create a strength of 50 to 120 kg, which increases the strength of K-wires enabling them to withstand enormous loading forces. Once the wire is tensioned, it is fixed to the ring with the help of bolt and the tensioner is then removed.

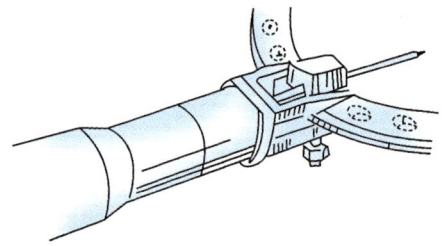

Fig. 19.122e

Wire Fixation Bolts

These are specially designed to fasten the K-wires to the rings. They are (i) slotted, so that the wire passes from the groove under the head of the bolt and (ii) cannulated, in which there is a 2 mm hole in the middle of the neck of the bolt through which the wire passes. These bolts have heads with 6 mm diameter and a 3 mm smooth neck which sinks into the ring holes.

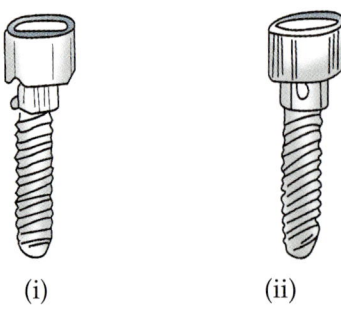

(i)   (ii)

Fig. 19.122f

Male and Female Posts

The male support has 13 mm long, standard threaded leg protruding from the butt end. The female post has no protruding rod, but 10 mm deep threaded hole at the butt end. This hole serves to connect bolts or rods. Their main advantages are that they can be placed virtually at any location, they can be turned 360° around their axis and they can be fixed in desirable position. They can be further modified, coupled together and converted into hinges as shown in the diagram.

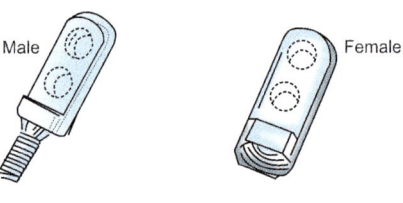
Male   Female

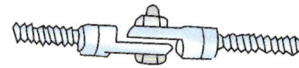

Fig. 19.122g

90° Femoral Arch (Italian Arch)

This is exclusively used for proximal femoral fixation. Schanz's pin can be fixed to this arch, with the help of bolts and posts, which is subsequently connected to the rings below by three-threaded rods, one at each end and other in the middle. Larger ones of 120° are also available.

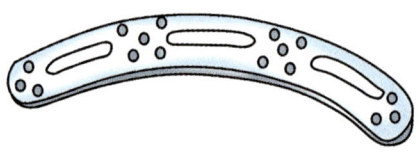

Fig. 19.122h

Oblique Support Connector

This helps in connecting the proximal and distal arches in the upper femoral fixation assembly.

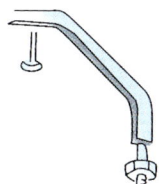

Fig. 19.122i

Proximal Femoral Fixation Assembly

The figure shows the use of Schanz's pins connected to the 90° half ring with the help of posts and the second half ring of 120°, which are interconnected by oblique connectors.

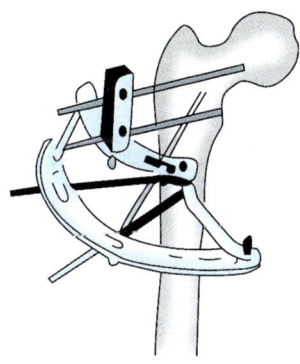

Fig. 19.123

This is an excellent assembly for the fixation of the upper third of the femur, i.e. the head, neck and subtrochanteric zone, which can be further connected down with the standard ring fixator. The above assembly circumvents the need to pass wires through the limb avoiding injury to important neurovascular structures.

Assembly Frame to Show Stabilization of Subtrochanteric and Shaft of Femur Fractures

Several half rings are used in the proximal part through which Shanz pins and K-wires are passed and subsequently connected to full rings below.

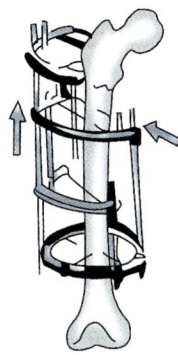

Fig. 19.124

Assembly for Communited Fracture of Tibia

This shows the utilization of several rings, at least two in the proximal and two in the distal fragment stabilizing the main fragments while the butterfly fragment is fixed and compressed utilizing olive wires which are passed through the fragments and fixed to the frame with the help of posts. The proximal and distal rings exert a vertical compression while the olive wires provide transverse interfragmentory compression.

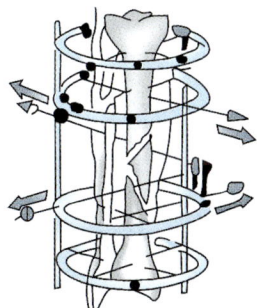

Fig. 19.125

Assembly Frame for Bone Transportation for Non-Union of Distal Tibia Fracture

This shows several rings, which are stabilized, in the main proximal and distal fragments by connecting long plate. A corticotomy is done in the proximal tibia and distraction between the second and third ring to produce neo-osteogenesis, while there is simultaneous compression between the fourth and fifth ring thereby managing the fracture non-union. This versatile frame can manage union, neo-osteogenesis as well as provides limb lengthening.

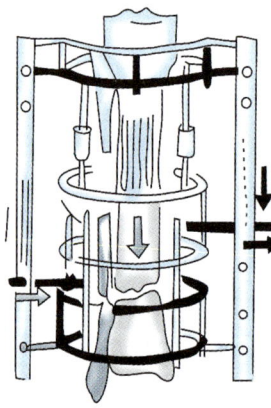

Fig. 19.126

Principle

- Distraction neo-osteogenesis which is mechanical induction of new bone between bony surfaces that are gradually pulled apart after corticotomy (cortex is cut, but medulla and its vessels are intact to a greater extent) as regenerate (new bone) forms.
- Compression to destroy infection, induce fracture healing in delayed and non-union.
- Stabilization of fracture so as to avoid POP cast or open reduction and internal fixation.

Indications

- Reduction of displaced, comminuted fractures.
- Limb lengthening, correction of deformity.
- Bone transport in bone loss for non-union, infection.
- Intra-articular, malunited fractures.
- Arthrodiastasis (stretching of the joint).
- Arthrodesis by compression.

Advantages

- Simultaneous correction of complex deformities.
- Early ambulation and joint mobilization.
- Light weight, high strength, radiolucent rings.
- Minimal surgical intervention.
- Secure and rigid fixation of fractures.

Disadvantages

- Cumbersome and heavy (new low weight carbon rings are available but very expensive).
- Time consuming.
- Difficult to arrange rings.
- Soft tissue management impossible.

Suture Materials

Characteristic of an ideal suture:
- It would consist of material which permits its use in any operation.
- It should handle comfortably and naturally to the surgeon.
- Tissue reaction stimulated should be minimal
- It should not create a situation favorably to bacterial growth
- The breaking strength should be high in small caliber.
- A knot should hold securely without fraying or cutting.
- It should be nonelectrolytic, noncapillary, nonallergenic and noncarcinogenic.

Type of Suture Materials

Suture can be conviently be divided into two broad groups: *absorbable and nonabsorbable.* Absorbable sutures can be associated as temporary, most nonabsorbable are permanent. Regardless of its nature, suture material is a foreign body to the human tissues in which it is implanted (See below).

Size and Tensile Strength

Size denote the diameter of the material, stated numerically, the more zeros (0) in the number, the smaller the size of the strand. As the number of 0's decreases, the size of strand increases. The 0's are designated as 5–0 for example, meaning 00000 which is smaller than a size 4–0.

The smaller the size, the less tensile strength the strand will have. Tensile strength of a suture is the measured force in pounds that the strands will withstand before it breaks when knotted.

Staples: In 1978, Ethicon, INC introduced the world's first reassembled disposable staging instrument. The staples are gently placed across the junction of the skin edges so they informally span the incision line. Approximately of the skin edges by stapling minimizes tissue compression. Skin staples are flexible in terms of their application.

Photographs Showing Staplers

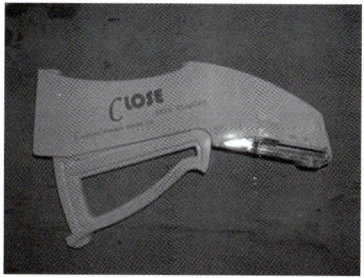

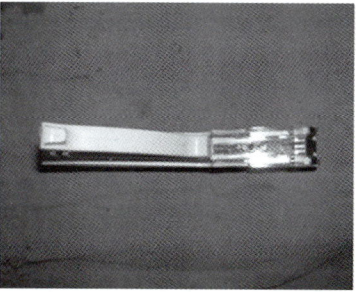

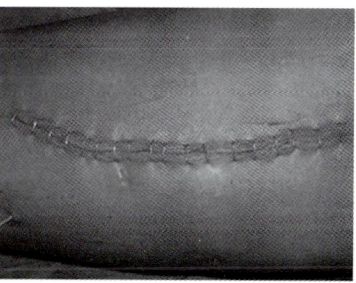

Fig. 19.127: Staplers

Suture materials

All suture material which is digested by body enzymes or hydrolyzed by tissue fluids is called ABSORBABLE	Tissue enzymes cannot dissolve some suture materials. These are called NON -ABSORBABLE

A further subdivision is useful: Monofilament and multifilament.

MONOFILAMENT	MULTIFILAMENT
• It is made of a single strand • It resists harboring microorganisms • It ties down smoothly	• It consist of several filaments twisted or braided together • This gives good handing and typing qualities

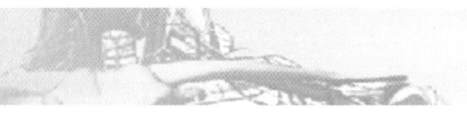

			Table 19.2: Suture materials commonly used in surgery		
Suture	*Types*	*Raw Material*	*Absorption rate*	*Contraindication*	*Uses*
Surgical Gut	Plain	Collagen derived from healthy mammals	Digested by body enzymes within 70 days	Should not be used in tissues that heal slowly and require support	Ligate superficial vessels;Sutures sub-cutaneous and other tissues that heal rapidly. Sometime used in presence of infection; ophthalmology
Surgical Gut	Chronic	Collagen derived from healthy mammals. Treated to resist digestion by body tissues	Digested by body enzymes within 90 days	Being absorbable should not be used where prolonged approximation of tissue under stress is required	May be used in presence of infection; Used in tissues that heals relatively slowly but intended for used as absorbable suture or ligature. Ophthalmology
Coated vicryl	Braided	Copolymer of lactide and glycolide coated with polyglactin -370 and calcium stearate	Minimal until about 40th day. Essentially complete between 60–90 days Absorbed by-slow hydrolysis	Being absorbable should not be used where prolonged approximation of tissue under stress is required	Ligate or suture tissues where an absorbable suture is desirable except where approximation under stress is required
PDS	Monofila-ment	Polyester polymer	Minimal until about 90th day. Essentially complete within 210 days absorbed by slow hydrolysis	Being absorbable should not be used where prolonged approximation of tissue under stress is required	Abdominal and thoracic closure. Subcutaneous tissue, colon and rectal surgery, can we in presence of infection, Orthopaedic plastic.
Surgical Silk	Braided	Natural protein fibres of raw silk spun by silk worm	Natural protein to found after two years	Should not be used for placement of vascular prosthesis and artificial heart valve	Most body tissues for ligating and suturing. General surgery, ophthal-mology and plastic surgery
Ethilon Nylon	Mono-filament	Polyamide polymer	Degrades at a rate of about 15–20% per year	None	Skin closure, retention, plastic surgery, ophthalmology and microsurgery
Mersilene	Braided	Polyester polyethylene terephthalate	Nonabsorbable: remains encap-sulated in body tissues	None	Cardiovascular general and plastic surgery, retention, ophthalmology
Prolene	Monofila-ment	Polymer of propylene	Nonabsorbable: remains encap-sulated in body tissues	None	General, plastic, cardiovascular surgery and skin closure; ophthalmology

Uses: They can be used virtually anywhere, regardless of the contour of the body they may be employed for routine skin closure in a wide variety operative procedure, to severe skin greater on burn patients, and for lacerations closed in the emergency department.

Contraindications: When it is not possible to maintain at least 5 mm from the stapled skin to underlying bones, vessels internal organs, the use of staples for skin closure is contraindicated.

STERILISATION AND AUTOCLAVING

Microorganisms are ubiquitous. Since they cause contamination, infection and decay, it becomes necessary to remove or destroy them from materials or from areas. This is the object of sterilization.

Sterilization is defined as the process by which an article, surface or medium is freed of all living microorganisms either in vegetative or spore state. Disinfection means the destruction or removal of all pathogenic organism, or organism capable of giving rise to infection.

Various agent used in sterilization can be classified as follows:

Physical

- Sunlight
- Drying
- Dry heat: Flaming, incineration, hot air
- Moist heat: Pasteurization, boiling, steam under normal pressure, steam under pressure
- Filtration: Candle, asbestos pads, membranes
- Radiation: Ionizing (X-rays, gamma rays and cosmic rays); Non-ionizing (infrared, ultraviolet radiation)
- Ultrasonic and sonic vibrations

Chemical

- Alcohols: Ethyl, isopropyl, trichlorobutanol
- Aldehydes: formaldehyde, glutaraldehyde
- Dyes
- Halogens
- Phenols
- Surface active agents
- Metallic salts
- Gases: Ethylene oxide, formaldehyde gas

The commonest mode which we across in OT is autoclaving. The principle of autoclave or steam sterilizer is that water boils when its vapour pressure equals that of the surrounding atmosphere. Hence, when pressure inside a closed vessel increases, the temperature at which water boils also increases.

Recommended temperature and duration for heat sterilization

Method	Temperature (°C)	Holding time (in min)
Autoclaving	121	15
	126	10
	134	3

Remember: Different method of sterilization for article used in day-to-day procedures in OT:

Material	Method
Skin	Tincture iodine
OT	Formaldehyde gas
Orthopaedics implants	Autoclaving
Suture material except catgut	Autoclaving
Catgut	Ionizing radiation (dose of 2.5 M rad)
Surgical instrument except sharp instrument	Autoclaving
Sharp instrument	5% cresol
Endoscope	Glutaraldehyde (cidex 2%) or ethylene oxide
Glass syringes	Hot air oven (180° C × 1 hr)
Disposable syringes	Ionizing radiation
Gloves, catheters	Autoclaving

20

Eponymic and Mnemonics

EPONYMIC (NAMED) FRACTURES

Barton's Fracture

Fracture of the distal end of the radius stable, oblique intra-articular fracture of the dorsal or ventral surface of the distal radius.

Bennett's Fracture

Fracture of the base of the first metacarpal, running into the carpo-metacarpal joint and complicated by subluxation.

Cotton's Fracture

Also called a tri-malleolar fracture. Refers to a combination of fractures involving medial malleolus, lateral malleolus and posterior lip of tibia.

Dupuytren's Fracture

Rupture of the deltoid ligament, fracture of medial malleolus, lateral subluxation of the talus and disruption of the distal tibiofibular syndesmosis with fracture of the distal fibula.

Essex-lopresti Fracture

Comminuted, impacted fracture of the radial head and neck with associated distal radioulnar joint dislocation.

Hutchinson's Fracture

Also called the **Chauffeurs fracture**, a sagittally oriented, intra-articular fracture of the distal radial styloid.

Jefferson Fracture

A burst fracture (compression) involving both anterior and posterior arches of the atlas.

Jones Fracture

Proximal diaphyseal fracture of the fifth metatarsal.

Lisfranc's Fracture

Fracture dislocation of the tarso-metatarsal joints (Lisfranc's joint).

Maisonnneuve's Fracture

Rupture of the deltoid ligament, lateral subluxation of the talus and disruption of the distal tibiofibular syndesmosis with fracture of the proximal fibula.

Malgaigne's Fracture

A supramalleolar transverse, oblique or comminuted fracture of the distal tibia. Also refers to fracture of the anterior and posterior pelvic arches on the same side.

Moore's Fracture

Fracture of distal radius with ulnar head dislocation and entrapment of the ulnar styloid beneath the annular ligament.

Pott's Fracture

It is a bimalleolar fracture with subluxation of talus.

FRACTURES WITH DESCRIPTIVE NAMES

Boxer's Fracture

A transverse fracture through the metacarpal neck, resulting in volar angulation of the head. The fracture name is derived from the common mechanism of injury, punching a solid object with a bare fist.

Bucket-handle Fracture

Fracture of the anterior and posterior pelvic arches on the opposite sides.

Bumper Fracture

Fracture of one or both legs caused by the impact of an automobile bumper, often occurs just below the knees and involves the tibial plateau.

Buttonhole Fracture

Perforation of the bone by a missile (bullet or other small, rapidly moving object).

Chance Fracture

Thoracolumbar distraction injury involving transverse fracture through the posterior elements, which may extend into the postero-superior or posteroinferior portion of the vertebral body.

Clay Shoveler's Fracture

Avulsion fracture of a spinous process, most often of the C 7 vertebra.

Fulcrum Fracture

Thoracolumbar distraction injury involving transverse fracture through the posterior elements and transverse fracture of the vertebral body.

Hangman's Fracture

Bilateral avulsion fractures through the pedicles of the axis C2 with or without subluxation of the C2 vertebra on the third.

Nutcraker Fracture

Crushing of the cuboid between the 4th and 5th metatarsal and the anterior calcaneus during lateral subluxation of the midtarsal joint (Chopart's joint).

Paratrooper Fracture

Fracture of the posterior articular margin of the tibia and/or of the medial/lateral.

Pilon Fracture

A comminuted fracture of the tibia involving the medial malleolus, lateral malleolus, anterior tibial lip and the distal tibia proximal to the articular surface. Its results from impact of the talus against the plafond. A hallmark of the pilon fracture is an anteriorly displaced fracture of the anterior tibial lip, often maintained in association with the talus.

Sprinter's Fracture

Avulsion fracture of the anterosuperior or anteroinferior iliac spine, caused by violent muscular action.

Straddle Fracture

Bilateral fracture of both pubic rami.

MNEMONICS

Chondrocalcinosis: "**Whip A Dog**"
 Wilson's disease
 Haemophilia
 Haemochromatosis
 Hyper parathyroidism
 Hypomagnesemia
 Idiopathic (Aging)

Psuedogout
Amyloidosis
Diabetes mellitus
Ochronosis
Gout

Secondary Osteoarthritis: "Not A Phowie"
Neurogenic arthropathy
Ochronosis
Trauma
Acromegaly, Avascular necrosis
Pseudogout
Haemochromatosis
Haemophilia
Occupational
Wilson's disease
Idiopathic
Erosive arthritis

Neuropathic Arthropathy: "6 D"
(Clinical features)
Distension (effusion)
Debris in the joint due to loose fragments
Dislocation due to joint instability
Disorganised joint
Destruction of articular surface
Density increased (sclerosis)

Protruso Acetabuli : "Port"
Daget's disease
Dsteomalacia
Dheumatoid arthritis
Drauma

Osteoblastic Secondaries: "5 Bees Lick Pollen"
Brain (medulloblastoma)
Bronchus
Breast
Bowel (carcinoid)
Bladder
Lymphoma
Prostate

Soap Bubble Appearance: "Fegnomashic"
Fibrous dysplasia
Enchondroma

Giant cell tumour
Non-ossifying fibroma
Osteoblastoma
Multiple myeloma, metastasis
Aneurysmal bone cyst
Simple bone cyst
Hyperthyroidism
Infections
Chondroblastoma

Aseptic Necrosis: "Aseptic"
Alcohol, arthrosclerosis, amyloidosis
Sickle cell anaemia, Storage diseases
Exogenous steroids
Pancreatitis, pregnancy, Perthes' disease
Trauma, radiation
Idiopathic
Caisson's disease

Generalized Sclerosis of Bone: "Marble"
Myelosclerosis, metabolic
(Hypervitaminosis d),
Anaemia (Sickle cell)
Renal osteodystrophy
Blastic metastasis, fluorosis
Lymphoma
Enigmas (Paget's disease, osteopetrosis)

Vertebral Collapse: "Fetish"
Fracture
Eosinophilic granuloma
Tumour (multiple myeloma, secondaries)
Infection
Steroids
Haemangioma

Diffuse Periosteal Reaction in Children: "Periosteal"
Pachydermoperiostosis
E Prostaglandin
Rickets (esp. Healing phase)
Idiopathic (Caffey's disease)
Osteoarthropathy (hypertrophic)
Syphilis, scurvy
Thyroid aeropachy
Excess flurorine (fluorosis)
A hypervitaminosis, abuse (child)
Leukaemia

Commonly Asked Questions

21

CHAPTERS 1, 2, 3, 15, 16, 17, 19: GENERAL ORTHOPAEDICS AND TRAUMATOLOGY

1. **Most common fracture in childhood is:**
   A. Femur
   B. Distal humerus
   C. Clavicle
   D. Radius

Ans. (B) Distal humerus

2. **Patients come with fracture femur in an acute accident, the first thing to do is:**
   A. Secure airway and treat the shock
   B. Splinting
   C. Physical examination
   D. X-ray

Ans. (A) Secure airway and treat the shock

3. **Most sensitive structure in a joints is:**
   A. Articular cartilage
   B. Synovium
   C. Fibrous capsule
   D. Bone

Ans. (C) Fibrous capsule

4. **Chemical synoviectomy is done by:**
   A. Osmic acid
   B. Chymopapain
   C. Chymotrypsin
   D. Trypsin

Ans. (A) Osmic acid

5. **Fat embolism is associated with:**
   A. Petechial hemorrhages
   B. Hemarthrosis
   C. Hematuria
   D. Bruise below the line of lesion

Ans. (A) Petechial hemorrhages

6. **Maximum weight used for skin traction is:**
   A. 5 kg   B. 7 kg
   C. 10 kg   D. 15 kg

Ans. (A) 5 kg

7. **K-wire is used in:**
   A. Circalage
   B. Fixing forearm bones
   C. Prior to plating
   D. All of the above

Ans. (D) All of the above

8. **The term orthopaedics was coined by:**
   A. Nicholas Andrey
   B. Hugh Owen Thomas
   C. Thoma Bryant
   D. Sir Rober Jones

Ans. (A) Nicholas Andrey

9. **Avascular necrosis of bone is most common is:**
   A. Scapula   B. Scaphoid
   C. Calcaneus   D. Cervical spine

Ans. **(B)** Scaphoid

10. **Which is not a principle of compound fracture treatment?**
    A. No tendon repair
    B. Aggressive antibiotics cover
    C. Wound debridement
    D. Immediate wound closure

Ans. **(D)** Immediate wound closure

11. **The structure responsible for longitudinal growth is:**
    A. Epiphysis
    B. Epiphyseal plate
    C. Metaphysis
    D. Diaphysis

Ans. **(B)** Epiphyseal plate

12. **The precartilaginous analogue to bone arises from:**
    A. Ectoderm
    B. Endoderm
    C. Mesenchyme
    D. None of the above

Ans. **(C)** Mesenchyme

13. **Fabella is:**
    A. Same as fibula
    B. An accessory projection from fibula
    C. A seasamoid bone
    D. None of the above

Ans. **(C)** A seasamoid bone

14. **The last step in the healing of a fracture is:**
    A. Hematoma formation
    B. Consolidation
    C. Remodeling
    D. Callus formation
    E. Demineralization of bones

Ans. **(C)** Remodeling

15. **Arthroplasty means:**
    A. The joint is made of plastic material
    B. The articulating parts of bones forming the joint are excised and made to fuse together
    C. The joint is excised and bones are so kept as to avoid fusion
    D. Any of the above

Ans. **(C)** The joint is excised and bones are so kept as to avoid fusion

16. **The characteristic of collagen is presence of:**
    A. Glycine
    B. Methionine
    C. Hydroxyproline
    D. None of the above

Ans. **(C)** Hydroxyproline

17. **Bone graft with maximum osteogenic potential is:**
    A. Fresh autograft
    B. Fresh cortical autograft
    C. Osteoperiosteal graft
    D. Vascular bone graft

Ans. **(B)** Fresh cortical autograft

18. **Distal femoral epiphysis is seen at the age of:**
    A. Just after birth   B. 10 weeks
    C. 20 weeks   D. 34 weeks

Ans. **(D)** 34 weeks

19. **Osteoblasts produce:**
    A. Collagen
    B. Calcium
    C. Pyrophosphate
    D. Monosodium urate

Ans. **(A)** Collagen

20. **Stress fracture are known to occur in the:**
    A. Metatarsals   B. Tibia
    C. Femur   D. Pelvis
    E. Radius and ulna   F. All except E

Ans. **(F)** All except E

21. **The most important factor in fracture healing is:**
   A. Good alignment
   B. Accurate reduction and 100% apposition of fractured fragments
   C. Immobilization
   D. Adequate calcium intake
   Ans. (C) Immobilization

22. **Spontaneous rupture of the Achilles tendon in an 18-year-old male it most likely to be due to excess stress beyond:**
   A. Tendon strength
   B. Bone strength
   C. Muscle strength
   D. Musculotendinous junction strength
   Ans. (A) Tendon strength

23. **Which of the following muscles are stance phase muscles?**
   A. Quadriceps
   B. Hamstring muscles
   C. Anterior tibial
   D. Peroneus longues
   E. Soleus-gastrocnemius
   F. All of the above
   Ans. (F) All of the above

24. **McMurray's osteotomy operation is based on the following principle:**
   A. Mechanical   B. Biological
   C. Bio-mechanical   D. None
   Ans. (C) Bio-mechanical

25. **Intramedullary nailing is contra-indicated in fracture shaft femur if:**
   A. The fracture is compound
   B. The fracture is near the knee joint
   C. The epiphysis have not fused
   D. Any of the above is present
   E. None of the above
   Ans. (E) None of the above

26. **The type of displacement of fractured fragment in which bone is not remodeled:**
   A. Anterior angulation
   B. Posterior angulation
   C. Lateral angulation
   D. Rotation
   Ans. (D) Rotation

27. **Most common cause of pathological fracture in a child is:**
   A. Malignancy
   B. Bone cyst
   C. Fibrous dysplasia
   D. Paget's disease
   Ans. (B) Bone cyst

28. **Normal bone remodeling in response to stress was described by:**
   A. Kuntscher
   B. Wolf
   C. Pauwels
   D. Hugh Owen Thomas
   Ans. (B) Wolf

29. **Cock-up splint is used in management of:**
   A. Ulnar nerve palsy
   B. Brachial plexus palsy
   C. Radial nerve palsy
   D. Combined ulnar and median nerve palsy
   Ans. (C) Radial nerve palsy

30. **Most common bone fracture in body is:**
   A. Radius   B. Clavicle
   C. Femur   D. Vertebra
   E. Pelvis
   Ans. (B) Clavicle

31. **Fracture which most often requires open reduction and internal fixation:**
   A. Lateral condyle of humerus
   B. Femoral condyle
   C. Distal tibial epipyseal separation
   D. Fracture both bones forearm
   Ans. (A) Lateral condyle of humerus

32. **Which of the following is best related to fat embolism:**
   A. 20% of polytrauma
   B. 40% of bilateral fracture femur
   C. 90% of trauma
   D. Only 15%
   Ans. (B) 40% of bilateral fracture femur

33. **Longitudinal bone growth is dependent on:**
    A. Metaphysis
    B. Diaphysis
    C. Epiphysis
    D. None

Ans. **(C)** Epiphysis

34. **Ideal site for bone graft harvesting:**
    A. Iliac crest
    B. Skull bones
    C. Femur cortex
    D. Tibial cortex

Ans. **(A)** Iliac crest

35. **Pathognomic sign of traumatic fracture:**
    A. Swelling
    B. Tenderness
    C. Redness
    D. Crepitus

Ans. **(D)** Crepitus

36. **Most common joint where arthroscopy is performed is:**
    A. Hip   B. Knee
    C. Ankle   D. Shoulder
    E. Elbow

Ans. **(B)** Knee

37. **Most common bone fracture during birth:**
    A. Scapula
    B. Humerus
    C. Clavicle
    D. Radius

Ans. **(C)** Clavicle

38. **Avascular necrosis occurs due to fracture of:**
    A. Medial femoral epicondyle
    B. Olecranon
    C. Talus
    D. Fibula

Ans. **(C)** Talus

39. **Common injury to baby is:**
    A. Fracture humerus
    B. Fracture clavicle
    C. Fracture radius:ulna
    D. Fracture femur

Ans. **(B)** Fracture clavicle

40. **Most common joint to undergo dislocation is:**
    A. Shoulder
    B. Radioulnar
    C. Hip
    D. Patellofemoral

Ans. **(A)** Shoulder

41. **Avascular necrosis is commonest one of the following fractures:**
    A. Garden 1 and 2 fracture of femoral neck
    B. Garden 3 and 4 fracture of femoral neck
    C. Sub-trochanteric fracture of femoral neck
    D. Basotrochanteric fracture

Ans. **(B)** Garden 3 and 4 fracture of femoral neck

42. **A man was diagnosed to have myositis ossificans progressive at the age of 20. yrs. He died 5 yrs later. What is the most probable cause of death?**
    A. Starvation and chest infection
    B. Myocarditis
    C. Hypercalcemia
    D. Hyperphosphatemia

Ans. **(A)** Starvation and chest infection

43. **Myositis ossificans is commonly seen at the ... joint.**
    A. Knee
    B. Elbow
    C. Shoulder
    D. Hip

Ans. **(B)** Elbow

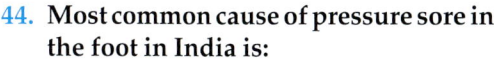

44. Most common cause of pressure sore in the foot in India is:
A. Diabetes
B. Syringomelia
C. Leprosy
D. Thorn prick

Ans. (C) Leprosy

45. Phalen's test is positive in:
A. Tennis elbow
B. de Quervain's disease
C. Carpal tunnel syndrome
D. Ulnar bursitis

Ans. (C) Carpal tunnel syndrome

46. Which of the following causes acute compartment syndrome most frequently?
A. Fractures
B. Postischemic swelling
C. Exercise initiated syndrome
D. Soft tissue injury

Ans. (A) Fractures

47. Pointing index is due to:
A. Ulnar nerve injury
B. Radial nerve injury
C. Medial nerve injury
D. Injury to flexor digitorum profundus tendon

Ans. (C) Medial nerve injury

48. A 15-year-old lady sustained a lacerated wound on the back of right thigh by the horn of a bull. The wound was sutured. Two months later she developed foot drop. The most likely diagnosis is:
A. Chronic ischaemic to limbs due to popliteal artery injury
B. Partial injury to sciatic nerve
C. Complete division of sciatic nerve
D. Injury to hamstring muscles

Ans. (C) Complete division of sciatic nerve

49. Diabetic Charcot's joint affect most commonly:
A. Knee   B. Ankle
C. Hip   D. Foot joint

Ans. (D) Foot joint

50. Which among the following benefits from cervical sympathectomy?
A. Sudeck's dystrophy
B. Compound palmar ganglion
C. Osteoarthritis of first MCP joint
D. deQuervain's tenosynovitis

Ans. (A) Sudeck's dystrophy

51. Most common type of shoulder dislocation:
A. Subcoracoid
B. Subglenoid
C. Posterior
D. Subclavicular

Ans. (A) Subcoracoid

52. Fracture surgical neck of humerus results in:
A. Wrist drop
B. Loss of sensations over forearm
C. Loss of roundness of shoulder
D. Clawhand

Ans. (C) Loss of roundness of shoulder

53. Treatment of fracture clavicle in an infant is best treated by:
A. Cuff and sling
B. Figure of 8 bandage
C. Open reduction
D. Shoulder cast

Ans. (B) Figure of 8 bandage

54. Anterior dislocation of shoulder causes all except:
A. Circumflex artery injury
B. Avascular necrosis head of humerus
C. Brachial plexus injury
D. Chip fracture scapula

Ans. (B) Avascular necrosis head of humerus

55. Nerve most commonly involved in fracture of surgical neck of humerus:
A. Radial N
B. Axillary N
C. Ulnar N
D. Median N

Ans. (B) Axillary N

56. Hill-Sachs lesion is:
A. Avulsion of glenoid labrum
B. Rupture of capsule near scapula
C. Bony defect in humeral head
D. Rupture of capsule near humerus

Ans. (C) Bony defect in humeral head

57. Most common cause for recurrent shoulder dislocation is:
A. Shallow glenoid labrum
B. Bankart lesion
C. Weakness of subscapularis muscle
D. Injury to humeral head

Ans. (B) Bankart lesion

58. Treatment of choice for fracture neck of humerus in a 70-year-old male:
A. Analgesic with arm sling
B. U-slap
C. Arthroplasty
D. Open reduction-Internal fixation

Ans. (A) Analgesic with arm sling

59. All are components of rotator cuff *except*:
A. Supraspinatus
B. Infraspinatus
C. Subscapularis
D. Teres major

Ans. (D) Teres major

60. Most commonly injured nerve in anterior dislocation shoulder is:
A. Nerve of bell
B. Axillary nerve
C. Radial nerve
D. Median nerve

Ans. (B) Axillary nerve

61. Treatment of anterior dislocation of shoulder is by:
A. Kocher's manoeuvre
B. Denis Browne splint
C. Barlow manoeuvre
D. Surgery

Ans. (A) Kocher's manoeuvre

62. Most common nerve damage in shoulder dislocation:
A. Radial nerve
B. Axillary nerve
C. Ulnar
D. Median

Ans. (B) Axillary nerve

63. Most common recurrent dislocation is seen with:
A. Shoulder
B. Patella
C. Elbow
D. Hip

Ans. (A) Shoulder

64. Luxatio erecta:
A. Tear of the glenoidal labium
B. Inferior dislocation of shoulder
C. Anterior dislocation of shoulder
D. Defect in humeral head

Ans. (B) Inferior dislocation of shoulder

65. Most common complication of clavicle fracture is:
A. Nonunion
B. Stiffness of finger
C. Vascular injury
D. Sudeck's dystrophy
E. None

Ans. (E) None

66. Ideal treatment with fracture neck of humerus in an old lady will be:
A. Triangular sling
B. Hemiarthroplasty
C. Chest arm bandage
D. Internal fixation

Ans. (A) Triangular sling

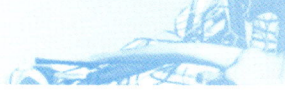

67. **Bankart lesion involves:**
   A. Anterior aspect of the head of humerus
   B. Anterior aspect of glenoid labrum
   C. Posterior aspect of glenoid labrum
   D. Posterior aspect of head of humerus

Ans. (B) Anterior aspect of glenoid labrum

68. **A patient with recurrent dislocation of shoulder presents to the hospital. The doctor tries to abduct his arm and to extend the elbow and external rotation, but the patient doesn't allow to do so. This test is called:**
   A. Duga's test
   B. Hamilton's test
   C. Callway's test
   D. Apprehension test

Ans. (D) Apprehension test

69. **If the greater tuberosity of the humerus is lost, which of the following movements will be affected:**
   A. Adduction and flexion
   B. Abduction and lateral rotation
   C. Medial rotation and adduction
   D. Flexion and medial rotation

Ans. (B) Abduction and lateral rotation

70. **All are related to recurrent shoulder dislocation except:**
   A. Hill-Sachs defect
   B. Bankart lesion
   C. Lax capsule
   D. Rotator cuff injury

Ans. (D) Rotator cuff injury

71. **Treatment of fracture head of radius in young patients:**
   A. Excision of head of radius
   B. Immobilization in cast
   C. Late excision after trial immobilization
   D. None of the above

Ans. (C) Late excision after trial immobilization

72. **In supracondylar fracture, the segment is often displaced:**
   A. Laterally
   B. Medially
   C. Anteriorly
   D. Posteriorly

Ans. (D) Posteriorly

73. **Tardy ulnar nerve palsy is due to:**
   A. Cubitus valgus
   B. Fixation of nerve in the groove by osteoarthritis
   C. Excision of elbow joint
   D. Fracture of internal condyle

Ans. (A) Cubitus valgus

74. **Tardy ulnar nerve palsy is seen in:**
   A. Cubitus valgus
   B. Dislocation of elbow
   C. Fracture scaphoid
   D. Supracondylar fracture of humerus

Ans. (A) Cubitus valgus

75. **In Volkmann's ischemia, surgery should be done:**
   A. Immediately
   B. After 6 hours
   C. 24 hours
   D. 72 hours

Ans. (A) Immediately

76. **Which fracture in children requires operative reduction:**
   A. Epiphyseal separation
   B. Both upper limb bones
   C. Dislocation of elbow
   D. Fracture humerus

Ans. (D) Fracture humerus

77. **Muscles involved in Volkmann's ischemic contracture:**
   A. Flexor policis longus
   B. Flexor digitorum profundus
   C. Flexor sublimes
   D. All
   E. A and B

Ans+. **(E)** A and B

78. **The cause of gun stock deformity is:**
    A. Supracondylar fracture
    B. Fracture both bones forearm
    C. Fracture surgical head of humerus
    D. Fracture fibula
Ans. **(A)** Supracondylar fracture

79. **True flexors of the elbow joint are:**
    A. Biceps   B. Brachialis
    C. Brachioradialis   D. Teres minor
    E. A, B and C
Ans. **(E)** A, B and C

80. **Myositis ossificans is most common around the ... joint.**
    A. Knee   B. Elbow
    C. Wrist   D. Hip
Ans. **(B)** Elbow

81. **The most important sign in Volkmann's ischemic contracture:**
    A. Pain
    B. Pallor
    C. Numbness
    D. Obliteration of radial pulse
Ans. **(A)** Pain

82. **Open reduction in children is done for:**
    A. Supracondylar fracture
    B. Forearm both bone fracture
    C. Femoral condyle fracture
    D. Lateral condyle of humerus fracture
Ans. **(D)** Lateral condyle of humerus fracture

83. **Triangular relation of elbow is maintained in:**
    A. Fracture ulna
    B. Anterior dislocation of elbow
    C. Posterior dislocation of elbow
    D. Supracondylar fracture
Ans. **(D)** Supracondylar fracture

84. **Treatment of acute myositis ossificans is:**
    A. Active mobilization
    B. Passive mobilization
    C. Infrared therapy
    D. Immobilization
Ans. **(D)** Immobilization

85. **Which fracture in children requires open reduction:**
    A. Fracture tibial epiphysis
    B. Fracture shaft of femur
    C. Fracture both bones forearm
    D. Fracture femoral condyle
Ans. **(A)** Fracture tibial epiphysis

86. **Tardy ulnar nerve palsy is seen with:**
    A. Lateral humeral condyle fracture
    B. Supracondyle fracture
    C. Medial humeral condyle fracture
    D. Fracture capitulum
Ans. **(A)** Lateral humeral condyle fracture

87. **Volkmann's ischemic contracture mostly involves:**
    A. Flexor digitorum superficialis
    B. Pronator teres
    C. Flexor digitorum produndus
    D. Flexor carpe radialis longus
Ans. **(C)** Flexor digitorum produndus

88. **Pulled elbow is:**
    A. Disarticulation of elbow
    B. Subluxation of distal radioulnar joint
    C. Subluxation of proximal radioulnar joint
    D. None of the above
Ans. **(C)** Subluxation of proximal radioulnar joint

89. **Open reduction for supracondylar fracture in a child is not preferred because of the fear of:**
    A. Injury to nerve and vessels in that region
    B. Myositis ossificans traumatica
    C. Permanent stiffness of the elbow
    D. Infection
Ans. **(C)** Permanent stiffness of the elbow

90. **Earliest sign of Volkmann's ischemic contracture is:**
    A. Pain during passive extension
    B. Pulselessness
    C. Necrosis of muscles
    D. Loss of adduction
Ans. **(A)** Pain during passive extension

91. **Treatment after removal of plaster for supracondylar fracture of humerus is:**
    - A. Active mobilization at elbow joint
    - B. Massage
    - C. No treatment
    - D. Passive movements at elbow joint

Ans. **(A)** Active mobilization at elbow joint

92. **Most common type of supracondylar fracture is:**
    - A. Extension type
    - B. Flexion type
    - C. Abduction type
    - D. Adduction type

Ans. **(A)** Extension type

93. **Excision of fractured fragment is practiced in all fractures *except*:**
    - A. Patella
    - B. Olecranon
    - C. Head of radius
    - D. Lateral condyle humerus

Ans. **(D)** Lateral condyle humerus

94. **Pulled elbow is due to:**
    - A. Fracture of radius
    - B. Fracture of ulna
    - C. Supracondylar fracture humerus
    - D. Subluxation of radial head

Ans. **(D)** Subluxation of radial head

95. **All the following requires open reduction and internal fixation almost always *except*:**
    - A. Lateral condyle of humerus
    - B. Olecranon
    - C. Patella
    - D. Volar Barton's fracture
    - E. B, C and D

Ans. **(E)** B, C and D

96. **Suspected medial epicondylar fracture of humerus in a 4-yr-old child requires:** **(PAL 96)**
    - A. X-ray both arms with elbow for comparison
    - B. X-ray same limb only

C. Examination under general anaesthesia
D. POP in full-flexed position

Ans. **(A)** X-ray both arms with elbow for comparison

97. **A young adult presenting with oblique, displaced fracture olecranon treatment of choice:**
    - A. Plaster cast
    - B. Percutaneous wiring
    - C. Tension ban wiring
    - D. Removal of displaced piece with triceps repair

Ans. **(C)** Tension ban wiring

98. **Earliest sign of Volkmann's ischemic contracture:**
    - A. On passive extension there is pain
    - B. Obliteration of radial pulse
    - C. Pale and cold hand
    - D. Warm and red hand

Ans. **(A)** On passive extension there is pain

99. **Carrying angle is decreased in:**
    - A. Cubitus varus
    - B. Cubitus valgus
    - C. Genu valgum
    - D. Genu varum

Ans. **(A)** Cubitus varus

100. **Treatment in the early stage of myositis ossifans is:**
    - A. Immobilization
    - B. Massage
    - C. Excision of the bone
    - D. Active joint movements

Ans. **(A)** Immobilization

101. **Volkmann's ischemic contracture the muscle commonly involved is:**
    - A. Palmaris longus
    - B. Flexor indicis
    - C. Flexor digitorum profundus
    - D. Flexor pollicis longus
    - E. C and D

Ans. **(E)** C and D

102. Osteotomy bone for malunited supracondylar fracture is:
  A. French
  B. Shan's
  C. McMurray's
  D. McAllister
Ans. (A) French

103. Earliest sign of Volkmann's ischemic contracture is:
  A. Pain
  B. Numbness
  C. Paresthesia
  D. Pallor
Ans. (A) Pain

104. The bestradiological view for fracture scaphoid is:
  A. AP
  B. PA
  C. Lateral
  D. Oblique
Ans. (D) Oblique

105. Carpal bone which fracture commonly:
  A. Scaphoid
  B. Lunate
  C. Hammate
  D. Pisiform
Ans. (A) Scaphoid

106. Complication of fracture scaphoid is:
  A. Injury to radial artery
  B. Avascular necrosis of proximal part
  C. Avascular necrosis of distal part
  D. Injury to radial nerve
Ans. (B) Avascular necrosis of proximal part

107. Dislocation of which one of the following carpal bones can present as median nerve palsy?
  A. Scaphoid
  B. Hamate
  C. Lunate
  D. Trapezium
Ans. (C) Lunate

108. The complication not common in Colles' fracture is:
  A. Malunion
  B. Nonunion
  C. Sudeck's atrophy
  D. Stiffness of wrist
Ans. (B) Nonunion

109. Oblique view is required to diagnose fracture of:
  A. Capitate
  B. Scaphoid
  C. Navicular
  D. Hamate
Ans. (B) Scaphoid

110. Most common site of fracture scaphoid:
  A. Waist
  B. Proximal third
  C. Distal third
  D. Tuberculosis
Ans. (A) Waist

111. In Colles' fracture not seen is:
  A. Proximal impaction
  B. Lateral rotation
  C. Dorsal angulation
  D. Medial rotation
Ans. (D) Medial rotation

112. Least common complication of Colles' fracture:
  A. Malunion
  B. Nonunion
  C. Stiffness of fingers
  D. Sudeck's dystrophy
Ans. (B) Nonunion

113. Most common complication of Colles' fracture:
  A. Nonunion
  B. Stiffness of fingers
  C. Vascular injury
  D. Sudeck's dystrophy
Ans. (B) Stiffness of fingers

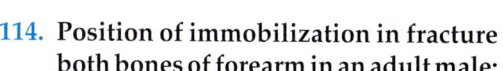

114. Position of immobilization in fracture both bones of forearm in an adult male:
    A. Prone
    B. Mid-prone
    C. Supine
    D. 10° supine
Ans. **(B)** Mid-prone

115. A lady presents with a history of fracture radius which was put on plaster of Paris cast for 4 weeks. After that she developed swelling of hands with shiny skin. What is the most likely diagnosis
    A. Rupture of extensor pollicic longus tendon
    B. Myostitis ossificans
    C. Reflex sympathetic dystrophy
    D. Malunion
Ans. **(C)** Reflex sympathetic dystrophy

116. Which one of the following statements is not correct regarding fracture of the scaphoid?
    A. It is the most commonly fracture carpal bone
    B. Persistent tenderness in the anatomical snuffbox is highly suggestive of fracture
    C. Immediated X-ray of hand may not reveal fracture line
    D. Malunion is a frequent complication
Ans. **(D)** Malunion is a frequent complication

117. Reduction of Bennett's fracture is difficult to keep in position due to the pull of:
    (AIIMS' 92)
    A. Abductor pollicis brevis
    B. Abductor pollicis longus
    C. Flexor pollicis longus
    D. Flexor pollicis brevis
Ans. **(B)** Abductor pollicis longus

118. In treatment of hand injuries, the greatest priority is:
    A. Repair of tendons
    B. Restoration of skin cover
    C. Repair of nerves
    D. Repair of blood vessels
Ans. **(B)** Restoration of skin cover

119. A Bennett's fracture is difficult to maintain in reduced position because of the pull of:
    A. Extensor pollicis longus
    B. Extensor pollicis brevis
    C. Abductor pollicis longus
    D. Abductor pollicis brevis
Ans. **(C)** Abductor pollicis longus

120. Most common complication of extracapsular fracture of neck of femur is:
    A. Nonunion
    B. Ischemic necrosis
    C. Malunion
    D. Pulmonary complications
Ans. **(C)** Malunion

121. Which fracture neck of femur has a poor prognosis?
    A. Intracapsular
    B. Extracapsular
    C. Both
    D. None
Ans. **(A)** Intracapsular

122. Histology of myositis ossificans mimics:
    A. Osteosarcoma
    B. Osteochondroma
    C. GCT
    D. Ewing's tumour
Ans. **(A)** Osteosarcoma

123. Avascular necrosis of head of femur can occur in:
    A. Sickle cell anaemia
    B. Caisson's disease
    C. Intracapsular fracture neck
    D. Trochanteric fracture
    E. A, B and C
Ans. **(E)** A, B and C

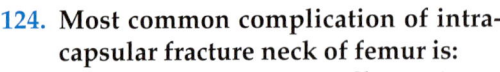

124. **Most common complication of intra-capsular fracture neck of femur is:**
    A. Osteoarthritis   B. Shortening
    C. Malunion   D. Nonunion
Ans. (D) Nonunion

125. **Avascular necrosis of the head of femur is not seen in:**
    A. Subcapital fracture
    B. Intertrochanteric fracture
    C. Transcervical fracture
    D. Central dislocation of hip
    E. B and D
Ans. (E) B and D

126. **In fracture neck of femur in a 64-year-old lady the treatment of choice is:**
    A. Prosthetic replacement of head of femur
    B. Conservative
    C. Austin Moore's pin
    D. SP nailing
Ans. (A) Prosthetic replacement of head of femur

127. **Fracture neck of femur in old persons is best treated by:**
    A. Replacement arthroplasty
    B. Thomas splint support
    C. No treatment
    D. Internal fixation with SP nail
Ans. (A) Replacement arthroplasty

128. **In 65-year-old male with history of fracture neck of femur 6 weeks old treatment of choice:**
    A. SP nailing
    B. McMurray's osteotomy
    C. Hemiarthroplasty
    D. None
Ans. (C) Hemiarthroplasty

129. **The most preferred treatment of fracture of neck of femur in young person is:**
    A. Hemiarthroplasty
    B. Total hip replacement
    C. Conservative treatment
    D. Closed reduction and internal fixation
Ans. (D) Closed reduction and internal fixation

130. **Bryant's triangle is useful in diagnosis of following *except*:**
    A. Supratrochanteric shortening
    B. Infratrochanteric shortening
    C. Anterior dislocation hip
    D. Posterior dislocation hip
Ans. (B) Infratrochanteric shortening

131. **The treatment of choice for nonunion of intracapsular fracture neck femur:**
    A. Hip spica
    B. Intramedullary nailing
    C. Internal fixation
    D. Compression plating
Ans. (C) Internal fixation

132. **Late complication of acetabular fracture:**
    A. Avascular necrosis of head of femur
    B. Avascular necrosis of iliac crest
    C. Fixed deformity of the hip joint
    D. Secondary osteoarthritis of hip joint
    E. A and D
Ans. (E) A and D

133. **In the case of 65-year-old person with fracture neck of femur the treatment of choice is:**
    A. Close reduction
    B. Close reduction with internal fixation
    C. Open reduction
    D. Replacement of head and neck of the femur with a prosthesis
Ans. (D) Replacement of head and neck of the femur with a prosthesis

134. **Most common type of dislocation of the hip is:**
    A. Anterior
    B. Posterior
    C. Central
    D. Dislocation with fracture of the shaft
Ans. (B) Posterior

135. **Most common dislocation of the hip is:**
   A. Posterior
   B. Anterior
   C. Central
   D. None
Ans. **(A)** Posterior

136. **The following is true in the treatment of posterior dislocation:**
   A. Closed reduction under anaesthesia
   B. Open reduction
   C. Skeletal traction
   D. Soft tissue release and then internal reduction in 2nd stage
Ans. **(A)** Closed reduction under anaesthesia

137. **Flexion, adduction and internal rotation is characteristic posture in:**
   A. Anterior dislocation of hip joint
   B. Posterior dislocation of hip joint
   C. Fracture of femoral head
   D. Fracture shaft of femur
Ans. **(B)** Posterior dislocation of hip joint

138. **Dashboard injury cases:**
   A. Anterior dislocation of the hip
   B. Posterior dislocation of the hip
   C. Central dislocation of hip
   D. Fracture neck femur
Ans. **(B)** Posterior dislocation of the hip

139. **Dislocation of hip joint palpable on per rectal examination:**
   A. Congenital dislocation of hip
   B. Posterior dislocation of hip
   C. Fracture neck of femur
   D. Anterior dislocation of hip
Ans. **(B)** Posterior dislocation of hip

140. **The pubic arch in females is above:**
   A. 60–70
   B. 70–75
   C. 100
   D. 130
Ans. **(C)** 100

141. **In comminuted fracture of the patella in an old lady the treatment is:**
   A. Excision of a small fragment
   B. Wire fixation
   C. Plaster cylinder
   D. Patellectomy
Ans. **(D)** Patellectomy

142. **Which of the following is correct in medial meniscus tear?**
   A. Rotation of femur on tibia
   B. Mensici do not heal
   C. Locking and unlocking episodes
   D. Menisci should be excised
   E. All of the above are correct
   F. A, C and D
Ans. **(F)** A, C and D

143. **Fracture femur in infants is best treated by:**
   A. Open reduction
   B. Closed reduction
   C. IM nailing
   D. Gallow's splinting
Ans. **(D)** Gallow's splinting

144. **Comminuted fracture of patella is treated by:**
   A. Tension wire bandage
   B. Surgery and immobilation
   C. Conservative
   D. Patellectomy
Ans. **(D)** Patellectomy

145. **Medial meniscus tear is more common than lateral meniscus because of its decreased:**
   A. Nerve supply
   B. Vascularity
   C. Mobility
   D. Fibroelasticity
Ans. **(C)** Mobility

146. **Medial meniscus is more vulnerable to injury because of:**
   A. Its fixity to tibial collateral ligaments
   B. Its semicircular shape
   C. Action of adductor magnus
   D. Its attachment to fibrous capsule
Ans. **(A)** Its fixity to tibial collateral ligaments

147. **Injury to the popliteal artery in fracture lower end of femur is often due to:**
    A. Distal fragment pressing the artery
    B. Proximal fragment pressing the artery
    C. Tight plaster
    D. Hematoma
Ans. **(A)** Distal fragment pressing the artery

148. **Recurrent dislocation of patella in an adolescent could be treated by:**
    A. Patellectomy
    B. Excision arthroplasty
    C. Puttipatt operation
    D. Lateral release
Ans. **(D)** Lateral release

149. **Recurrent dislocation of patella is most often associated with:**
    A. Abnormally high patella
    B. Abnormally low patella
    C. Bowleg
    D. Quadriceps contracture
Ans. **(A)** Abnormally high patella

150. **Drawer sign is diagnostic for injuries of:**
    A. Neck femur
    B. Shaft femur
    C. Collateral ligaments of knee
    D. Cruciate ligaments of knee
Ans. **(D)** Cruciate ligaments of knee

151. **Treatment of choice for old nonunited fracture of shaft of femur:**
    A. Compression plating
    B. Bone grafting
    C. Nailing
    D. Compression plating with bone grafting
Ans. **(D)** Compression plating with bone grafting

152. **Stiffness in knee is maximum when traction is at:**
    A. Skin
    B. Lower end femur

    C. Upper end tibia
    D. Calcaneum
Ans. **(C)** Upper end tibia

153. **Most common cause of hemarthrosis knee joint is:**
    A. Hemophilia
    B. Anterior cruciate ligament tear
    C. Medial meniscus tear
    D. Lateral meniscus tear
Ans. **(C)** Medial meniscus tear

154. **A positive pivot shift test in the right knee joint of an athlete is suggestive of injury to:**
    A. Lateral meniscus injury
    B. Medial meniscus injury
    C. Injury to anterior cruciate ligament
    D. Injury to posterior cruciate ligament
Ans. **(C)** Injury to anterior cruciate ligament

155. **A football player while playing twists his knee over the ankle. He still continues to play. After 2 days the noticed painful swelling of the knee joint. The diagnosis is:**
    A. Medial meniscus tear
    B. Anterior cruciate ligament tear
    C. Medial collateral ligament injury
    D. Posterior cruciate ligament injury
Ans. **(A)** Medial meniscus tear

156. **Medial meniscus is more prone for injury because:**
    A. It is semilunar in shape
    B. Medial portion is thicker
    C. Medial collateral ligaments is attached to it
    D. Avascular
Ans. **(C)** Medial collateral ligaments is attached to it

157. **Best diagnostic procedure for ant cruciate ligament injury is:**
    A. Lachman test
    B. Pivot shift test
    C. Anterior drawer test
    D. McMurray's test
Ans. **(A)** Lachman test

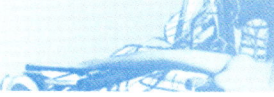

158. Infarction of the distal epiphyses of the second metatarsal bone is:
- A. Kienböck's disease
- B. Köhler's disease
- C. Freiberg's disease
- D. Perthes' disease

Ans. (C) Freiberg's disease

159. Which joint is not fused in triple arthrodesis:
- A. Tibiotalar
- B. Calcaneocuboid
- C. Talanavicular
- D. Talocalcaneal

Ans. (A) Tibiotalar

160. Fall on heel with fracture os calcis is associated with commonly:
- A. Fracture clavicle
- B. Fracture vertebra
- C. Fracture femur
- D. Any of the above

Ans. (B) Fracture vertebra

161. The most common cause of a sprained ankle is injury of:
- A. Deltoid ligament
- B. Lateral ligament
- C. Inferior tibiofibular ligament
- D. Anterior talofibular ligament

Ans. (D) Anterior talofibular ligament

162. Transverse fracture of medial malleolus is caused by:
- A. Abduction
- B. Adduction
- C. Rotation of foot
- D. Dorsiflexion of foot

Ans. (C) Rotation of foot

163. After a fall from a height calcaneal fracture is associated with fracture of:
- A. Tibia
- B. Vertebra
- C. Pelvis
- D. Femur

Ans. (B) Vertebra

164. Most common ligament injured in ankle sprain:
- A. Anterior talofibular
- B. Posterior talofibular
- C. Deltoid
- D. Spring ligament

Ans. (A) Anterior talofibular

165. A segmental compound fracture tibia with 1 cm skin wound is classified as:
- A. Type I
- B. Type II
- C. Type III A
- D. Type III B

Ans. (A) Type I

166. Traction injury to epiphyses of the vertebra is know as:
- A. Osgood–Schlatter disease
- B. Sinding–Larsen disease
- C. Scheuermann's disease
- D. Sever's disease

Ans. (C) Scheuermann's disease

167. Commonest cause of paraplegia is:
- A. Tuberculosis
- B. Trauma
- C. Secondaries
- D. Trasverse myelitis

Ans. (B) Trauma

168. Most commone intramedullary spinal tumours is:
- A. Secondaries
- B. Neurofibroma
- C. Ependymoma
- D. None of the above

Ans. (C) Ependymoma

169. Most common site of prolapse is:
- A. C_5-C_6
- B. T_8-T_9
- C. L_4-L_5
- D. L_5-S_1
- E. A and C

Ans. (E) A and C

170. **The following is true of spondy-lolisthesis:**
    A. Slipping of SI over L5
    B. Posterior arch defect
    C. Congenital defect
    D. More in pregnancy
    E. B and C
Ans. **(E)** B and C

171. **Intervertebal disc prolapse is treated chemically by:**
    A. Hyalse
    B. Chymotrypain
    C. Chymopapain
    D. Elastase
Ans. **(C)** Chymopapain

172. **Vertebra plana occurs in:**
    A. TB spine
    B. Secondaries in spine
    C. Pyogenic osteomyelitis
    D. Eosinophilic granulomas
Ans. **(D)** Eosinophilic granulomas

173. **Vertebra plana is caused by:**
    A. Malignancy
    B. Tuberculosis
    C. Syphilis
    D. Eosinophilic granuloma
Ans. **(D)** Eosinophilic granulomas

174. **When a person reports with vertebral fracture hemiplegia and urinary retention the acute measure to be taken is:**
    A. Suprapubic cystostomy
    B. Catheteriation
    C. Hot fomentation
    D. Condom drainage
Ans. **(B)** Catheteriation

175. **Local application of the following drug is used for eradication of *Pseudomonas* infection from the wound:**
    A. Acriflavine solution
    B. Eusol paraffin
    C. Acetic acid
    D. Tincture iodine
Ans. **(C)** Acetic acid

176. **Tetanus is noticed usually in:**
    A. Burn cases
    B. Wounds contaminated with faecal matter
    C. Open fractures
    D. Gunshot wounds
    E. All of the above
Ans. **(E)** All of the above

177. **Organism causing osteomyelitis in Sickle cell anaemia:**
    A. *Salmonella*
    B. *Staphylococcus*
    C. *Pneumonia*
    D. *Streptococcus*
    E. A and B
Ans. **(E)** A and B

178. **Tuberculosis of the spine is known as:**
    A. Pott's disease
    B. Scheuermann's disease
    C. Perthes' disease
    D. Freiberg's disease
Ans. **(A)** Pott's disease

179. **Tuberculous arthritis in advanced cases lead to:**
    A. Bony ankylosis
    B. Fibrous ankylosis
    C. Loose joint
    D. Charcot's joint
    E. A and B
Ans. **(E)** A and B

180. **Tuberculosis of the spine starts in:**
    A. Vertebral body
    B. Nucleous pulposus
    C. Annulus
    D. Fibrosis
    E. Paravertebral fascia
Ans. **(A)** Vertebral body

181. **Treatment of triple deformity is:**
    A. ATT
    B. ATT + immobilization
    C. ATT + immobilization + debridement
    D. None
Ans. **(D)** None

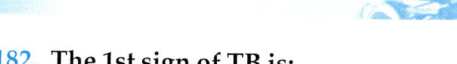

182. The 1st sign of TB is:
A. Narrowing of intervertebral space
B. Rarefaction of vertebral bodies
C. Destruction of laminae
D. Fusion of spinous processes
Ans. **(A)** Narrowing of intervertebral space

183. The ideal surgical treatment for Pott's paraplegia is:
A. Laminectomy and decompression
B. Anterior decompression
C. Anterolateral decompression
D. Costotransversectomy
Ans. **(C)** Anterolateral decompression

184. Earliest fracture of TB vertebra:
A. Decreased joint space
B. Soft tissue swelling
C. Decreased movements
D. Pain
Ans. **(D)** Pain

185. Most important pathology in clubfoot is:
A. Congenital talonavicular dislocation
B. Tightening of tendo-Achilles
C. Calcaneal fracture
D. Lateral derangement
Ans. **(A)** Congenital talonavicular dislocation

186. Treatment of clubfoot should begin:
A. As soon as possible after birth
B. 1st month after birth
C. 1st year after birth
D. None of the above
Ans. **(A)** As soon as possible after birth

187. Treatment of CTEV should start at the age of:
A. 2 weeks B. 1 month
C. Soon after birth D. 9 months
Ans. **(A)** 2 weeks

188. In congenital dislocation of knee deformity seen is:
A. Varus B. Valgus
C. Flexion D. Extension
Ans. **(D)** Extension

189. Most common deformity in congenital dislocation of hip:
A. Small head of femur
B. Angle of torsion
C. Decreased neck shaft angle
D. Shallow accetabulum
Ans. **(D)** Shallow accetabulum

190. Osteoblastic bone secondary is usually from:
A. Ovary B. Kidney
C. Breast D. Prostate
E. C and D
Ans. **(E)** C and D

191. Most radiosensitive bone tumour is:
A. Chondrosarcoma
B. Osteoclastoma
C. Ewing's sarcoma
D. Osteosarcoma
Ans. **(C)** Ewing's sarcoma

192. Most common benign bone tumour is:
A. Osteochondroma
B. Chondrosarcoma
C. Osteoid osteoma
D. Osteosarcoma
Ans. **(A)** Osteochondroma

193. Commonest benign bone tumour is:
A. Bone cyst B. Chondroma
C. Chordoma D. Osteoma
Ans. **(B)** Chondroma

194. Which of the following is a true tumour?
A. Bone cyst
B. Fibrous dysplasia
C. Osteochondroma
D. Brodie's tumour
E. None
Ans. **(E)** None

195. Which tumour does not arise from cartilage?
A. Osteoblastoma
B. Osteochondroma
C. Chondrosarcoma
D. Enchondroma
Ans. **(A)** Osteoblastoma

196. **Malignant growth involving the vault of the skull include:**
   A. Osteitis fibrosa cystica
   B. Osteoclastoma
   C. Myeloid epulis
   D. Adamantinoma
   E. Nephroblastoma
   F. B and E
   Ans. (F) B and E

197. **Physaliphorous cells (large vacuolated cells) on histopathology are characteristic of:**
   A. Osteosarcoma
   B. Osteoclastoma
   C. Liposarcoma
   D. Chondrosarcoma
   E. Chordoma
   Ans. (E) Chordoma

198. **Osteoclastoma is common in age group of:**
   A. Below 10 years
   B. 10–20 years
   C. 20–40 years
   D. All age groups
   Ans. (C) 20–40 years

199. **Which is the most common site of osteoclastoma?**
   A. Lower end of femur
   B. Upper end of tibia
   C. Lower humerus
   D. Upper radius
   Ans. (A) Lower end of femur

200. **True statement regarding osteogenic sarcoma is:**
   A. Affects middle-aged people
   B. X-ray shows honeycombing
   C. Can be a complication of Paget's disease of bone
   D. All of the above
   Ans. (C) Can be a complication of Paget's disease of bone

201. **Most common benign tumour under 21 yrs of age:**
   A. Aneurysmal bone cyst
   B. Osteochondroma
   C. Giant cell tumour
   D. Osteoid talus
   Ans. (D) Osteoid talus

202. **Multiple exostosis usually presents at:**
   A. Birth   B. Puberty
   C. After 21 yrs   D. At 5 yrs of age
   Ans. (D) At 5 yrs of age

203. **Densely calcified metastatic shadows are found in:**
   A. Synovial cell carcinoma
   B. Osteosarcoma
   C. Chondrosarcoma
   D. Chondroblastoma
   Ans. (B) Osteosarcoma

204. **Most common mode of metastasis in osteogenic sarcoma:**
   A. Subperiosteal spread
   B. Hematogenous
   C. Lymphatic
   D. Transcortical
   Ans. (B) Hematogenous

205. **In an 8-year-old child the least common cause of lytic bone lesion in proximal femur:**
   A. Plasmacytoma
   B. Histiocytoma
   C. Metastasis
   D. Brown tumour
   Ans. (A) Plasmacytoma

206. **Aneurysmal bone cysts:**
   A. Are true aneurysms of nutrient arteries
   B. Occur only in flat bones
   C. Are the same as osseous haemangiomas
   D. Manifest as osteolytic lesions in long bones
   Ans. (D) Manifest as osteolytic lesions in long bones

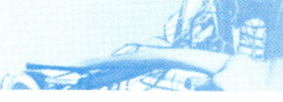

207. **Most common site of eosinophilic granuloma:**
   A. Radius
   B. Femur
   C. Skull
   D. Lumber vertebrae
Ans. **(C)** Skull

208. **Bone dysplasia is due to:**
   A. Faulty nutrition
   B. Faulty development
   C. Vitamin deficiency
   D. Hormonal imbalance
Ans. **(B)** Faulty development

209. **Rare site of metastasis in bone:**
   A. Skull
   B. Spine
   C. Upper end of humerus
   D. Below elbow and knee
Ans. **(D)** Below elbow and knee

210. **Most reliable method for detecting bony metastases is:**
   A. MRI   B. CT scan
   C. Radiography D. SPECT
   E. None
Ans. **(E)** None

211. **A 50-year-old patient presents with a lesion in the midline involving the sacrum which is sclerotic what is the likely diagnosis:**
   A. Osteosarcoma
   B. Chordoma
   C. Metastasis
   D. Osteoclastoma
Ans. **(C)** Metastasis

212. **A 70-year-old lady presented with mild low back pain and tenderness in L3 vertebra. On examination Hb 8 gm ESR 110 mm/1hr, A/G ratio of 2:4 likely diagnosis is:**
   A. Waldenström's
   B. Multiple myeloma
   C. Bone secondaries
   D. None
Ans. **(B)** Multiple myeloma

213. **Bamboo spine is seen in:**
   A. Ankylosing spondylitis
   B. Rheumatoid arthritis
   C. Scheuermann's disease
   D. Pott's spine
Ans. **(A)** Ankylosing spondylitis

214. **The cause of rheumatoid arthritis is:**
   A. Familial
   B. Immunological
   C. Infective
   D. Traumatic
   E. A, B and C
Ans. **(E)** A, B and C

215. **Joint least affected by neuropathy:**
   A. Shoulder   B. Hip
   C. Wrist   D. Elbow
   E. None
Ans. **(E)** None

216. **Epiphyseak widening may be seen in:**
   A. Rheumatoid arthritis
   B. Juvenile rheumatoid arthritis
   C. Osteoarthritis
   D. Gouty arthritis
Ans. **(B)** Juvenile rheumatoid arthritis

217. **Therapeutic programme for gout could include administration of:**
   A. Heavy dose of vit C
   B. Phenyl butazone
   C. Furadatin
   D. Gold therapy
Ans. **(B)** Phenyl butazone

218. **Most common degenerative joint disease in:**
   A. Gout   B. Osteoporosis
   C. Rheumatoid
      arthritis   D. Osteoarthritis
Ans. **(D)** Osteoarthritis

219. **In rheumatoid arthritis, the pathology starts in:**
   A. Articular cartilage
   B. Synovium
   C. Capsule
   D. Muscles
Ans. **(B)** Synovium

220. **Para-articular erosions are most commonly seen in:**
    A. Osteoarthritis
    B. Rheumatoid arthritis
    C. Gout
    D. Acute suppurative arthritis
Ans. **(B)** Rheumatoid arthritis

221. **In osteoarthritis, following is not a predisposing factor:**
    A. Diabetes mellitus
    B. Defective joint position
    C. Weight bearing joints
    D. Incongruity of articular surfaces
    E. Old age
    F. None
Ans. **(F)** None

222. **Treatment of osteoarthritis include all *except*:**
    A. Graded muscle exercises
    B. Replacement of articular surfaces
    C. Correction of deformities
    D. Increase the weight bearing by the affected joint
    E. Rest to the joint in acute phase
Ans. **(D)** Increase the weight bearing by the affected joint

223. **Treatment of rheumatoid arthritis include all *except*:**
    A. Give rest to the joint
    B. Correction of deformities
    C. Synovectomy
    D. Excercises
    E. Immunosuppressive drugs
Ans. **(A)** Give rest to the joint

224. **Osteoarthritis involves all *except*:**
    A. Hip joint
    B. Knee joint
    C. Distal interphalangeal joint
    D. Metacarpophalangeal joint of thumb
Ans. **(D)** Metacarpophalangeal joint of thumb

225. **Calcification of menisci is seen in:**
    A. Hyperparathyroidism
    B. Pseudogout

C. Renal osteodystrophy
    D. Acromegaly
Ans. **(B)** Pseudogout

226. **Osteitis fibrosa cystica is seen in:**
    A. Hyperparathyroidism
    B. Hypoparathyroidism
    C. Hypothroidism
    D. Hyperthyroidism
Ans. **(A)** Hyperparathyroidism

227. **Menisci calcification is a feature of:**
    A. Gout
    B. Hyperparathyroidism
    C. Pseudogout
    D. Ankylosing spondylitis
Ans. **(C)** Pseudogout

228. **Absence of lamina dura in the alveolus occurs in:**
    A. Rickets
    B. Osteomalacia
    C. Deficiency of vitamin C
    D. Hyperparathyroidism
Ans. **(D)** Hyperparathyroidism

229. **A finding of phosphoethanolamine in the urine is highly suggestive of:**
    A. Renal osteodystrophy
    B. Hypophosphatasia
    C. Urinary phosphate excretion
    D. Serum calcium level
Ans. **(D)** Serum calcium level

230. **Not a complication of menopause:**
    A. Fracture spine
    B. Colles' fracture
    C. Fracrure neck of femur
    D. Supracondylar fracture humerus
Ans. **(D)** Supracondylar fracture humerus

231. **Soft tissue calcification occurs in all *except*:**
    A. Hyperparathyroidism
    B. Scleroderma
    C. Hyperthyroidism
    D. Hypervitaminosis
Ans. **(C)** Hyperthyroidism

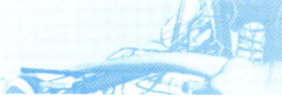

232. Treatment of hypercalcemia is all *except*:
A. Rizdol
B. Plicamycin
C. Ritodrinate
D. Gallium nitrate
Ans. **(A)** Rizdol

233. Calcium content of bone is increased in:
A. Prolonged immobilisation
B. Glucocorticoid administration
C. Hyperparathyroidism
D. Estrogen supplementation in post-menopausal women
Ans. **(D)** Estrogen supplementation in post-menopausal women

234. What is the diagnostic radiological finding skeletal fluorosis:
A. Sclerosis of sacroiliac joint
B. Interosseous membrane ossification
C. Osteosclerosis of vertebral body
D. Ossification of ligaments of knee joint
Ans. **(B)** Interosseous membrane ossification

235. Rocker bottom foot results from:
A. Congenital vertical talus
B. Poliomyelitis
C. Clubfoot over correction
D. Spina bifida
E. A and C
Ans. **(E)** A and C

236. Sclerotic lesions in the bone is seen in all *except*:
A. Osteitis fibrosa
B. Osteopetrosis
C. Melorheostosis
D. Caffey's disease
Ans. **(A)** Osteitis fibrosa

237. Recurrent clubfoot is due to failure of development of:
A. Tendocalcaneus
B. Peroneal muscles
C. Plantar fascia
D. Tibialis anterior
Ans. **(B)** Peroneal muscles

238. Housemaid's knee is inflammation of bursa:
A. Subpatellar
B. Suprapatellar
C. Infrapatellar
D. Prepatellar
Ans. **(D)** Prepatellar

239. Arthrodesis of which is not done to correct flatfoot:
A. Talus
B. Cuboid
C. Navicular
D. Calcaneum
Ans. **(B)** Cuboid

240. Weaver's bottom is:
A. Eczematous lesions over buttocks of weavers due to their sedentary position
B. Ischiogluteal bursitis
C. Coccydynia
D. None of the above
Ans. **(B)** Ischiogluteal bursitis

241. Trigger finger is most likely to be associated with:
A. Diabetes
B. Trauma
C. Gout
D. Rheumatoid arthritis
Ans. **(D)** Rheumatoid arthritis

242. All of following may be cause of flexible flatfoot *except*:
A. In elderly
B. In children
C. In obese
D. In congenital vertical talus
Ans. **(D)** In congenital vertical talus

243. In hallus valgus surgery, the patients who are likely to bee most satisfied are:
A. Those with pain
B. Those with hammer toe
C. Those with metatarsus primus varus
D. Young age
Ans. **(D)** Young age

244. **The long-flexor tendon of the thumb can be advanced for more than 1 cm for repair in Zone 1 because:**
   A. Paratendinous adhesions are fewer following advancement than following free tendon graft
   B. Only two annular pulleys bind the tendon to bone
   C. Vascularity of the tendon is not compromised because vinculum is absent
   D. The tendon is long enough to allow easy advancement
   E. A and C
Ans. **(E)** A and C

245. **Earliest changes in Perthes' disease is seen in:**
   A. X-ray
   B. CT
   C. MRI
   D. US
   E. Nuclear scan
Ans. **(E)** Nuclear scan

246. **Accessory navicular is called:**
   A. Os trigonum
   B. Os tibiale internum
   C. Os tibiale externum
   D. Os navicular
Ans. **(C)** Os tibiale externum

247. **Sever's disease refers to:**
   A. Calcaneum
   B. Radius
   C. Talus
   D. Capitulum
Ans. **(A)** Calcaneum

248. **Dysplasia epiphysis hemimelica is:**
   A. Trevor's disease
   B. Blount's disease
   C. Streeter's dysplasia
   D. Leri's disease
Ans. **(A)** Trevor's disease

249. **Adventitious bursa is:**
   A. Found normally over any joint
   B. Due to degeneration of connective tissue over a joint
   C. Found over bony prominences
   D. Can turn into malignancy
Ans. **(C)** Found over bony prominences

250. **Osteochondritis dissecans occurs at:**
   A. Lateral surface lateral condyle
   B. Medial surface of lateral condyle
   C. Medial surface medial condyle
   D. Lateral surface medial condyle
Ans. **(D)** Lateral surface medial condyle

251. **Engelmann's disease is:**
   A. Multiple epiphyseal dysplasia
   B. Infantile cortical hyperostosis
   C. Cleidocranial dysplasia
   D. Progressive diaphyseal dysplasia
Ans. **(D)** Progressive diaphyseal dysplasia

252. **Sprengels' shoulder is due to deformity of:**
   A. Scapula
   B. Humerus
   C. Clavicle
   D. Vertebra
Ans. **(A)** Scapula

253. **Subperiosteal new bone formation is seen in all *except*:**
   A. Scurvy
   B. Osteosarcoma
   C. Osteomyelitis
   D. Eosinophilic granuloma
Ans. **(D)** Eosinophilic granuloma

254. **Most common cause of loose bodies in joints in adults:**
   A. Tuberculous tenosynovitis
   B. Rheumatoid arthritis
   C. Osteoarthritis
   D. Osteochondritis dissecans
Ans. **(C)** Osteoarthritis

255. **Trouser leg appearance on an ascending myelogram is suggestive of tumour:**
   A. Extradural
   B. Extramedullary
   C. Intramedullary
   D. None of the above
Ans. **(C)** Intramedullary

256. **Myositis ossificans is commonly seen at the ... joint.**
   A. Knee
   B. Elbow
   C. Shoulder
   D. Hip
Ans. **(B)** Elbow

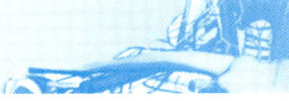

257. **Pectus excavatum is seen in:**
   A. Cretinism
   B. Senile osteoporosis
   C. Osteogenesis imperfecta
   D. Chronic asthma
Ans. **(D)** Chronic asthma

258. **Tissue most sensitive to radiation is:**
   A. Osteoblast
   B. Cartilage
   C. Epiphysis
   D. Metaphysis
Ans. **(C)** Epiphysis

259. **The cause of short fourth metacarpal bone is:**
   A. Down syndrome
   B. Edward's syndrome
   C. Turner's syndrome
   D. Pseudohypo-parathyroidism
   E. C and D
Ans. **(E)** C and D

260. **Increased density of skull vault is seen in:**
   A. Hyperparathyroidism
   B. Multiple myeloma
   C. Fluorosis
   D. Renal osteodystrophy
   E. C and D
Ans. **(E)** C and D

261. **Soft tissue calcification around the knee is seen in:**
   A. Scurvy
   B. Scleroderma
   C. Hyperparathyroidism
   D. Pseudogout
   E. B, C and D
Ans. **(E)** B, C and D

262. **Increased density in metaphysis is seen in:**
   A. Hypervitaminosis
   B. Healed rickets
   C. Congenital syphilis
   D. Perthes' disease
Ans. **(A)** Hypervitaminosis

263. **Meyer's operation is done for:**
   A. Dislocation of patella
   B. Fracture neck of femur
   C. Dislocation of shoulder
   D. Fracture fibula
Ans. **(B)** Fracture neck of femur

264. **Bleeding into joint cavities is not common in:**
   A. Hemophilia
   B. ITP
   C. Christmas disease
   D. None of the above
Ans. **(B)** ITP

265. **Battle sign is seen in:**
   A. Fracture middle cranial fossa
   B. Fracture base of skull
   C. Fracture anterior cranial fossa
   D. All of the above
   E. A and B
Ans. **(E)** A and B

266. **Duga's test is helpful in:**
   A. Dislocation of hip
   B. Scaphoid fracture
   C. Fracture neck of femur
   D. Anterior dislocation of shoulder
Ans. **(D)** Anterior dislocation of shoulder

267. **Trendelenburg sign is not seen in:**
   A. Tuberculous arthritis
   B. Rheumatoid arthritis
   C. Posterior dislocation hip
   D. Tom Smith arthritis
Ans. **(D)** Tom Smith arthritis

268. **Gaenslen's test is positive in:**
   A. Tennis elbow
   B. deQuervain's disease
   C. Carpal tunnel syndrome
   D. Ulnar bursitis
   E. None
Ans. **(E)** None

269. **Bone growth is influenced maximally by:**
   A. Estrogen   B. Thyoxine
   C. Growth hormone   D. Testosterone
Ans. **(C)** Growth hormone

270. **Cartilage is quite vascular in:**
    A. Embryonic life
    B. Early chldhood
    C. Early adulthood
    D. Old age
Ans. **(A)** Embryonic life

271. **A recessive form of osteogenesis imperfecta may closely resemble:**
    A. Alkaptonuria
    B. Cretinism
    C. Hypophosphatasia
    D. Homocystinuria
Ans. **(C)** Hypophosphatasia

272. **Who is acclaimed worldwide for total joint replacement?**
    A. Paul Brand
    B. John Charnley
    C. Paul Harrington
    D. Huckstep
Ans. **(B)** John Charnley

273. **Ossification in foetus starts in:**
    A. 1st week of intrauterine life
    B. 2nd week of intrauterine life
    C. 5th week of intrauterine life
    D. 5th month of intrauterine life
Ans. **(C)** 5th week of intrauterine life

274. **During the surgical procedure:**
    A. Tendons should be repaired before nerve
    B. Nerve should be repaired before tendons
    C. Tendons should not be repaired at the same time
    D. None is true
Ans. **(B)** Nerve should be repaired before tendons

275. **Which of the following is NOT true regarding synovial fluid?**
    A. Contains HCO_3 and CI ions more than plasma
    B. Contains minerals ions less than plasma
    C. Contains uric acid more than plasma
    D. Contains fibrinolysin
Ans. **(C)** Contains uric acid more than plasma

276. **Which of the following is NOT found normally in synovial membrane:**
    A. Two layers of lymphatics
    B. Pacinian corpuscle
    C. Basement membrane
    D. A fibrocollagenous layer
Ans. **(C)** Basement membrane

277. **Bilateral symmetrical idiopathic fractures are most commonly seen in:**
    A. Osteoporosis
    B. Osteogenesis imperfecta
    C. Polytrauma
    D. Stress fracture
Ans. **(B)** Osteogenesis imperfecta

278. **Synovial tissue is seen earliest in a developing point at the age of:**
    A. 8th week of intrauterine life
    B. 12th week of intrauterine life
    C. 15th week of intrauterine life
    D. 28th week of intrauterine life
Ans. **(B)** 12th week of intrauterine life

279. **Adult bone trabeculae are differentiated from foetal bone trabaeculae histologically by the presence of:**
    A. Haversian system
    B. Lamellar structure
    C. Certain special staining chartacterisitics
    D. Different type of bone cells in each
Ans. **(B)** Lamellar structure

280. **The tensions resistance of normal fascia per square inch, such as the fascia lata, has been determined to be:**
    A. 550 pounds
    B. 1000 pounds
    C. 2000 pounds
    D. 5000 pounds
    E. 7000 pounds
Ans. **(E)** 7000 pounds

281. **Macewen's osteotomy is performed in cases of:**
    A. Coxa vara
    B. Tibia vara
    C. Genu valgum
    D. Tom Smith disease
Ans. **(C)** Genu valgum

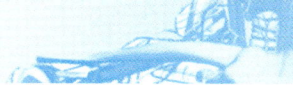

282. Infection in ring finger in acute teno-synovitis is most likely to spread to:
A. Dorsum of hand
B. Thenar space
C. Parona's space
D. Mid palmar space
Ans. (D) Mid palmar space

283. Sclerosis of bone is seen in all *except*:
A. Fluorosis
B. Osteopetrosis
C. Secondaries from prostate
D. Hyperparathyroidism
Ans. (D) Hyperparathyroidism

284. Triple deformity of knee is seen in:
A. Polio
B. Tuberculosis
C. Villonodular synovitis
D. Rheumatoid arthritis
E. A, B and D
Ans. (E) A, B and D

285. Cause of painful limb are all *except*:
A. Perthes' disease
B. Congenital coxa vara
C. Slipped femoral epiphysis
D. TB hip
Ans. (B) Congenital coxa vara

286. Phocomelia is best described is:
A. Defect in development of long bones
B. Defect in development of flat bones
C. Defect of intramembranous ossification
D. Defect of cartilage replacement by bone
Ans. (A) Defect in development of long bones

287. Pseudoarthrosis of tibia is best treated by:
A. Internal fixation
B. Internal fixation and bone grafting
C. Above knee POP cast
D. Below knee POP cast
Ans. (B) Internal fixation and bone grafting

288. Viscosity of synovial fluid depends on:
A. Chondroitin sulphate
B. Keratosulphate

C. Hyaluronic acid
D. Heparin sulphate
Ans. (C) Hyaluronic acid

289. Triple deformity is a complication of:
A. Rheumatoid arthritis
B. Tuberculosis
C. Osteoarthritis
D. Septic arthritis
E. A and B
Ans. (E) A and B

290. Epiphyseal enlargement is a manifestation of:
A. Rickets
B. Ankylosing spondylitis
C. Spondylo-epiphyseal dysgenesis
D. Scurvy
Ans. (A) Rickets

291. Limb salvage primarily depends on:
A. Vascular injury
B. Skin cover
C. Bone injury
D. Nerve injury
Ans. (A) Vascular injury

292. Maximal shortening of lower limb is with:
A. Posterior dislocation
B. Central dislocation
C. Fracture neck of femurs
D. Trochanteric fracture
Ans. (A) Posterior dislocation

293. One of the following fracture requires plaster of Paris cast with equines position:
A. Distal fracture both bones leg
B. Distal fracture fibula
C. Bimalleolar
D. Fracture talus
Ans. (D) Fracture talus

294. Pathological changes in Caisson's disease is due to:
A. N_2 B. O_2
C. CO_2 D. CO
Ans. (A) N_2

295. **Treatment based on "Gate theory" is:**
    A. Short wave diatherapy
    B. Ultrasound
    C. Electrical nerve stimulation
    D. Infrared therapy
    Ans. **(C)** Electrical nerve stimulation

296. **Osteophytes developing at the joint at Luscka characteristically compresses spinal nerve at:**
    A. Intervertebral foramen
    B. Anterior part of body
    C. Posteior part of body
    D. Paradural areas
    Ans. **(A)** Intervertebral foramen

297. **Schmorl's node is:**
    A. Radiological findings; protruded nucleus pulposus into the vertebral body
    B. Soft tissue tumour in relation to the vertebral body
    C. A tumour in the intervertebral disc
    D. None of the above
    Ans. **(A)** Radiological findings; protruded nucleus pulposus into the vertebral body

298. **Osteosclerotic rim is seen in:**
    A. Growing epiphysis
    B. Gaint cell tumour
    C. Enchondroma
    D. Old people
    Ans. **(A)** Growing epiphysis

299. **Least correction in remodelling of bone in children is seen in:**
    A. Fracture shaft of humerus
    B. Fracture shaft of femur
    C. Subtrochanteric fracture
    Ans. **(A)** Fracture shaft of humerus

300. **Steinmann pin is used for all *except*:**
    A. Joint dislocation
    B. Ligament laxity
    C. Osteoporosis
    D. Blue sclera
    Ans. **(D)** Blue sclera

301. **Ortolani's test is done for:**
    A. Congenital dislocation of hip
    B. Congenital dislocation of knee
    C. Acquired dislocation of hip
    D. Acquired dislocation of knee
    Ans. **(A)** Congenital dislocation of hip

302. **On measurement, the base of Bryant's triangle on the left side is found to the short by 2 cm as compared to the right side. This indicates:**
    A. Fracture of the neck of the femur
    B. Fracture of the shaft of the femur
    C. Osteoarthritis of hip joint
    D. Rheumatoid arthritis of the hip joint
    Ans. **(A)** Fracture of the neck of the femur

303. **Actinomycosis is commonly seen in:**
    A. Tibia
    B. Mandible
    C. Scapula
    D. Femur
    Ans. **(B)** Mandible

304. **Meyer's operation is done for:**
    A. Recurrent dislocation of patella
    B. Dislocation of shoulder joint
    C. Dislocation of hip joint
    D. # Scaphoid
    E. None
    Ans. **(E)** None

305. **Resorption of the terminal phalanx is not seen in:**
    A. Hyperparathyroidism
    B. Reiter's syndrome
    C. Scleroderma
    D. Psoriasis
    Ans. **(B)** Reiter's syndrome

306. **Short wave diathermy is used for all of the following *except*:**
    A. Back pain
    B. Haemophiliac joint
    C. Osteoarthritis
    D. Sprain
    Ans. **(B)** Haemophiliac joint

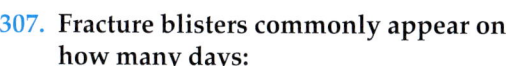

307. **Fracture blisters commonly appear on how many days:**
   A. 1–3 days
   B. 3–5 days
   C. 5–7 days
   D. 5–9 days
Ans. **(A)** 1–3 days

308. **Hourglass contaction of hip on X-ray is seen in:**
   A. Achondroplasia
   B. Congenital dislocation hip
   C. Strongyloid infection
   D. Rickets
Ans. **(A)** Achondroplasia

309. **Minimal intradiscal pressure in vertebral column is seen when a person is:**
   A. Standing
   B. Sitting
   C. Lying flat
   D. Lying on one side
Ans. **(A)** Lying flat

310. **A 3-yr-old child falls from 2 m height. On X-ray no abnormality of lower leg was seen. After 2 years, the child presents with calcaneal valgus. Probable cause is:**
   A. Undiagnosed
   B. Tibial epiphyseal plate injury
   C. Vascular necrosis of talus
   D. Rocker bottom foot
Ans. **(B)** Tibial epiphyseal plate injury

311. **Young man with # tibia of left side 2 months ago, is having popliteal cast. Now needs mobilization with single crutch. Which will be the preferred site?**
   A. Left sided crutch
   B. Right sided
   C. Any side
   D. Both sides
Ans. **(B)** Right sided

CHAPTER 4: METABOLIC BONE DISEASES

1. **Triradiate pelvis is seen in:**
   A. Paget's disease
   B. Rickets
   C. Osteomalacia
   D. Chondroma
Ans. **(C)** Osteomalacia

2. **Pseudo-fracture or looser's zone is seen in:**
   A. Osteoporosis
   B. Osteomalacia
   C. Hypoparathyroidism
   D. Pseudohypoparathyroidism
Ans. **(B)** Osteomalacia

3. **In Burton's disease there is:**
   A. Scurvy and rickets
   B. Scurvy and syphilis
   C. Syphilis and rickets
   D. Scurvy and pellagra
Ans. **(A)** Scurvy and rickets

4. **Senile osteoporosis is radiologically manifest only when ..... of skeleton has been lost.**
   A. 20%
   B. 30%
   C. 40%
   D. 80%
Ans. **(B)** 30%

5. **Fish-head appearance of the vertebral bodies is seen in:**
   A. Paget's disease
   B. Rickets
   C. Osteomalacia
   D. Osteoporosis
Ans. **(D)** Osteoporosis

6. **Increased bone density occurs in:**
   A. Cushing's syndrome
   B. Hypoparathyrodism
   C. Fluorosis
   D. Hyperthyroidism
Ans. **(C)** Fluorosis

7. **Most common site of fracture in senile osteoporosis is:**
   A. Neck of femur
   B. Shaft of femur
   C. Radius
   D. Vertebra
Ans. **(D)** Vertebra

8. **Drug of choice for senile osteoporosis is:**
   A. Estrogens
   B. Androgens
   C. Calcitonin
   D. Ethidronate
Ans. **(D)** Ethidronate

9. **Metaphyseal fracture is commonly seen in:**
   A. Osteogenesis imperfecta
   B. Scurvy
   C. Rickets
   D. None
Ans. **(B)** Scurvy

10. **In long-term therapy in vitamin D-resistant rickets, the best guide to safe treatment is:**
    A. Urinary phosphate excretion
    B. Urinary calcium excretion
    C. Serum alkaline phosphatase
    D. Serum phosphate level
    E. Serum calcium level
Ans. **(D)** Serum phosphate level

11. **All of following conditions may be responsible for osteoporosis *except*:**
    A. Steroid therapy
    B. Prolonged weightlessness in space-ship
    C. Hyperparathyroidism
    D. Hypoparathyroidism
Ans. **(D)** Hypoparathyroidism

12. **Marker for bone formation:**
    A. Osteocalcin
    B. TRAP
    C. 5 mucleotidase
    D. Parathormone
Ans. **(A)** Osteocalcin

13. **Most common site of fracture in osteoporosis:**
    A. Fracture neck femur
    B. Vertebra
    C. Hip bone
    D. Humerus
Ans. **(B)** Vertebra

CHAPTER 5: INFECTIONS

1. **Bony ankylosis result from:**
   A. Pyogenic arthritis
   B. TB arthritis
   C. Osteoarthritis
   D. Rheumatic arthritis
   E. A and B
Ans. **(E)** A and B

2. **The joint commonly involved in symphilitis arthritis is:**
   A. Hip
   B. Shoulder
   C. Wrist
   D. Knee
Ans. **(D)** Knee

3. **Most common organism causing osteomyelitis in children under 3 years is:**
   A. *Haemophilus*
   B. Staphylococcal
   C. Streptococcal
   D. *Salmonella*
Ans. **(B)** Staphylococcal

4. **Most common site for acute osteomyelitis in infant is:**
   A. Hip joint
   B. Tibia
   C. Femur
   D. Radial
Ans. **(B)** Tibia

5. **Osteomyelitis of the spine is mostly cause:**
   A. *Salmonella*
   B. Pneumcoccus
   C. Tubercle bacilli
   D. *Staphylococcus*
Ans. **(C)** Tubercle bacilli

6. **Osteomyelitis in a case of Sickle cell anaemia is caused by:**
   A. *Salmonella*
   B. Pneumococcus
   C. *Streptococcus*
   D. *Haemophilus*
   Ans. **(A)** *Salmonella*

7. **Acute hematogenous osteomyelitis is treated with all *except:***
   A. Antibiotics
   B. Splinting
   C. Analgesics
   D. Surgery
   E. None
   Ans. **(E)** None

8. **Which is true regarding acute osteomyelitis?**
   A. *Staphylococcus* is the usual organism
   B. Rest and elevation relieves pain
   C. Parental antibiotics are given
   D. Surgery is the only treatment
   E. A, B and C
   Ans. **(E)** A, B and C

9. **What is Brodie's abscess?**
   A. Long-standing localized pyogenic abscess in the bone
   B. Cold abscess
   C. Subperiosteal abscess
   D. Soft tissue abscess
   Ans. **(A)** Long-standing localized pyogenic abscess in the bone

10. **Brodie's abscess usually involves:**
    A. Long bones
    B. Short bones
    C. Pelvic bones
    D. Flat bones
    Ans. **(A)** Long bones

11. **Viral osteomyelitis seen usually is due to vaccination for:**
    A. Smallpox virus infection
    B. Influenza virus infection
    C. Coxsackievirus infection
    D. Dengue fever
    Ans. **(A)** Smallpox virus infection

12. **When osteomyelitis disseminates by haematogenous way the most affected part bone is?**
    A. Metaphyses
    B. Epiphyses
    C. Diaphyses
    D. Any of the above
    Ans. **(A)** Metaphyses

13. **Tom Smith arthritis manifest as:**
    A. Increase hip mobility and unstability
    B. Hip stiffness
    C. A and B
    D. Shortening of limb
    E. A and D
    Ans. **(E)** A and D

14. **Most common cause of hematogenous osteomyelitis:**
    A. *Streptococcus*
    B. *Staph aureus*
    C. *Salmonella*
    D. *H. influenzae*
    Ans. **(B)** *Staph aureus*

15. **Actinomycosis is commonly seen in:**
    A. Tibia
    B. Mandible
    C. *Scaoula*
    D. Femur
    Ans. **(B)** Mandible

16. **All are seen in chronic osteomyelitis *except*:**
    A. Sequestrum
    B. Amyloidosis
    C. Myositis ossificans
    D. Metastatic abscess
    Ans. **(C)** Myositis ossificans

17. **Acute osteomyelitis can best be distinguished from soft tissue infection by:**
    A. Clinical examination
    B. X-ray
    C. CT scan
    D. MRI
    Ans. **(A)** Clinical examination

18. **Most common site of skeletal tuberculosis is:**
    A. Tibia
    B. Radius
    C. Humerus
    D. Vertebrate
Ans. (D) Vertebrate

19. **Earliest manifestation of spinal TB is:**
    A. Cold abscess formation
    B. Paraplegia
    C. Gibbus
    D. Muscle spasm
Ans. (D) Muscle spasm

20. **Most common site of TB spine is:**
    A. C8–T2
    B. T2–T6
    C. T10–L1
    D. L1–L4
Ans. (C) T10–L1

21. **Earliest sign in X-ray in TB spine:**
    A. Paravertebral shadow
    B. Narrowing of disc space
    C. Gibbus
    D. Straightening of the spinal curves
Ans. (B) Narrowing of disc space

22. **The early feature of Pott's paraplegia is:**
    A. Flexor spas
    B. Increased tendon jerk
    C. Ankle clonus
    D. Sensory loss
Ans. (C) Ankle clonus

23. **Recovery in TB spine is delayed in children be cause of:**
    A. Inadequate rest
    B. Fragile bone
    C. More cartilage
    D. Increased vascularity
Ans. (A) Inadequate rest

24. **Most common site of TB spine:**
    A. Dorso lumber
    B. Lumber
    C. Sacral
    D. Cervical
Ans. (A) Dorso lumber

1. **The following is false of achondroplasia:**
    A. Autosomal dominant
    B. Mental retardation
    C. Due to gene mutation
    D. Shortening of limbs present
Ans. (B) Mental retardation

2. **Shepherd's Crook deformity is seen in:**
    A. Achondroplasia
    B. Gaucher's disease
    C. Hypothroidism
    D. Fibrous dysplasia
Ans. (B) Gaucher's disease

3. **Trident hand is seen in:**
    A. Achondroplasia
    B. Scurvy
    C. Mucopolysaccharidosis
    D. None
Ans. (A) Achondroplasia

4. **All are seen in osteogenesis imperfecta** *except*:
    A. Joint dislocation
    B. Ligament laxity
    C. Osteoporosis
    D. Blue sclera
Ans. (C) Osteoporosis

5. **Not associated with osteogenesis imperfecta is:**
    A. Blue sclera
    B. Cataract
    C. Deafness
    D. Fractures
Ans. (B) Cataract

6. **Marble bone disease is also known as:**
    A. Osteogenesis imperfecta
    B. Osteopetrosis
    C. Perthes' disease
    D. Ochoronosis
Ans. (B) Osteopetrosis

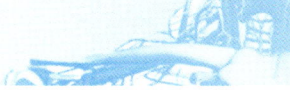

7. **Multiple bone fracture in a newborn is seen in:**
   A. Scurvy
   B. Syphilis
   C. Osteogenesis imperfecta
   D. Morquio's syndrome
   Ans. (C) Osteogenesis imperfecta

8. **Musculoskeletal abnormalities in neurofibromatosis is:**
   A. Hypertrophy of limb
   B. Scoliosis
   C. Pseudo arthrosis
   D. All of the above
   Ans. (D) All of the above

9. **Bilateral symmetrical idiopathic fractures are most commonly seen in:**
   A. Osteogenesis imperfecta
   B. Stress fracture
   C. Polytrauma
   D. Osteoporosis
   Ans. (A) Osteogenesis imperfecta

CHAPTER 7: DISEASES OF JOINTS

1. **Heberden's nodes are seen in:**
   A. Osteoarthritis
   B. Rheumatoid arthritis
   C. Rheumatic arthritis
   D. Psoriatic arthritis
   Ans. (A) Osteoarthritis

2. **HLA B27 is associated with:**
   A. Rheumatoid arthritis
   B. Ankylosing spondylitis
   C. Rheumatic arthritis
   D. Gouty arthritis
   Ans. (B) Ankylosing spondylitis

3. **Bamboo spine is seen in:**
   A. Tuberculosis
   B. Rheumatoid arthritis
   C. Ochronosis
   D. Ankylosing spondylitis
   Ans. (D) Ankylosing spondylitis

4. **The following is involved in rheumatoid arthritis:**
   A. Synovial fluid
   B. Synovial membrane
   C. Cartilage
   D. Subchondral bone
   Ans. (B) Synovial membrane

5. **Gaenslen's operation is done for:**
   A. Cervical spondylosis
   B. Recurrent shoulder dislocation
   C. TB arthritis of knee joint
   D. Sacroiliac subluxation
   Ans. (D) Sacroiliac subluxation

6. **Bouchard's nodes are seen in:**
   A. Proximal IP joints
   B. Distal IP joints
   C. Sternoclavicular joints
   D. Knee joints
   Ans. (A) Proximal IP joints

7. **Most common cause of neuropathic joints:**
   A. Diabetes
   B. Leprosy
   C. Syphilis
   D. Rheumatoid arthritis
   Ans. (A) Diabetes

8. **Osteo-arthritis does not affect:**
   A. Knee joint
   B. Hip joint
   C. Interphalangeal joint
   D. Metacarpophalangeal joint
   E. Shoulder joint
   Ans. (D) Metacarpophalangeal joint

9. **Positivity of HLA B 27 in ankylosing spondylitis:**
   A. 10%
   B. 96%
   C. 78%
   D. 100%
   Ans. (B) 96% (it is around 85% so the most appropriate option would be 96%)

10. **Earliest visible change in osteoarthritis is:**
    A. Loss of water
    B. Fibrillation
    C. Decreased collagen content
    D. Decreased hyaluronic acid level
    Ans. (B) Fibrillation

11. **Distal interphalangeal joint is not involved in:**
    A. Rheumatoid arthritis
    B. Osteoarthritis
    C. Psoriatic arthropathy
    D. Multiple histocytosis
Ans. **(A)** Rheumatoid arthritis

12. **Disease where distal interphalangeal joint is:**
    A. Psoriatic arthritis
    B. Rheumatoid
    C. SLE
    D. Gout
Ans. **(A)** Psoriatic arthritis

13. **The factor/ responsible for viscocity of synovial fluid:**
    A. Chondritin sulfate
    B. Hyaluronic acid
    C. Heparin sulfate
    D. All of the above
Ans. **(B)** Hyaluronic acid

14. **In Haemophillia pseudotumour is found in:**
    A. Gastrocnemius
    B. Quadriceps
    C. Ilio psoas
    D. Semimembranous
Ans. **(C)** Ilio psoas

CHAPTER 10:
ORTHOPAEDIC NEUROLOGY

1. **Clawhand is seen in:**
   A. Ulnar nerve injury
   B. Carpal tunnel syndrome
   C. Syringomyelia
   D. Cervical rib
   E. A, C and D
Ans. **(E)** A, C and D

2. **Pointing index sign is seen in ... nerve palsy.**
   A. Ulnar   B. Radial
   C. Median   D. Axillary
Ans. **(C)** Median

3. **Nerve abscess is seen in the ... nerve.**
   A. Median
   B. Ulnar
   C. Lateral fibular
   D. Sciatic
Ans. **(B)** Ulnar

4. **Most common cause of wrist drop is:**
   A. Intramuscular injection
   B. Fracture humerus
   C. Dislocation of elbow
   D. Dislocation of shoulder
Ans. **(B)** Fracture humerus

5. **The lesion of Klumpke's paralysis is in:**
   A. Cervical plexus
   B. Lower brachial
   C. Upper brachial
   D. Sacral plexus
Ans. **(B)** Lower brachial

6. **Dorsum of middle finger is supplied by:**
   A. Radial nerve
   B. Median nerve
   C. Ulnar nerve
   D. A and B
   E. A, B and C
Ans. **(E)** A, B and C

7. **Sensory supply of the tip of the ring finger is:**
   A. Radial nerve
   B. Median nerve
   C. Ulnar nerve
   D. Posterior interosseous nerve
   E. B and C
Ans. **(E)** B and C

8. **Which nerve repair has worst prognosis?**
   A. Ulnar
   B. Radial
   C. Median
   D. Lateral popliteal
Ans. **(A)** Ulnar

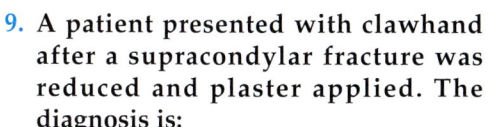

9. A patient presented with clawhand after a supracondylar fracture was reduced and plaster applied. The diagnosis is:
   A. Median nerve injury
   B. Volkmann's ischaemic contracture
   C. Ulnar nerve injury
   D. Dupuytren's contracture
   E. B and C
Ans. **(E)** B and C

10. Phalen's test is positive in:
    A. Ulnar bursitis
    B. Tennis elbow
    C. Carpal tunnel syndrome
    D. deQuervain's disese
Ans. **(C)** Carpal tunnel syndrome

11. Total clawhand is caused by injury to:
    A. Radial nerve
    B. Ulnar and radial nerve
    C. Ulnar and medial nerve
    D. Radian and median nerve
Ans. **(C)** Ulnar and medial nerve

12. Radial nerve injury above elbow lead to:
    A. Ape thumb   B. Trigger finger
    C. Wrist drop   D. Clawhand
Ans. **(C)** Wrist drop

13. Peripheral nerves can withstand ischemia up to:
    A. 30 minutes   B. 1 hour
    C. 2 hours   D. 4 hours
    E. None
Ans. **(E)** None

14. Axillary nerve injury at its origin leads to paralysis of:
    A. Deltoid and teres minor
    B. Deltoid
    C. Deltoid and teres major
    D. Latissimus dorsi and deltoid
Ans. **(A)** Deltoid and teres minor

15. Radial nerve injury of the type recovers with conservative management:
    A. Neurotmesis
    B. Crush injury
    C. Neuropraxia
    D. Chemical injury
Ans. **(C)** Neuropraxia

16. Polio paralysis differs from paralysis due to other causes:
    A. Weakness
    B. Deformity of limbs
    C. No sensory loss
    D. Full recovery is possible
Ans. **(C)** No sensory loss

17. Tendon transfer in polio is done at age of:
    A. Less than 6 months
    B. 5 months to 1 year
    C. 2 years
    D. 5 years
Ans. **(D)** 5 years

18. The 'Card Test' tests the function of:
    A. Median nerve   B. Ulnar nerve
    C. Axillary nerve   D. Radial nerve
Ans. **(B)** Ulnar nerve

19. Injury of median nerve at wrist is best detected by:
    A. Action of abductor pollicis brevis
    B. Action of flexor pollicis brevis
    C. Loss of sensation of radial half of palm
    D. Loss of sensation of tip of ring finger
Ans. **(A)** Action of abductor pollicis brevis

20. Weber–Fechnar law is:
    A. Magnitude of sensation is proportional to number of receptor stimulated
    B. Magnitude of sensation is proportional amplitude of action potential or receptor
    C. Magnitude of sensation is proportional to logarithm of intensity of stimulus
    D. Intensity of frequency of stimulus
Ans. **(C)** Magnitude of sensation is proportional to logarithm of intensity of stimulus

21. **Brachialis is supplied by:**
    A. Radial and ulnar nerve
    B. Median and musculocutaneous nerve
    C. Radial and musculocutaneous nerve
    D. Radial and median nerve

Ans. (C) Radial and musculocutaneous nerve

22. **Nerve which responds best to repair is:**
    A. Median
    B. Ulnar
    C. Sciatic
    D. Radial

Ans. (D) Radial

23. **Extension of the metacarpophalangeal joint is lost in jury to:**
    A. Radial nerve
    B. Ulnar nerve
    C. Median nerve
    D. Posterior interosseous nerve
    E. A and D

Ans. (E) A and D

24. **Clumsiness of the hand in case of leprosy is due to involvement of:**
    A. Interosseous muscle
    B. Abductor pollicis longus
    C. Extensor carpi ulnaris
    D. Flexor carpi ulnaris

Ans. (A) Interosseous muscle

CHAPTER 11: REGIONAL ORTHOPAEDIC

1. **Most common cause of scoliosis in children is:**
   A. Unequal limb length
   B. Post-poliomyelitis
   C. Hemivertebrae
   D. Marfan's syndrome

Ans. (B) Post-poliomyelitis

2. **Fracture dislocation injury of the spine is caused by:**
   A. Flexion only
   B. Rotation
   C. Extension
   D. Flexion and rotation

Ans. (D) Flexion and rotation

3. **Slipped femoral epiphysis is commonly seen in the:**
   A. 1st decade
   B. 2nd decade
   C. 3rd decade
   D. 4th decade

Ans. (B) 2nd decade

4. **Pes cavus is caused by:**
   A. Weakness of intrinsic muscles of the foot
   B. Excessive tone of intrinsic muscles
   C. Collapse of the arch
   D. Fracture of calcaneum

Ans. (A) Weakness of intrinsic muscles of the foot

5. **Coxa vara is found in:**
   A. Perthes' disease
   B. Tuberculosis
   C. Rickets
   D. Rheumatoid arthritis
   E. A and C

Ans. (E) A and C

6. **Painful are syndrome is due to:**
   A. Chronic supraspinatus tendonitis
   B. Subacromial bursitis
   C. Fracture greater tubercle
   D. All of the above

Ans. (D) All of the above

7. **Which is true about Perthes' disease?**
   A. Not painful
   B. It manifests at puberty
   C. Involves head of femur
   D. Viral etiology

Ans. (C) Involves head of femur

8. **Earliest changes in Perthes' disease is seen by:**
   A. X-ray
   B. CT
   C. MRI
   D. US
   E. Nuclear scan

Ans. (E) Nuclear scan

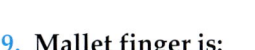

9. **Mallet finger is:**
   A. Avulsion fracture of extensor tendon of distal phalanx
   B. Fracture of distal phalanx
   C. Fracture of middle phalanx
   D. Fracture of proximal phalanx
   Ans. **(A)** Avulsion fracture of extensor tendon of distal phalanx

10. **Dupuytren's contracture is:**
    A. Thickening of palmar fasia
    B. Base of little finger involved first
    C. Seen in cirrhotics
    D. Seen in epileptics on hydantoin
    E. All of the above
    F. A, C and D
    Ans. **(F)** A, C and D

11. **Dupuytren's contracture is fibrosis of:**
    A. Palmar fascia
    B. Forearm muscles
    C. Sartorius fascia
    D. None
    Ans. **(A)** Palmar fascia

12. **Beheaded Scottish terrier sign is seen in:**
    A. Disc prolapse
    B. Sacarlisation of L5
    C. Spondylosis
    D. Spondylolisthesis
    Ans. **(D)** Spondylolisthesis

CHAPTER 12: CONGENITAL ANOMALIES

1. **Clubfoot seen in a 15-year-old could be treated successfully by:**
   A. Appropriate footwear
   B. Soft tissue operation
   C. Triple arthrodesis
   D. Quardriple fusion
   Ans. **(C)** Triple arthrodesis

2. **Clubfoot in a newborn is treated by:**
   A. Surgery
   B. Manipulation by the mother
   C. Denis Browne splint
   D. Strapping
   Ans. **(B)** Manipulation by the mother

3. **Treatment of CTEV should begin:**
   A. Soon after birth
   B. After discharge from hospital
   C. After one month
   D. At 2 years
   Ans. **(A)** Soon after birth

4. **Clubfoot CTEV should be treated at the age of:**
   A. 10–12 years of age of child
   B. From the day of birth
   C. 2–3 years of age of child
   D. After epiphyseal fusion
   Ans. **(B)** From the day of birth

5. **Treatment of chronic cases of clubfoot is:**
   A. Triple arthrodesis
   B. Dorso medial release
   C. Amputation
   D. None
   Ans. **(A)** Triple arthrodesis

6. **In correction of clubfoot by manipulation which deformity should be corrected first:**
   A. Forefoot adduction
   B. Varus
   C. Equines
   D. Internal tibial torsion
   Ans. **(A)** Forefoot adduction

7. **Child aged 3¼ years is treated for CTEV by:**
   A. Triple arthrodesis
   B. Posteromedial soft tissue release
   C. Lateral wedge resection
   D. Tendo Achilles lengthening and posterior capsulotomy
   Ans. **(B)** Posteromedial soft tissue release

8. **Which of the following is seen in bilateral congenital dislocation of hip?**
   A. Waddling gait
   B. Shenton's line is broken
   C. Trendelenburg test positive
   D. Telescopy not positive
   E. A and B
   Ans. **(E)** A and B

9. In a newborn child abduction and internal rotation produces a click sound. It is known as:
   A. Ortolani's sign
   B. Telescoping sign
   C. McMurray's sign
   D. Lachman sign
   Ans. (A) Ortolani's sign

10. Sprengel's deformity of scapula is:
    A. Undescended/elevated scapula
    B. Undescended neck of scapula
    C. Exostosis scapula
    D. None of the above
    Ans. (A) Undescended/elevated scapula

11. Cleidocranial dysostosis may show:
    A. Wide foramen magnum
    B. Absence of clavicles
    C. Coxa vara
    D. All of the above
    Ans. (B) Absence of clavicles

12. Phocomelia is caused by ingestion of ... during pregnancy.
    A. Steroids
    B. Tetracycline
    C. Thalidomide
    D. Barbiturates
    Ans. (C) Thalidomide

CHAPTER 13: BONE TUMOURS

1. Ivory osteoma commonly arises in the
   A. Skull   B. Ribs
   C. Pelvis   D. Vertebra
   Ans. (A) Skull

2. Most common site of multiple myeloma:
   A. Skull
   B. Ribs
   C. Vertebra
   D. Long bones
   E. Pelvis
   Ans. (C) Vertebra

3. Most common site of chondro-blastoma:
   A. Epiphysis

B. Diaphysis
C. Metaphysis
D. Soft tissues
E. Periosteum
Ans. (A) Epiphysis

4. Osteoblastic secondaries can arise from:
   A. Carcinoma prostate
   B. Thyroid carcinoma
   C. Renal carcinoma
   D. Breast carcinoma
   E. A and D
   Ans. (E) A and D

5. Most common benign tumour of the bone is:
   A. Osteoma
   B. Osteochondroma
   C. Osteoid osteoma
   D. Chondroma
   Ans. (B) Osteochondroma

6. Sunray appearance is seen in:
   A. Osteogenic sarcoma
   B. Ewing's sarcoma
   C. Multiple myeloma
   D. Osteoclastoma
   Ans. (A) Osteogenic sarcoma

7. Tumour arising from diaphysis:
   A. Osteogenic sarcoma
   B. Ewing's sarcoma
   C. Multiple myeloma
   D. Osteoclastoma
   Ans. (B) Ewing's sarcoma

8. Tumour most sensitive to radio-therapy is:
   A. Osteogenic sarcoma
   B. Ewing's sarcoma
   C. Multiple myeloma
   D. Osteoclastoma
   Ans. (B) Ewing's sarcoma

9. Enchondroma commonly arises from:
   A. Ribs   B. Vertebra
   C. Tibia   D. Phalanges
   Ans. (D) Phalanges

10. **Osteogenic sarcoma can develop in:**
    A. Osteoblastoma
    B. Paget's disease
    C. Osteoid osteoma
    D. All of the above
Ans. **(B)** Paget's disease

11. **The treatment of enchodroma is:**
    A. Amputation
    B. Irradiation
    C. Local excision
    D. Curettage and bone chip filling
Ans. **(D)** Curettage and bone chip filling

12. **Onion peel appearance in X-ray suggest:**
    A. Osteogenic sarcoma
    B. Ewing's sarcoma
    C. Osteoclastoma
    D. Chondrosarcoma
Ans. **(B)** Ewing's sarcoma

13. **Soap bubble appearance in X-ray suggests:**
    A. Osteogenic sarcoma
    B. Ewing's sarcoma
    C. Osteoclastoma
    D. Chondrosarcoma
Ans. **(C)** Osteoclastoma

14. **Involvement of regional lymph nodes is seen in:**
    A. Osteogenic sarcoma
    B. Synovial sarcoma
    C. Osteoclastoma
    D. Fibrosarcoma
Ans. **(B)** Synovial sarcoma

15. **Pain in osteoid osteoma is specifically relieved by:**
    A. Salicylates
    B. Nacrotic analgesics
    C. Radiation
    D. Splinting
Ans. **(A)** Salicylates

16. **Osteogenic sarcoma metastasizes to … commonly:**
    A. Liver
    B. Lung
    C. Brain
    D. Regional lymph nodes
Ans. **(B)** Lung

17. **Most common bone tumour are:**
    A. Osteosarcoma
    B. Osteoclastoma
    C. Secondaries
    D. Multiple myeloma
Ans. **(C)** Secondaries

18. **Osteosarcoma have a very poor prognosis because:**
    A. Highly malignant
    B. Resistant to radiotherapy
    C. Inoperable
    D. Spreads to lung very fast
Ans. **(D)** Spreads to lung very fast

19. **In carcinoma prostate with metastasis which is raised:**
    A. ESR
    B. Alkaline phosphatase
    C. Acid phosphatase
    D. Bilirubin
Ans. **(C)** Acid phosphatase

20. **Which of the following arises from epiphysis?**
    A. Osteogenic sarcoma
    B. Ewing's sarcoma
    C. Osteoclastoma
    D. Multiple myeloma
Ans. **(C)** Osteoclastoma

21. **Multiple myeloma is most frequently encountered in the … decade.**
    A. Third
    B. Fourth
    C. Fifth
    D. Seventh
Ans. **(D)** Seventh

22. **Most common site of bone cyst:**
    A. Upper end of humerus
    B. Lower end of tibia
    C. Lower end of femur
    D. Upper end of femur
Ans. **(A)** Upper end of humerus

23. Most common site for osteogenic sarcoma is:
    A. Upper end of femur
    B. Lower end of femur
    C. Upper end of tibia
    D. Lower end of tibia
Ans. (B) Lower end of femur

24. Most common site of osteoclastoma is:
    A. Upper end of femur
    B. Lower end of femur
    C. Upper end of tibia
    D. Lower end of tibia
Ans. (B) Lower end of femur

25. In multiple myeloma which of the following is seen:
    A. Raised serum calcium
    B. Raised alkaline phosphatase
    C. Raised acid phosphatase
    D. All
Ans. (A) Raised serum calcium

26. Most common tumour arising from the metaphysis is:
    A. Osteoclastoma
    B. Osteosarcoma
    C. Ewing's sarcoma
    D. Synovial sarcoma
Ans. (B) Osteosarcoma

27. Treatment of solitary bone cyst is:
    A. Curettage
    B. Excision
    C. Curettage and bone grafting
    D. Irradiation
Ans. (C) Curettage and bone grafting

28. Age group of osteogenic sarcoma is:
    A. 1–10   B. 10–20
    C. 20–30   D. 30–40
Ans. (B) 10–20

29. The lytic lesion in the epiphysis in children is seen:
    A. Osteogenic sarcoma
    B. Osteoclastoma
    C. Aneurysmal bone cyst
    D. Chondroblastoma
Ans. (D) Chondroblastoma

30. In which of the following tumour of the extremity of limb is excision of regional lymph node done?
    A. Adamantinoma
    B. Osteoclastoma
    C. Ewing's sarcoma
    D. Synovial cell sarcoma
Ans. (D) Synovial cell sarcoma

31. Bone cysts most commonly occur in:
    A. Spine
    B. Humerus
    C. Femur
    D. Tibia
Ans. (B) Humerus

32. Most common site of ivory osteoma:
    A. Orbit
    B. Maxilla
    C. Frontal sinus
    D. Mandible
Ans. (C) Frontal sinus

33. Fibrous dysplasia of bone with precocious puberty and pigmentation is seen in:
    A. Adrenal hypoplasia
    B. Achondroplasia
    C. Albright's syndrome
    D. Gardner's syndrome
Ans. (C) Albright's syndrome

34. Most common site of aneurysmal bone cyst is:
    A. Lower end of humerus
    B. Pelvic bones
    C. Radius
    D. Upper end of tibia
Ans. (D) Upper end of tibia

35. The most confirmatory test for myeloma is:
    A. Aspiration of the lesion and histology
    B. Bence Jones protein in urine
    C. Serum electrophoresis
    D. Technitium –99m radionuclide bone scan
Ans. (C) Serum electrophoresis

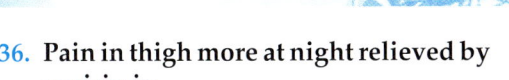

36. Pain in thigh more at night relieved by aspirin is:
  A. Osteosarcoma
  B. Osteoclastoma
  C. Ewing's tumour
  D. Osteoid osteoma
Ans. (D) Osteoid osteoma

37. Bone tumour metastasising to bone is:
  A. Giant cell tumour
  B. Ewing's sarcoma
  C. Chondrosarcoma
  D. Osteosarcoma
Ans. (B) Ewing's sarcoma

38. Vertical striations on vertebral bodies are seen in:
  A. Haemangioma
  B. Paget's disease
  C. Vertebral metastasis
  D. Osteoporosis
Ans. (A) Haemangioma

39. Most reliable method for detecting bone metastases:
  A. MRI
  B. CT scan
  C. Radiography
  D. SPECT
  E. None
Ans. (E) None

40. A boy presenting with swelling at lower end of femur with calcified nodular shadow in lung has:
  A. Osteosarcoma
  B. Osteochondroma
  C. Tuberculosis femur lower end
  D. Osteomyelitis
Ans. (B) Osteochondroma

41. Ewing's tumour arises from:
  A. Mesothelial cell
  B. Endothelial cell
  C. Squamous cell
  D. None of the above
Ans. (D) None of the above

42. Most common lesion of hand is:
  A. Endochondroma
  B. Synovioma
  C. Exostosis
  D. Osteoclastoma
Ans. (A) Endochondroma

43. A child with upper leg swelling with pulmonary nodule most probable diagnosis is:
  A. Osteoclastoma
  B. Chondrosarcoma
  C. Osteosarcoma
  D. Chondroblastoma
Ans. (C) Osteosarcoma

44. An 8-year-old child has a swelling in diaphysis of femur. Histology reveals small clear round symmetrical cells minimum cytoplasm, necrotic areas, minimum osteoid and chondroid material cells. Most likely, it contains:
  A. Mucin
  B. Lipid
  C. Iron
  D. Glycogen
Ans. (D) Glycogen

45. Kachrumal, a 46-year-old man has expensive growth metaphysis with endosteal scalloping and dense punctate calcification. Most likely bone tumour is:
  A. Osteosarcoma
  B. Chondrosarcoma
  C. Oteoclastoma
  D. Osteoid osteoma
Ans. (B) Chondrosarcoma

46. Most common site of tumours of bone is:
  A. Femur
  B. Tibia
  C. Humerus
  D. Vertebral column
Ans. (A) Femur

CHAPTER 13: AMPUTATION

1. **Distance from elbow in forearm amputation … inches.**
   A. 5   B. 7
   C. 8   D. 9
   Ans. (B) 7

2. **Distance from the acromian in arm amputation is … inches.**
   A. 5   B. 7
   C. 8   D. 9
   Ans. (C) 8

3. **Distance from the lip of greater trochanter in thigh amputation is … inches.**
   A. 5   B. 7
   C. 9   D. 11
   Ans. (D) 11

4. **Distance from the knee joint in below knee amputation is … inches:**
   A. 4   B. 5.5
   C. 6   D. 7
   Ans. (B) 5.5

5. **Complications of an amputation stump may be:**
   A. Phantom limb
   B. Stump neuroma
   C. Ring sequestrum
   D. All the above
   Ans. (D) All the above

6. **Syme's amputation is contraindicated in:**
   A. Malignancy of big toe
   B. Diabetic foot
   C. Madura mycosis foot
   D. Crush injury
   E. None
   Ans. (E) None

CHAPTER 14: MISCELLANEOUS DISEASES

1. **Pain in Paget's disease is relieved best by:**
   A. Simple analgesic
   B. Narcotic analgesics
   C. Radiation
   D. Calcitonin
   Ans. (D) Calcitonin

2. **The complications of Paget's disease is:**
   A. Osteogenic sarcoma
   B. Deafness
   C. Heart failure
   D. All of the above
   Ans. (D) All of the above

3. **Deafness in cases of Paget's disease is due to:**
   A. Thickened cranium
   B. Narrowing of foramina of skull
   C. Brain compression
   D. Otosclerosis
   Ans. (D) Otosclerosis

4. **The following are radiological signs of Paget's disease of bone *except*:**
   A. "Cotton Wool" appearance
   B. "Picture Window Frame" appearance
   C. "Hair-on-end" appearance
   D. "Blade of grass" appearance
   Ans. (C) "Hair-on-end" appearance

5. **Following are features of Paget's disease *except*:**
   A. Deformity of bones
   B. Secondary osteosarcoma
   C. Lowered serum alkaline phosphatase
   D. Increased urinary excretion of hydroxyproline
   Ans. (C) Lowered serum alkaline phosphatase

6. **Drug therapy of Paget's disease (Osteitis deformans):**
   A. Alendronate
   B. Etidronate
   C. Calcitonin
   D. Plicamycin
   Ans. (D) Plicamycin

7. **Caffey's disease occur in:**
   A. Infants below 6 months
   B. Above 5 years
   C. Above 10:20 years
   D. 20–40 years
   Ans. (A) Infants below 6 months

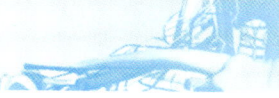

8. **Treatment of choice for Caffey's disease:**
   A. Multiple drilling
   B. Tetracycline
   C. Penicillin
   D. Curettage
   Ans. **(C)** Penicillin

9. **Hand–Schüller–Christian disease, which is correct:**
   A. Proliferation of reticulo-endothelial cells
   B. Foam cells seen
   C. Punched out lesions in X-ray
   D. Diabetes insipidus and exophthalmos present
   E. All are correct
   Ans. **(E)** All are correct

10. **Osteomyelitis of jaw is seen in:**
    A. Osteomalacia
    B. Osteopoikilosis
    C. Osteoporosis
    D. Caffey's disease
    Ans. **(D)** Caffey's disease

CHAPTER 17: SPLINTS

1. **Non-dynamic splint is:**
   A. Banjo
   B. Opponens
   C. Cock-up
   D. Brand
   Ans. **(C)** Cock-up

2. **Aeroplane splint is used for:**
   A. Brachial plexus palsy
   B. Volkmann's ischaemic contracture
   C. Myositis ossificans
   D. Fracture talus
   Ans. **(A)** Brachial plexus palsy

3. **Von Rosen splint in used in:**
   A. CTEV
   B. CDH
   C. Fracture shaft of femur
   D. Fracture tibia
   Ans. **(B)** CDH

4. **Milwaukee brace is used in:**
   A. Scoliosis
   B. Fracture skull
   C. Fracture tibia
   D. CTEV
   Ans. **(A)** Scoliosis

CHAPTER 20: EPONYMIC AND MNEUMONICS

1. **Shoveller's fracture is:**
   A. Stress fracture of spinous processes
   B. Fracture of forearm bones
   C. Fracture of the body of atlas
   D. Fracture dislocation of axis vertebrae
   Ans. **(A)** Stress fracture of spinous processes

2. **March fracture affects:**
   A. Neck of 2nd metatarsal
   B. Body of 2nd metatarsal
   C. Neck of 1st metatarsal
   D. Fracture of lower end of tibia
   E. Fracture of lower end of fibula
   Ans. **(A)** Neck of 2nd metatarsal

3. **March fracture is:**
   A. Stress fracture of neck of second metatarsal
   B. Stress fracture of neck of talus
   C. Compression fracture of calcaneum
   D. Fracture lower end of fibula
   Ans. **(A)** Stress fracture of neck of second metatarsal

4. **Jefferson fracture occurs at:**
   A. C1
   B. C2
   C. C1, C2
   D. C2, C3
   Ans. **(A)** C1

5. **Lisfranc's dislocation is:**
   A. Tarsometatarsal dislocation
   B. Lunate dislocation
   C. Scaphoid dislocation
   D. Posterior dislocation of elbow
   Ans. **(A)** Tarsometatarsal dislocation

6. **Bennett's fracture is fracture dislocation of base of ... metacarpal.**
   A. 4th
   B. 3rd
   C. 2nd
   D. 1st
   Ans. **(D)** 1st

Index

331

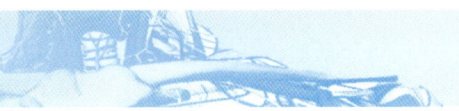

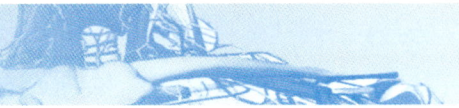

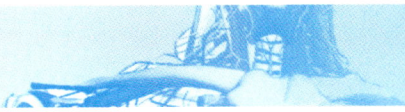